# Autoimmune (IgG4-related) Pancreatitis and Cholangitis

Michael J. Levy • Suresh T. Chari
Editors

# Autoimmune (IgG4-related) Pancreatitis and Cholangitis

Springer

*Editors*
Michael J. Levy
Division of Gastroenterology and Hepatology
Mayo Clinic
Rochester, MN, USA

Suresh T. Chari
Division of Gastroenterology and Hepatology
Internal Medicine
Mayo Clinic College of Medicine
Rochester, MN, USA

ISBN 978-1-4419-6429-8 ISBN 978-1-4419-6430-4 (eBook)
DOI 10.1007/978-1-4419-6430-4
Springer New York Heidelberg Dordrecht London

Library of Congress Control Number: 2013941882



Printed on acid-free paper

Springer is part of Springer Science+Business Media (www.springer.com)

# Preface

It is not very often that a new disease entity is discovered. While autoimmune pancreatitis was christened in 1995, it is only in the last few years that the terms type 2 autoimmune pancreatitis and IgG4-related disease have been coined to describe new disease entities. So it is with great pleasure that we present this book titled IgG4-related disease (IgG4-RD). Our goal is to provide a timely overview of this disease entity with particular emphasis on its most well-described manifestations, namely, autoimmune pancreatitis (AIP) and IgG4-related sclerosing cholangitis (IgG4-SC).

As gastroenterologists, this effort grew out of our interest in AIP and IgG4-SC. As worldwide experience has grown, AIP and IgG4-SC are now recognized as manifestations of a multiorgan disease process termed IgG4-related disease (IgG4-RD). While there is much overlap in terms of the clinical, serological, histological, and imaging features among the various organs involved, there are also key differences. Clearer understandings of the overlapping and disparate features have substantially aided patient care and are reviewed in detail throughout this book.

Initial efforts around the world occurred in isolation producing often conflicting evaluation and management strategies, leading to confusion and uncertainty among physicians. Recent multinational collaborative efforts have enhanced our understanding of the pathogenesis as well as clinical, laboratory, and imaging findings associated with IgG4-RD. This combined effort has led to the adoption of a broadly accepted nomenclature and helped standardize the diagnostic and therapeutic approach. However, in this book we do elaborate on key differences that remain throughout the world, thereby allowing clinicians and researchers to tailor their practice and studies accordingly. This book offers a manageable understanding of key aspects of the disease while providing in-depth information that should well serve those seeking a deeper understanding of this unique disorder.

We would like to acknowledge the renowned team of experts that we feel fortunate to have worked with, and we appreciate their hard work and devotion to this project. We have found this journey of discovery to be rewarding and hope you will as well.

Rochester, MN, USA

Michael J. Levy
Suresh T. Chari

# Contents

# Contributors

**Edward Alabraba** NIHR Pancreas Biomedical Research Unit, Royal Liverpool University Hospital, Liverpool, UK

**Shameena Bharucha** NIHR Pancreas Biomedical Research Unit, Royal Liverpool University Hospital, Liverpool, UK

**Einar S. Björnsson** Landspitali University Hospital, Reykjavik, Iceland

Department of Internal Medicine, Division of Gastroenterology, The National University Hospital of Iceland, Reykjavik, Iceland

**William R. Brugge** Harvard Medical School, Massachusetts General Hospital, Boston, MA, USA

**Suresh T. Chari** Division of Gastroenterology and Hepatology, Internal Medicine, Mayo Clinic College of Medicine, Rochester, MN, USA

**Clancy J. Clark** Wake Forest Baptist Health, Medical Center Blvd., Winston-Salem, NC, USA

**Lynn D. Cornell** Laboratory Medicine and Pathology, Mayo Clinic, Rochester, MN, USA

**Vikram Deshpande** Department of Pathology, Massachusetts General Hospital, Boston, MA, USA

**Michael B. Farnell** Mayo Clinic, Rochester, MN, USA

**Carlos Fernandez-del Castillo** Department of Surgery, Massachusetts General Hospital, Boston, MA, USA

**Chris E. Forsmark** Division of Gastroenterology, Hepatology, and Nutrition, University of Florida, Gainesville, FL, USA

**Luca Frulloni** Department of Medicine, University of Verona, Verona, Italy

**Timothy B. Gardner** Gastroenterology and Hepatology, Dartmouth Medical School, Lebanon, NH, USA

**Phil A. Hart** Division of Gastroenterology and Hepatology, Internal Medicine, Mayo Clinic College of Medicine, Rochester, MN, USA

**Gideon M. Hirschfield** Centre for Liver Research, NIHR Biomedical Research Unit, University of Birmingham, Institute of Biomedical Research, Birmingham, UK

**Atsushi Irisawa** Department of Gastroenterology, Fukushima Medical University Aizu Medical Center, Aizuwakamatsu, Japan

**Evangelos Kalaitzakis** Department of Gastroenterology, Skåne University Hospital, Lund, Sweden

**Terumi Kamisawa** Department of Internal Medicine, Tokyo Metropolitan Komagome Hospital, Honkomagome, Bunkyo-ku/Tokyo, Japan

**Ali D. Karaosmanoglu** Department of Radiology, Massachusetts General Hospital (ADK, DS), Boston, MA, USA

**Myung-Hwan Kim** Department of Internal Medicine, University of Ulsan College of Medicine, Asan Medical Center, Seoul, South Korea

**Günter Klöppel** Department of Pathology, University Hospital, University of Kiel, Munich, Bavaria, Germany

**Markus M. Lerch** Department of Medicine, University Hospital Greifswald, Greifswald, Germany

**Michael J. Levy** Division of Gastroenterology and Hepatology, Mayo Clinic, Rochester, MN, USA

**Keith D. Lindor** Gastroenterology and Hepatology, Mayo Clinic, Rochester, MN, USA

**Daniel S. Longnecker** Department of Pathology, Geisel School of Medicine at Dartmouth, Dartmouth-Hitchcock Medical Center, Lebanon, NH, USA

**Sung-Hoon Moon** Department of Internal Medicine, Hallym University Sacred Heart Hospital, Hallym University College of Medicine, Anyang-si, South Korea

**Kazuichi Okazaki** Department of Gastroenterology and Hepatology, Kansai Medical University, Hirakata, Osaka, Japan

**Jay H. Ryu** Division of Pulmonary and Critical Care Medicine, Mayo Clinic College of Medicine, Rochester, MN, USA

**Raghuwansh P. Sah** Internal Medicine, Mayo Clinic Rochester, Rochester, MN, USA

**Dushyant V. Sahani** Department of Radiology, Massachusetts General Hospital (ADK, DS), Boston, MA, USA

**Hiroshi Sekiguchi** Division of Pulmonary and Critical Care Medicine, Mayo Clinic Rochester, Rochester, MN, USA

**Tooru Shimosegawa** Department of Gastroenterology, Hohoku University Hospital, Sendai, Miyagi, Japan

**Thomas C. Smyrk** Department of Pathology, Mayo Clinic, Rochester, MN, USA

**Robert Sutton** NIHR Pancreas Biomedical Research Unit, Royal Liverpool University Hospital, Liverpool, UK

**Naoki Takahashi** Department of Radiology, Mayo Clinic, Rochester, MN, USA

**Kazushige Uchida** Department of Gastroenterology and Hepatology, Kansai Medical University, Hirakata, Osaka, Japan

**Penny Watson** Department of Veterinary Medicine, Queen's Veterinary School Hospital, University of Cambridge, Cambridge, Cambs, UK

**George Webster** GI Services, University College London Hospitals, London, UK

**Eunhee S. Yi** Department of Laboratory Medicine and Pathology, Mayo Clinic, Rochester, MN, USA

**Giuseppe Zamboni** Servizio di Anatomia-Istologia Patologica, Università di Verona, Ospedale S.Cuore-Don Calabria, Negrar-Verona, Italy

**Lizhi Zhang** Department of Laboratory and Anatomic Pathology, Mayo Clinic, Rochester, MN, USA

# Background and Perspective

1

Daniel S. Longnecker

## Introduction

The recognition and characterization of autoimmune pancreatitis (AIP) and $IgG_4$-related disease ($IgG_4$-RD) has evolved over the course of more than 50 years. The possibility and probability that chronic pancreatitis was sometimes caused by autoimmune mechanisms was mentioned in several publications beginning in 1959, but the recognition of characteristic clinical, imaging, and histopathologic features for such patients was not recorded until the 1990s as noted below. The characterization of AIP continues to be refined as reflected in the other chapters of this book. The recognition of $IgG_4$-related disease ($IgG_4$-RD) was an outgrowth of study of autoimmune pancreatitis, so our first focus is on the recognition of AIP.

## Recognition of Autoimmune Pancreatitis

AIP is a rare disease with an estimated annual incidence in the range of 0.82 per 100,000 in Japan [1]. There is currently no reason to think that its prevalence is higher in Western nations although there are no data bearing on this assumption [2, 3]. Because of the low incidence, most clinicians, radiologists, and pathologists are likely to see only occasional cases. As might be expected, this low incidence delayed the recognition of AIP. There is also evidence that the incidence of AIP has risen dramatically during the past two decades [4]. This provides a further basis for the relatively recent recognition of the disease.

Because AIP may cause pancreatic enlargement that is often localized in the head, patients are likely to be referred to tertiary care centers for diagnosis and treatment. Many patients with these inflammatory masses have undergone pancreatectomy because of a preoperative clinical diagnosis of a pancreatic neoplasm and then been diagnosed after resection as having pancreatitis by the surgical pathologist. Experience with such cases is the basis for the histopathologic diagnosis of AIP. Retrospective studies in specialized centers in the USA indicate that 2.2–2.5 % of pancreatectomies were done because of mass-forming AIP [5–7]. These data reflect a period before there was emphasis on the clinical diagnosis of AIP. With improved understanding and recognition of AIP, reducing the rate of such resections is an obvious goal [8].

The survival of patients with AIP is reported to be similar to that of the general population of the same age [9], although one finds reference to patients that progress to a stage of cachexia and death in older literature [10]. Since AIP is rarely fatal, at least in the current era, it is rarely the focus of an autopsy. We can anticipate that

D.S. Longnecker, M.D. (✉)
Department of Pathology, Geisel School of Medicine at Dartmouth, Dartmouth-Hitchcock Medical Center, One Medical Center Drive, Lebanon, NH 03756, USA
e-mail: Daniel.S.Longnecker@Dartmouth.EDU

M.J. Levy and S.T. Chari (eds.), *Autoimmune (IgG4-related) Pancreatitis and Cholangitis*,
DOI 10.1007/978-1-4419-6430-4_1, 

end-stage AIP would be encountered at a low incidence in autopsies done following death from other causes, but we do not really know if AIP would be distinguished from end-stage chronic pancreatitis of other causes. Suda described early- and late-stage AIP, the latter based on prominent loss of acinar cells [11]. All specimens were from pancreatic resection or biopsy, and all contained inflamed ducts. Although the late-stage patients ($n = 11$) were about 2.5 years older than the early-stage group ($n = 17$) at disease onset, the age difference was not significant. The degree of lymphoplasmacytic infiltration was more variable, and venulitis was less frequent in the late stage, but it is not obvious that the late-stage group should be regarded as end stage.

Because AIP is now diagnosed and treated nonoperatively, it is possible that patients with a well-supported clinical diagnosis of AIP will be followed until death and autopsied—allowing characterization of the sequelae ("end stage") of AIP. Because of the likelihood that such patients will have been treated with corticosteroids, even this approach may not reveal the natural course of the disease.

## Recognition of Autoimmune Etiology

There are several early literature references to a possible autoimmune etiology of pancreatitis. In 1959, Thal et al. reported pancreatic autoantibodies in a patient with chronic pancreatitis [12] and subsequently commented that "The finding of true auto-antibodies in this case raised the interesting possibility that his disease was either precipitated by or aggravated by an auto-immunizing mechanism" [13]. In 1961, Sarles reported a group of patients having "primary inflammatory sclerosis" of the pancreas stating that "It appears in later life (average age of onset, 61.4 years) and is found as often in women as in men" [10]. The authors mention a lymphoplasmacytic infiltrate, perilobular fibrosis, and lobular sclerosis in one pancreas patient and hypergammaglobulinemia in two patients. These findings are supportive of a diagnosis of AIP, although the clinical and pathologic data are not adequate to allow a firm retrospective diagnosis of AIP for all patients in the group. The following statement appears in the last lines of the summary: "It is thus possible to put forward the hypothesis that this type of pancreatitis is an inflammatory, noninfectious disease that is caused by phenomena of self-immunization" [10].

Autoimmune pancreatitis ("Autoimmunpankreatitis") is explicitly mentioned as a possible cause of chronic sclerosing pancreatitis in a 1979 review by Putzke [14]. The prominence of interstitial lymphoplasmacytic infiltrates and perilobular, intralobular, and periductal fibrosis was noted in some pancreases—consistent with our current histopathologic criteria for the diagnosis of AIP. The dominant view regarding the pathogenesis of immune-mediated pancreatitis at that time centered on humoral immunity. This view was based in part on studies in which animals were immunized with and developed antibodies against pancreas-derived fractions and subsequently developed pancreatic fibrosis [15]. Thal stated "It is not yet clear whether these circulating antibodies are merely a side result of a more important reaction of the delayed hypersensitivity type occurring at the cellular level" [15]. A central role for antibody-mediated injury was supported by a later study in which diffuse interstitial pancreatitis developed in mice treated with antiserum from guinea pigs immunized with pancreatic fractions [16]. In fact, one still finds the statement that it is unclear whether autoimmune antibodies that yield elevations of IgG and IgG4 in AIP patients represent an epiphenomenon or play a role in the pathogenesis of disease [17].

The central role of cell-mediated immunity in the pathogenesis of other autoimmune diseases was recognized later beginning in 1974 [18]. Its role was specifically supported as a possible mechanism in AIP by the demonstration of high numbers of T lymphocytes in infiltrates in the pancreas [19, 20] and experimentally by the induction of pancreatitis in rats by adoptive transfer of CD4(+) T cells sensitized to a pancreatic epitope [21].

In the literature from Western nations, the 1997 paper by Ectors et al. stands out because a pattern of chronic pancreatitis that was clearly different than chronic alcoholic pancreatitis was identified in a group of resected pancreases from nonalcoholic patients [19]. The name "chronic nonalcoholic duct destructive pancreatitis" was suggested for this type of pancreatitis. Some of these patients (4/12) had autoimmune disease manifest in other organs, and autoimmune etiology for the ductal lesions in the pancreas was carefully considered although the pancreatitis was ultimately classified as idiopathic.

Yoshida is credited with introducing the term "autoimmune pancreatitis," citing 11 cases including one of their own and 10 others reported from 1961 to 1991 [22]. This appears to be the first use of the term in English literature. There were numerous reports from Japanese centers that characterized AIP during the following decade. However, it is clear that the concept of autoimmune-mediated pancreatic injury emerged in several centers and several countries over multiple decades. Acceptance of the term (AIP) and an increasing focus on diagnosis, characterization, and treatment of the disease are evident in a search for publications on the topic in sequential time periods (Table 1.1).

**Table 1.1** Publications on AIP listed in sequential searches for "autoimmune pancreatitis" using the MEDLINE database for 1950–2010

| Years | No.[a] | Comment |
|---|---|---|
| 1950–1978 | 0 | Several clinical and experimental papers during this period focused on immune-mediated pancreatic disease (see text) |
| 1979–1994 | 1 | "Autoimmunpankreatitis" is mentioned in a German review [14] |
| 1995 | 1 | First use of "autoimmune pancreatitis" in an English publication [22] |
| 1996–2000 | 17 | Eleven of these papers were from Japan |
| 2001–2005 | 170 | In 2003, 21/28 listings were from Japan |
| 2006–2010 | 538 | In 2010, 99 listings originated in 14 countries |

[a]Number of journal references listed in the Ovid MEDLINE database for 1950–2010 using the term "autoimmune pancreatitis.mp" as keyword and the Ovid MEDLINE database on Jan. 5, 2011

## Recognition of Subtypes

Heterogeneity in the pathology of AIP resection specimens also delayed its recognition. This heterogeneity has now resolved into the recognition of at least two subtypes of AIP as discussed in Chap. 3. Early descriptions focused on the prominence of mixed infiltrates of lymphocytes and plasma cells in some cases of chronic pancreatitis [23]. The first use of the descriptive diagnosis "lymphoplasmacytic sclerosing pancreatitis," now often referred to as LPSP, or type 1 AIP, appears to have been in 1991 [23].

Another report focused on ductal inflammation, sometimes resulting in duct destruction, and it was noted that intraductal aggregates of neutrophilic granulocytes were commonly associated with duct destructive lesions [19]. Variation in the number of granulocytic leukocytes (neutrophils and eosinophils) was noted among cases of AIP [24]. The neutrophilic aggregates were called granulocytic epithelial lesions (GEL) [25], and it is now recognized that GEL are a characteristic of type 2 AIP [26]. A matter of passing interest focuses on the acronym applied to type 2 AIP, often referred to as IDCP. The basis for this acronym is ambiguous, being defined variously as "idiopathic duct centric pancreatitis" [3, 27] and alternately as "idiopathic duct-centric pancreatitis" [20, 28].

## Recognition of $IgG_4$-Related Disease ($IgG_4$-RD)

The recognition of the possible role of IgG4 in the pathogenesis of type 1 AIP [29] and subsequently of $IgG_4$-related disease (called IgG4-related sclerosing disease [30] and IgG4-related systemic diseases [3]) evolved as follows. AIP was noted in early reports cited above to occur in patients coincident with several other autoimmune diseases [19, 22]. Overall, it appears that there is evidence of involvement of other organs by autoimmune processes in a quarter to more than half of AIP patients in various series.

A variety of autoantibodies were detected in patients with AIP [22]. Hypergammaglobulinemia was documented in some patients [10, 22], leading to the examination of immunoglobulin subclasses and recognition in 2001 that IgG4 was elevated in the serum of most Japanese patients with AIP [31]. Later, increased numbers of IgG4-positive plasma cells were demonstrated in a high fraction of pancreases with AIP [29], and finally similar elevations of IgG4-positive cells were identified in other involved organs [29]. This led to the proposal that AIP was part of an IgG4-associated systemic autoimmune disease [29, 30]. A MEDLINE search for IgG4-related sclerosing disease yielded 55 listings with the first appearing in 2006 [30]. In a 2008 review, Kamisawa states that "This disease includes AIP, sclerosing cholangitis, cholecystitis, sialadenitis, retroperitoneal fibrosis, tubulointerstitial nephritis, interstitial pneumonia, prostatitis, inflammatory pseudotumor and lymphadenopathy, all IgG4-related" [32].

## Concluding Comments

As the literature for AIP is reviewed, it is necessary to consider what is included under the term AIP in each report. It is typical for series from Japan to be composed entirely or predominantly of type 1 AIP patients—the type of AIP that is seen in $IgG_4$-related disease. Accordingly, we find that as many as 95 % of the patients have elevated serum IgG4 in series from Japan [31]. In contrast, in Western literature it is likely that series of patients are composed of mixtures of type 1 and type 2 AIP with the latter comprising fewer than half of most series. In series from the USA and Europe, the fraction of patients with elevation of IgG4 is reported as 53–76 %, depending on cutoff level, in various series [33, 34]. This seems to reflect the inclusion of type 2 AIP patients who typically do not have elevation of serum IgG4 [9]. In a recent discussion of $IgG_4$-related diseases, it seems clear that the authors include both LPSP and IDCP when they discuss AIP although AIP subtypes are specifically mentioned [17].

The reason for the higher fraction of AIP type 1 patients in Japan than in the West is not known, but emerging information at the molecular and genetic level regarding the causes of autoimmune disease seems relevant. The Fc receptor, FcgRIIa, has been identified as an inflammatory mediator in rheumatoid arthritis and systemic lupus erythematosus [35]. FcgRIIa binds immunoglobulins of several classes including IgG4 with varying affinity. IgG4 has recently been reported in immune complexes deposited within pancreases with AIP [36]. This Fc receptor has been found to have several polymorphisms. One of these, FcgRIIa H131, has a higher affinity for IgG2 than FcgRIIa R131 [37]. FcgRIIa H131 is more prevalent in Japanese and Chinese than among Americans [38]. While there are no specific data to tie this polymorphism to the pathogenesis of AIP, these observations illustrate the type of genetic variation that could cause differences in the incidence and type of AIP occurring in different racial and geographic groups.

Although most AIP can be classified on the basis of histopathology as type 1 or type 2 by expert pathologists when a resection specimen is available [27], some cases are difficult to classify by the current criteria. We do not know if these are simply examples of type 1 or type 2 AIP that are atypical, perhaps due to differences in stage or degree of involvement, or whether they might represent yet other rarer subtypes of the disease. Recognition of rare subtypes of a rare disease will be very difficult and may depend on finding new genetic or immunologic markers.

**Acknowledgment** The author thanks William F. Hickey, Günter Klöppel, and Thomas Smyrk for suggestions during the preparation of this chapter.

## References

1. Nishimori I, Tamakoshi A, Otsuki M. Research Committee on Intractable Diseases of the Pancreas, Ministry of Health, Labour, and Welfare of Japan. Prevalence of autoimmune pancreatitis in Japan from a nationwide survey in 2002. J Gastroenterol. 2007;42(Suppl 18):6–8.
2. Pannala R, Chari ST. Autoimmune pancreatitis. Curr Opin Gastroenterol. 2008;24(5):591–6.

3. Sugumar A, Chari S. Autoimmune pancreatitis: an update. Expert Rev Gastroenterol Hepatol. 2009;3(2):197–204.
4. Kojima M, Sipos B, Klapper W, et al. Autoimmune pancreatitis: frequency, IgG4 expression, and clonality of T and B cells. Am J Surg Pathol. 2007;31(4):521–8.
5. Abraham SC, Wilentz RE, Yeo CJ, et al. Pancreaticoduodenectomy (Whipple resections) in patients without malignancy: are they all 'chronic pancreatitis'? Am J Surg Pathol. 2003;27(1):110–20.
6. Hardacre JM, Iacobuzio-Donahue CA, Sohn TA, et al. Results of pancreaticoduodenectomy for lymphoplasmacytic sclerosing pancreatitis. Ann Surg. 2003;237(6):853–8.
7. Weber SM, Cubukcu-Dimopulo O, Palesty JA, Suriawinata A, Klimstra D, Brennan MF, Conlon K. Lymphoplasmacytic sclerosing pancreatitis: inflammatory mimic of pancreatic carcinoma. J Gastrointest Surg. 2003;7(1):129–37.
8. Hughes DB, Grobmyer SR, Brennan MF. Preventing pancreaticoduodenectomy for lymphoplasmacytic sclerosing pancreatitis: cost effectiveness of IgG4. Pancreas. 2004;29(2):167.
9. Sah RP, Pannala R, Chari ST, et al. Prevalence, diagnosis, and profile of autoimmune pancreatitis presenting with features of acute or chronic pancreatitis. Clin Gastroenterol Hepatol. 2010;8(1):91–6.
10. Sarles H, Sarles JC, Muratore R, Guien C. Chronic inflammatory sclerosis of the pancreas—an autonomous pancreatic disease? Am J Dig Dis. 1961;6:688–98.
11. Suda K, Nishimori I, Takase M, Oi I, Ogawa M. Autoimmune pancreatitis can be classified into early and advanced stages. Pancreas. 2006;33(4):345–50.
12. Thal AP, Egner W, Murray MJ. Circulating antibodies in chronic pancreatitis. Surg Forum. 1959;10:240–3.
13. Murray MJ, Thal AP. The clinical significance of circulating pancreatic antibodies. Ann Intern Med. 1960;53:548–55.
14. Putzke HP. Morphology of acute and chronic pancreatitis. Z Gesamte Inn Med. 1979;34(10):266–71.
15. Thal AP. The occurrence of pancreatic antibodies and the nature of the pancreatic antigen. Surg Forum. 1960;11:367–9.
16. Freytag G, Kloppel G. Experimental pancreatitis and inflammation of the islets after treatment with immune sera against extract of pancreas of varying degrees of purity. Beitr Pathol Anat. 1969;139(2):138–60.
17. Narula N, Vasudev M, Marshall JK. IgG4-related sclerosing disease: a novel mimic of inflammatory bowel disease. Dig Dis Sci. 2010;55(11):3047–51.
18. Gonatas NK, Howard JC. Inhibition of experimental allergic encephalomyelitis in rats severely depleted of T cells. Science. 1974;186(4166):839–41.
19. Ectors N, Maillet B, Aerts R, et al. Non-alcoholic duct destructive chronic pancreatitis. Gut. 1997;41(2):263–8.
20. Notohara K, Burgart LJ, Yadav D, Chari S, Smyrk TC. Idiopathic chronic pancreatitis with periductal lymphoplasmacytic infiltration: clinicopathologic features of 35 cases. Am J Surg Pathol. 2003;27(8):1119–27.
21. Davidson TS, Longnecker DS, Hickey WF. An experimental model of autoimmune pancreatitis in the rat. Am J Pathol. 2005;166(3):729–36.
22. Yoshida K, Toki F, Takeuchi T, Watanabe S, Shiratori K, Hayashi N. Chronic pancreatitis caused by an autoimmune abnormality. Proposal of the concept of autoimmune pancreatitis. Dig Dis Sci. 1995;40(7):1561–8.
23. Kawaguchi K, Koike M, Tsuruta K, Okamoto A, Tabata I, Fujita N. Lymphoplasmacytic sclerosing pancreatitis with cholangitis: a variant of primary sclerosing cholangitis extensively involving pancreas. Hum Pathol. 1991;22(4):387–95.
24. Pearson RK, Longnecker DS, Chari ST, et al. Controversies in clinical pancreatology: autoimmune pancreatitis: does it exist? Pancreas. 2003;27(1):1–13.
25. Zamboni G, Luttges J, Capelli P, et al. Histopathological features of diagnostic and clinical relevance in autoimmune pancreatitis: a study on 53 resection specimens and 9 biopsy specimens. Virchows Arch. 2004;445(6):552–63.
26. Kloppel G, Detlefsen S, Chari ST, Longnecker DS, Zamboni G. Autoimmune pancreatitis: the clinicopathological characteristics of the subtype with granulocytic epithelial lesions. J Gastroenterol. 2010;45(8):787–93.
27. Chari ST, Kloeppel G, Zhang L, Notohara K, Lerch MM, Shimosegawa T. Autoimmune Pancreatitis International Cooperative Study Group (APICS). Histopathologic and clinical subtypes of autoimmune pancreatitis: the Honolulu consensus document. Pancreas. 2010;39(5):549–54.
28. Shimosegawa T, Kanno A. Autoimmune pancreatitis in Japan: overview and perspective. J Gastroenterol. 2009;44(6):503–17.
29. Kamisawa T, Funata N, Hayashi Y, et al. A new clinicopathological entity of IgG4-related autoimmune disease. J Gastroenterol. 2003;38(10):982–4.
30. Kamisawa T, Okamoto A. Autoimmune pancreatitis: proposal of IgG4-related sclerosing disease. J Gastroenterol. 2006;41(7):613–25.
31. Hamano H, Kawa S, Horiuchi A, et al. High serum IgG4 concentrations in patients with sclerosing pancreatitis. N Engl J Med. 2001;344(10):732–8.
32. Kamisawa T, Okamoto A. IgG4-related sclerosing disease. World J Gastroenterol. 2008;14(25):3948–55.
33. Ghazale A, Chari ST, Smyrk TC, et al. Value of serum IgG4 in the diagnosis of autoimmune pancreatitis and in distinguishing it from pancreatic cancer. Am J Gastroenterol. 2007;102(8):1646–53.
34. Frulloni L, Scattolini C, Falconi M, et al. Autoimmune pancreatitis: differences between the focal and diffuse forms in 87 patients. Am J Gastroenterol. 2009;104(9):2288–94.
35. Tan Sardjono C, Mottram PL, Hogarth PM. The role of FcgammaRIIa as an inflammatory mediator in rheumatoid arthritis and systemic lupus erythematosus. Immunol Cell Biol. 2003;81(5):374–81.
36. Detlefsen S, Bräsen J, Zamboni G, Capelli P, Klöppel G. Deposition of complement C3c, immunoglobulin (Ig)G4 and IgG at the basement membrane of

pancreatic ducts and acini in autoimmune pancreatitis. Histopathology. 2010;57:825–35.
37. Pradhan V, Patwardhan GK. Fc gamma receptor polymorphisms in systemic lupus erythematosus and their correlation with the clinical severity of the disease. Indian J Hum Genet. 2008;14(3):77–81.
38. van Schie RC, Wilson ME. Evaluation of human FcgammaRIIA (CD32) and FcgammaRIIIB (CD16) polymorphisms in Caucasians and African-Americans using salivary DNA. Clin Diagn Lab Immunol. 2000;7(4):676–81.

# Part I

# Autoimmune Pancreatitis

# 2 Immune Pathogenesis

Edward Alabraba, Shameena Bharucha, Penny Watson, and Robert Sutton

Autoimmune pancreatitis (AIP) can present as acute pancreatitis, but is typically recognised as a distinct form of chronic pancreatitis. Key features include pancreatic lymphoplasmacytic infiltration, chronic inflammatory storiform fibrosis and hypergammaglobulinaemia [1, 2]. Heavy infiltration of the pancreas by lymphocytes targeting acinar and/or duct cells may lead to severe damage, which is to a varying extent reversible with steroid therapy. Two predominant patterns of AIP have been identified, namely, lymphoplasmacytic sclerosing pancreatitis (LPSP or type 1; see Fig. 2.1) and idiopathic duct-centric pancreatitis (IDCP or type 2; see Fig. 2.2), that both share some common histopathological features. LPSP characteristically shows the hallmark periductal lymphoplasmacytic infiltrate, high levels of serum and tissue $I_gG4$-positive plasma cells, storiform fibrosis and obliterative phlebitis [1A]. In contrast, IDCP is typified by intense neutrophilic infiltration in the lobule and duct, referred to as granulocyte epithelial lesions (GEL) that may lead to ductal destruction. Some use the term '$I_gG_4$-related sclerosing cholangitis ($I_gG_4$-SC)' in reference to the bile duct disease frequently associated with AIP [3, 4]. Little is known regarding the triggers of AIP or why the pancreatic and bile ducts become targets of immune-mediated damage. There are, however, a number of intriguing clues that provide early insight, including genetic predisposition, the number of candidate pancreatic autoantigens bearing structural similarity to microbial pathogens (attacked by molecular mimicry), animal forms of AIP that offer further insight, the roles of TGF-β and complement activation by immune complexes, as well as potential triggers for AIP including *H. pylori* [1A].

## Pancreaticobiliary Anatomy and Histological Features of AIP

Intercalated ducts are the first tier of pancreatic ducts that receive acinar secretions and gradually coalesce into larger ducts which terminate in the main pancreatic duct, contributing to and

E. Alabraba, Ph.D., MRCS, MBChB
S. Bharucha, MBChB, MRCP
R. Sutton, D.Phil., FRCS (✉)
NIHR Liverpoool Pancreas Biomedical Research Unit, Institute of Translational Medicine, University of Liverpool, Royal Liverpool University Hospital, Daulby Street, Liverpool L69 3GA, UK
e-mail: r.sutton@liverpool.ac.uk

P. Watson, M.A., VetMD, CertVR, DSAM, DipECVIM
Department of Veterinary Medicine, Queen's Veterinary School Hospital, University of Cambridge, Cambridge, Cambs, UK

M.J. Levy and S.T. Chari (eds.), *Autoimmune (IgG4-related) Pancreatitis and Cholangitis*, DOI 10.1007/978-1-4419-6430-4_2, © Springer Science+Business Media New York 2013

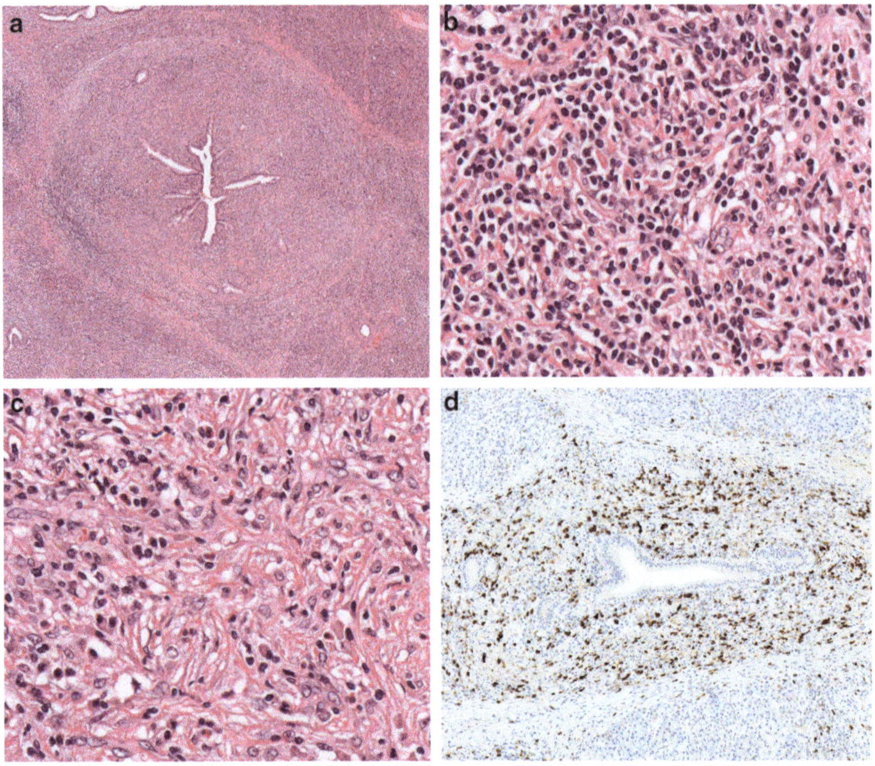


**Fig. 2.1** *Lymphoplasmacytic sclerosing pancreatitis, or 'type 1 AIP'*. (**a**) Low-power view of diffuse lymphoplasmacytic infiltration with (**b**) higher-power view of storiform fibrosis with (**c**) some areas of myofibroblast predominance. Pancreatic acini are not in evidence, having been replaced by inflammation and fibrosis, although these may be preserved in other areas. The inflammation clearly surrounds the ducts but leaves the ductal epithelium and lumen largely intact (A-C, H and E). (**d**) Immunohistochemical demonstration of characteristically dense infiltration by $I_gG4$ plasma cells

draining exocrine secretion into the duodenum. Centroacinar cells lining the acinar lumen continue into the intercalated and intralobular ducts as cuboidal epithelium, while the epithelial lining of the larger interlobular ducts varies with their size. The biliary ducts are lined by cuboidal or columnar epithelial cells and are surrounded by capillary plexuses arising from the hepatic artery.

Pancreatic arterial supply arises from the celiac trunk and superior mesenteric artery, and venous blood drains to the portal vein. A third of lobular terminal arterioles supply islets before reaching acinar capillary beds although the functional significance is unclear [5, 6]. Abundant lymphatics around lobular blood vessels drain interstitial fluid to peripancreatic nodes and subsequently to lymph nodes draining the pancreas [7, 8].

In human AIP, pancreatic lymphoplasmacytic infiltrates co-localise with macrophages and myofibroblasts [9], likely contributing to AIP through cell-cell crosstalk. AIP distorts lobular anatomy, and secondary inflammation around the pancreatic ducts causes a severe obliterating periductal fibrosis [10–12]; small veins show obliterative phlebitis, and there is enlargement of peripancreatic and peribiliary lymph nodes [13]. Although the intrapancreatic portion of the extrahepatic bile duct is affected in AIP involving the head of the pancreas, medium- to large-sized interlobular ducts are usually targeted [10, 12, 13] and lymphoplasmacytic sclerosing cholecystitis is also reported [14]. Around the extrahepatic and intrahepatic large bile duct exist peribiliary glands which contain exocrine acini and express pancreatic exocrine enzymes and

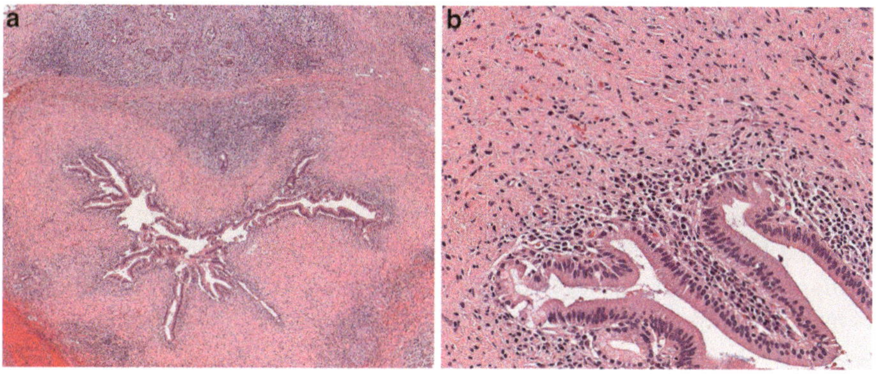


**Fig. 2.2** *Idiopathic duct-centric pancreatitis, or 'type 2 AIP'*. (**a**) Low-power view showing inflammatory cell infiltrate extending to the ductal epithelium, which has been destroyed in parts. (**b**) Higher-power view of (**a**) showing infiltrate directly beneath the ductal epithelium that is damaged at one point. Beyond this, there is extensive fibrosis (H and E)

lactoferrin, a non-enzymatic secretory protein; the presence of these glands has been proposed to account for similar pathology arising from the bile duct and the pancreas [15]. These peribiliary glands are also targets of immune destruction in AIP [15]. Biliary and pancreatic ductal epithelial cells of affected ducts in AIP may be relatively spared despite being surrounded by fibrosis [15].

Although pancreatic infiltration by eosinophils was not seen in the relatively smaller number of specimens analysed by Wang et al. [16], larger studies [17, 18] showed prominent pancreatic eosinophil infiltration. Eosinophils also exist in GELs, which typify the IDCP form or AIP, although neutrophils predominate in these lesions [12]. Some studies have shown sustained reversal of peripheral eosinophilia following steroid therapy [16, 19], while others have reported variable responses [18].

Islet autoantibodies are uncommon and islets are not infiltrated by $I_gG_4$ cells [20, 21]. Fibrosis does occur around islets, but the total islet mass is relatively preserved in AIP [22], helped by islet differentiation from ductal precursor cells overexpressing insulin promoter factor-1 (IPF-1) [23] or by the protective effect of infiltrating macrophages [24]. Nevertheless, diabetes mellitus is observed in some cases, and epitope spreading (see next section) including to islet antigens does occur in experimental AIP [1].

A less well-studied leukocyte subset in AIP is eosinophils although peripheral eosinophilia is reported in patients with AIP [16–18].

## General Overview of Immunity

A concise overview of critical components of immunity, many of which are featured in AIP, is included here to assist the general reader. Responses to invading microbes may be innate or adaptive (acquired). The innate immune response detects and alerts the host to the presence of invading pathogens and generates adaptive immune responses. The innate immune system comprises mononuclear phagocytes (monocytes, macrophages, dendritic cells), granulocytes (neutrophil, eosinophils, basophils), mast cells and natural killer (NK) cells [25].

Pathogens bear pathogen-associated molecular patterns (PAMPs) which immune cells recognise via pattern recognition receptors (PRRs), such as Toll-like receptors (TLRs) [26]. Ligation of cell-expressed TLRs leads to activation of immune cells, which secrete inflammatory cytokines via downstream signalling pathways. A well-known PRR is TLR4, which is expressed by all innate immune cells and recognises the bacterial PAMP, lipopolysaccharide (LPS). TLRs expressed by pancreatic stellate and endothelial cells contribute to the role of these cells in immune responses.

The innate response activates the complement system to generate several immunologically active products including C3b, C3a, C4a, C5a, C5a and the membrane-attack complex, which act as opsonins, cell activators, chemoattractants and inducers of cell lysis.

Phagocytic clearance of pathogen-derived molecules by neutrophils and monocytes/macrophages causes these immune cells to become activated and secrete inflammatory cytokines, part of innate immunity driving adaptive immunity. Dendritic cells (DC) function as antigen-presenting cells (APC) which present antigen to T cells in association with major histocompatibility complex (MHC) molecules thus initiating acquired immune responses in secondary lymphoid tissues such as local draining lymph nodes [27]. The MHC genes are present in most vertebrates and code for cell-surface proteins named the human leukocyte antigens (HLA) in man. MHC molecules exist as class I via which self-peptides are presented to $CD8^+$ T cells and class II for presentation of exogenous peptides to $CD4^+$ T cells. There exists three subsets of MHC class I molecules, namely, HLA-A, HLA-B and HLA-C, and of class II molecules, namely, HLA-DP, HLA-DQ and HLA-DR. Antigen recognition is specific because the T cell receptor (TCR) is only able to recognise antigenic peptides linked with MHC molecules. A similar process occurs for B cells and is mediated by the B cell receptor (BCR). Lymphocytes only recognise small parts of antigens (epitopes), owing to the much smaller size of lymphocyte receptors relative to antigens. Haptens are antigens that are too small to elicit immune responses unless they are coupled to larger immunogenic molecules called carriers.

Effective MHC-mediated antigen presentation necessitates contact between APCs and lymphocytes and co-stimulatory activation of lymphocytes. Stable cell contact is maintained by binding of APC-expressed intercellular adhesion molecule 1 (ICAM-1) to lymphocyte-expressed lymphocyte function-associated antigen 1 (LFA-1), and co-stimulatory signals for lymphocyte activation are generated by the respective ligations of APC-expressed CD80/CD86 and CD40 by lymphocyte-expressed CD28 and CD154. Ligation of CD80/86 by lymphocyte-expressed cytotoxic T lymphocyte-associated antigen 4 (CTLA-4) instead of CD28 downregulates lymphocyte activation and may promote tolerance [28, 29].

Autoimmunity can be initiated by unique aberrations of antigen processing, namely, epitope spreading and molecular mimicry. In epitope spreading, collateral tissue damage induced by pathogen-specific T cells causes release of self-epitopes that become targets for lymphocyte attack as a result of bearing homology to the immunodominant sequence of pathogens [30] or may occur because non-self-target antigens happen to be linked with bystander self-antigens in complexes [20]. Molecular mimicry occurs when pathogen peptides share sequence or structural similarities with self-antigens and thus trigger the production of immune cells and antibodies that cross-react with these self-proteins.

Terminally differentiated B cells called plasma cells produce immunoglobulins ($I_g$) which are antigen-specific antibodies. Individual B cells evolve to express only one specific antibody. Plasma-cell precursors are generated in germinal centres that arise in lymphoid tissue during the immune response [31]. Following antigen recognition, clones of B cells with high affinity and specificity for an antigen undergo proliferation and produce large quantities of antigen-specific antibody. Antibodies are composed of two identical heavy chains and two identical light chains joined by disulfide bonds. The termini of the heavy and light chains that are not involved in antigen binding form the constant region and define the class and subclass of the antibody. There exist five classes of $I_g$ determined by the constant region of the heavy chains, namely, $I_gG$, $I_gA$, $I_gM$, $I_gD$ and $I_gE$. $I_gG$ is further split into four subclasses, $I_gG_{1–4}$.

Unlike innate responses, adaptive responses become more efficient on subsequent exposure(s) to antigens because during the primary immune response when antigen is first encountered, memory lymphocytes are generated. For instance, memory B cells produce larger amounts of antibody with greater affinity for the antigen on subsequent exposure to antigens compared to the primary response. Functions of antibodies include classic complement pathway activation and antibody-dependent cellular cytotoxicity towards target cells.

## T Cells in Inflammation

The T cell subset repertoire is ever expanding, but key subsets are $CD4^+$, $CD8^+$ and regulatory T cells (which can express $CD4^+$, $CD8^+$ and other characteristic molecules), all contributing to inflammatory responses.

$CD4^+$ helper T cells secrete cytokines that facilitate immune responses. $CD4^+$ T helper ($T_h$) cells may be $T_h0$, $T_h1$, $T_h2$ or $T_h17$ cells. $T_h0$ cells are uncommitted naïve cells capable of differentiating into other functional phenotypes depending on the prevailing cytokine milieu. Differentiation of $T_h1$ cells is stimulated by interferon gamma (IFN-γ) and interleukin-12 (IL-12), of $T_h2$ cells by IL-4 and of $T_h17$ cells by TGF-β and IL-6 or IL-23. $T_h1$ cells produce IFN-γ, IL-2 and IL-12; $T_h2$ cells produce IL-4, IL-5, IL-6 and IL-10; $T_h17$ cells produce IL-17A, IL-17F, IL-21 and IL-22 [32, 33]. $T_h1$ cytokines activate macrophages and promote T cell-mediated cytotoxicity, while $T_h2$ cytokines promote humoral immunity (mediated by B cell-produced antibodies). $T_h17$ cells have effector functions distinct from those of $T_h1$ and $T_h2$ cells, primarily clearing pathogens that are not adequately handled by $T_h1$ or $T_h2$ cells. $T_h17$ cells amplify immune responses at sites of inflammation and are implicated in chronic inflammation and autoimmune disease [34]. $T_h17$ cytokine IL-17 promotes germinal centre formation and autoantibody secretion [35], while IL-21 induces proliferation of B cells and their differentiation into $I_g$-producing plasma cells [36].

$CD8^+$ cytotoxic or killer T cells eliminate virally infected cells following detection via MHC I-linked viral peptides. Cytotoxic $CD8^+$ T cells kill target cells via the granzyme-perforin or the Fas-FasL pathways. In the granzyme-perforin pathway, granzyme serine proteinases released from activated $CD8^+$ T cells are passed into the target cell via pores in the target-cell membrane created by perforins, also released by activated $CD8^+$ T cells. Granzymes cleave granzyme A, granzyme B, caspases, and Bcl2-interacting domain, inducing apoptosis of the target cell. FasL-bearing $CD8^+$ T cells can bind the Fas molecule on target cells thus activating caspases within and inducing apoptosis of target cells.

Regulatory, suppressor T cells ($T_{regs}$) are typically $CD4^+$ $CD25^+$ T cells that express the transcription factor forkhead box P3 (Foxp3). $T_{regs}$ may occur naturally in the thymus or may be induced in peripheral lymphoid organs. $T_{regs}$ are also identifiable by high level of expression of CD45RO, CTLA4 and glucocorticoid-induced tumour necrosis factor receptor (GITR), as well as low levels of CD127 and CD45RA. $T_{regs}$ suppress activation, proliferation and effector functions of T cells, NK cells, B cells and a range of APCs. Suggested mechanisms by which $T_{regs}$ induce suppressor activity include CTLA4-mediated suppression of APCs, contact-induced suppression of effector T cells and secretion of TGF-β and IL-10. The translational potential of harnessing the suppressive effect of $T_{regs}$ is under investigation in clinical trials of autoimmune diseases [37] where impaired $T_{reg}$ response is implicated [38]; such an approach may be applicable to AIP. T cell differentiation is tightly regulated as naïve T cells stimulated with TGF-β differentiate into $T_{regs}$, but into $T_h17$ cells in the presence of both TGF-β and IL-6 [33].

## B Cells in Inflammation

B cell responses to antigenic stimulation may be T cell dependent or independent. In T cell-dependent responses, antigen taken up by B cells is processed and presented to T cells via MHC II in secondary lymphoid organs. Naïve B cells subsequently mature and undergo clonal expansion, somatic hypermutation, and class-switch recombination. Naïve B cells are of $I_gM$ and $I_gD$ isotypes. Class-switch recombination of $I_g$ heavy chain permits B cells to produce antigenic-specific antibodies of different isotypes, while somatic mutation of $I_g$ gene rearrangements increases the antigen binding affinity of the B cell receptor (BCR). As well as maturing into $I_g$-secreting plasma cells, naïve antigen-specific B cells also mature into memory B cells, allowing rapid induction of high levels of high affinity $I_gG$, $I_gA$ and $I_gE$ antibodies to be generated after a secondary antigen challenge. Class-switch recombination is important for memory B cell generation and relies on interactions between T cell-expressed CD40L and B cell-expressed CD40.

T cell-independent responses are induced by polymeric antigens such as LPS which activate B cells by cross-linking surface $I_g$ molecules [39]. Most T cell-independent antibody responses do not involve somatic mutation, resulting in weak immune memory to T cell-independent antigens. The emergence of self-reactive clones of B cells is prevented by processes such as clonal deletion, receptor editing to less self-reactive ones and clonal anergy. Autoimmune responses by self-reactive B cells can also be inhibited by macrophage-secreted IL-6 and CD40L. Failings at these checkpoints allow expansion of memory B cell pools that promote autoimmunity [40–43]. B cells promote autoimmunity by producing pathogenic autoantibodies, presenting antigen to autoreactive T cells, forming tissue-damaging immune complexes, secreting proinflammatory cytokines such as IL-2 and IFN-γ, as well as by ectopic neo-lymphogenesis [44]. Ectopic neo-lymphogenesis is de novo formation and maintenance of germinal centres in ectopic tissue sites thus amplifying local disease [45], frequently observed in AIP. B cells function as autoantigen-presenting cells in diabetic NOD mice [46]. B cell depletion by targeting the CD20 antigen, expressed by B cells at almost all stages of differentiation, is therapeutically beneficial in NOD mice with autoimmune diabetes [47] or in patients with rheumatoid arthritis [48]. B cells are also capable of inhibiting immune responses by producing IL-10 and TGF-β or promoting differentiation of $T_{regs}$ [49].

## Specific Changes of Autoimmunity in AIP

Evidence of autoimmune injury in AIP includes the presence of autoantibodies, lymphocyte infiltration, association with specific HLA haplotypes and associations with other immune inflammatory diseases. Unlike classic autoimmune diseases, AIP affects males more commonly than females, and as previously mentioned, identified autoantibodies are not completely specific for AIP. Rodent and dog models have increased our understanding of the immune process underlying AIP. Because of the clinical focus on antibodies in AIP with blood being far easier to sample than pancreatic tissue, $I_gG_4$ and autoantibodies are discussed first, even though it may be that T cell responses have a predominating role in the pathogenesis of AIP. A diagrammatic representation of the immune mechanisms that may contribute to AIP is given in Fig. 2.3.

## $I_g$G4 in AIP

Serum and pancreatic tissue elevations of $I_gG_4$ occur in AIP [50–52]. The $I_gG_4$ subclass accounts for only 3–6 % of total serum $I_gG$ in normal subjects and has significantly higher concentrations in men than women [53]. The elevation of $I_gG_4^+$ cells in AIP patients may be due to a global increase in the total number of infiltrating plasma cells (see Fig. 2.3) and not a preferential increase of $I_gG_4^+$ plasma cells alone [54].

Unlike other $I_gG$ subclasses, $I_gG_4$ cannot bind C1q and is unable to activate the classic complement pathway [55]. Classic complement pathway activation, however, does occur in patients with AIP and is associated with elevated serum $I_gG_1$ [56]. Kawa et al. showed $I_gG_4$ can undergo Fc-Fc binding interactions with $I_gG$ subtypes 1–3, which induces aggregation of $I_g$ to form complexes; they speculated that the easier clearance of aggregate complexes terminates the inflammatory process

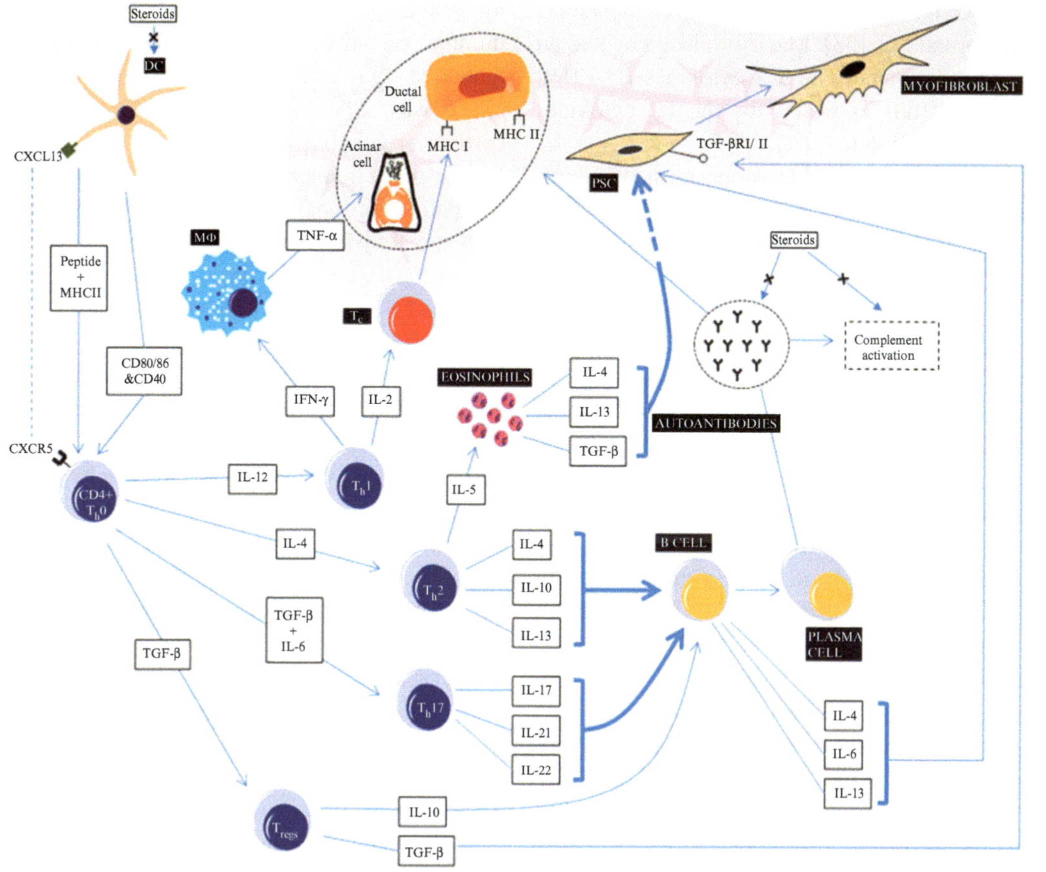


**Fig. 2.3** *Schematic representation of immune events in AIP*. Autoimmune attack on pancreatic acinar and ductal cells in AIP begins with uncommitted CD4+ T helper cells (*$T_h0$*) experiencing an MHC-complexed autoantigen presented by antigen-presenting cells such as dendritic cells (*DC*) in association with appropriate co-stimulatory signals. CXCL13-expressing DC may attract and undergo cognate interactions with CXCR5-expressing lymphocytes in AIP. $T_h0$ cells become activated and differentiate into $T_h1$, $T_h2$, $T_h17$, or $T_{regs}$ depending on the nature of the antigen and the cytokines prevalent in the pancreatic microenvironment. $T_h1$, $T_h2$, $T_h17$, and $T_{regs}$ are induced by IL-12, IL-4, TGF-β and IL-6 and TGF-β alone, respectively. These $T_h$ subsets drive immune reactions that are partly driven by the cytokines they produce. $T_h2$ cells drive B cell differentiation into autoantibody-producing plasma cells by producing IL-4, IL-10, and IL-13. Plasma cells produce autoantibodies directed against endocrine pancreatic antigens, thus acinar and ductal cells (*highlighted* within pancreas by *ellipse with dashed outline*). Production of antibodies by plasma cells leads to complement activation. $T_h2$ cytokine IL-5 promotes recruitment of eosinophils which may themselves secrete pro-fibrotic cytokines such as IL-4, IL-13, and TGF-β. The $T_h1$ cytokine IFN-γ activates macrophages to secrete TNF-α which may activate acinar or endothelial cells, and IL-2 promotes differentiation of cytotoxic T cells (*$T_c$*). Aberrant MHC expression by pancreatic ductal cells renders them more susceptible to attack by $T_c$, particularly CD8+ T cells via granzyme-perforin or Fas-FasL pathways. $T_h17$ cells produce IL-17A, IL-17F, IL-21 and IL-22 which promote germinal-centre formation, autoantibody secretion, induce B cell proliferation and differentiation into $I_g$-producing plasma cells. $T_{regs}$ oppose the proinflammatory actions of other T cells and promote fibrosis by activating pancreatic stellate cells (PSC) to myofibroblasts via secreted TGF-β which binds to TGF-βRI/II expressed by PSC. Steroids treat AIP by inhibiting DCs, complement activation and antigen-specific antibody production

[57]. $I_gG_1$ is itself elevated in AIP, even in patients with normal $I_gG_4$ [58]. $I_gG_4$ is produced by human B cells stimulated with $T_h2$ cytokines IL-4 [59] and IL-13 [60], as well as by the $T_{reg}$ cytokines IL-10 and TGF-β [61, 62].

$I_gG_4$ is uniquely able to perform 'Fab-arm exchange' in which random swapping of heavy and light chain pairs between $I_gG_4$ molecules occurs leading to bi-specific antibodies (enabling cross-linking of non-identical antigens) which are anti-inflammatory [63]. $I_gG_4$ antibodies generated in $I_gE$-mediated allergic responses are usually associated with tolerance-inducing mechanisms [64]. Bi-specific antibodies formed by 'Fab-arm exchange' are functionally monovalent (cannot cross-link identical antigens) despite being structurally hetero-bivalent and are thus less likely to form large immune complexes and have a low potential for inducing inflammation. If large numbers of target and effector cells are present, binding by high levels of bi-specific antibodies can lead to immunopathology as may occur in Wegener's granulomatosis [65] and bullous pemphigoid [66]. There are no data to support a causative role for $I_gG_4$ in AIP, and expression of the pro-fibrotic cytokines TGF-β and PDGF-B is not affected by the $I_gG_4$ status of AIP patients [9]. $I_gG_4$ autoantibodies may simply be generated as a result of chronic autoimmune inflammation and may not actually cause injury, but based on evidence to date including work that has shown $I_gG_4$ in AIP can be an autoantibody [68], the possibility that $I_gG_4$ either exacerbates or reduces the pathology of AIP cannot be discounted.

## Autoantibodies in Human AIP

The targeting of inflammatory damage to pancreaticobiliary ducts in AIP suggests antigens expressed by ductal epithelium are recognised by the immune system. Immune responses are elicited following in vivo alteration of rat pancreatic ductal antigens by ductal infusion of trinitrobenzene sulfonic acid (TNBS) which acts as a hapten [67]. The presence of organ-specific autoantibodies in the serum of AIP patients is demonstrated by increased $I_gG_4$ expression in normal tissue immunoreacted with sera from AIP patients, the increased $I_gG_4$ expression being attenuated if serum was obtained from patients treated with corticosteroids [68].

The most frequent autoantibodies detected in AIP patients are anti-lactoferrin (anti-LF) and anti-carbonic anhydrase type II and/or IV (anti-CA-II or anti-CA-IV), which detect the candidate target antigens LF and CA [69–72]. A recent series of 26 Japanese patients with AIP was reported in which 90 % of patients' sera were positive for either anti-CA-II or anti-LF and 30 % positive for both [73]. Carbonic anhydrase is also expressed by salivary glands and kidneys and lactoferrin by breast, bronchial, salivary and gastric glands. Neither is specific for AIP as either or both can be detected in Sjögren's syndrome [69], ulcerative colitis [74] and primary sclerosing cholangitis [75].

Other autoantigens implicated in AIP are α-Fodrin and serine protease inhibitor Kazal-type 1 (SPINK-1, also known as pancreatic secretory trypsin inhibitor or PSTI, mutations of which predispose to chronic pancreatitis). α-Fodrin expression is limited to AIP patients with associated Sjögren syndrome or sclerosing cholangitis [76], also an autoantigenic marker of Sjögren syndrome [77]. Autoantibodies to SPINK1 detected in patients with AIP are of $I_gG1$ subclass [73]. Screening of a human pancreas cDNA library with serum from a patient with AIP revealed clones identical to amylase α-2A [78] and heat shock protein 10 (HSP 10) cDNA [79]. Autoantibodies against amylase α-2A [78] and HSP 10 [79] have been detected in Japanese patients with AIP, and serum autoantibody titres were reduced by steroid therapy.

In a recently published study undertaken by Löhr et al. [80], a comprehensive genomics and proteomics approach to AIP extended our understanding through the finding that acinar cells and their protein components are targeted by the inflammatory process. The loss of acinar cells was associated with elevated autoantibody titres against cationic and anionic trypsinogens (PRSS1 and PRSS2) and SPINK-1; there was no difference in the findings between both subtypes of AIP. These autoantibodies were found to have a

**Table 2.1** Autoantibodies identified in patients with AIP

| Autoantibody | References |
|---|---|
| Anti-lactoferrin (anti-LF) | [69] |
| Anti-carbonic anhydrase II or IV anti-CA-II or anti-CA-IV) | [68–71] |
| Anti-α-Fodrin | [75] |
| Anti-amylase α -2A | [77] |
| Anti-heat shock protein 10 (anti-HSP 10) | [78] |
| Anti-cationic trypsinogen (anti-PRSS1) | [79] |
| Anti-anionic trypsinogen (anti-PRSS2) | [79] |

predictive accuracy of 80 % for distinguishing patients with AIP from those with non-AIP chronic pancreatitis, and an accuracy of 86 % for AIP patients versus healthy controls. The detection of these antibodies by ELISA may help to distinguish AIP from other types of pancreatitis such as alcoholic pancreatitis.

All the autoantigens identified so far are expressed by pancreatic ducts and acini, in keeping with the histological injury observed in AIP. A list of the autoantibodies is given in Table 2.1. These autoantibodies may arise from cell destruction or by epitope spreading of initial autoantigens.

## Cellular Responses in Human AIP

MHC class I (HLA-ABC) and II antigens (HLA-DR and HLA-DQ) are focally expressed by pancreatic ductal epithelium in AIP [81–83]. Aberrant expression of MHC I and MHC II by pancreatic ducts is seen in chronic pancreatitis [84–87]. In AIP, pancreatic duct cells may act as APC alongside dendritic cells to present MHC-complexed autoantigenic peptides to T cells. The chemokine CXCL13 and its receptor CXCR5 are expressed by cells in periductal and parenchymal areas of the pancreata of patients with AIP [54]. In tissues affected by autoimmune disease, CXCL13-expressing follicular dendritic cells and CXCR5-expressing naïve B or memory $CD4^+$ T cells are known to undergo cognate interactions crucial for maintaining lymphocytic infiltrates and supporting germinal centres of lymphoid follicles [88].

Polyclonal lymphocyte populations are detected in most patients with AIP, suggesting the immune response targets numerous antigens or numerous antigenic epitopes generated by epitope spreading [51]. Similar polyclonal B cell activation producing $I_gM$, $I_gG_1$, $I_gG_2$ and $I_gG_4$ plasma cells occurs in AIRE-deficient NOD mice with AIP [89].

In patients with AIP and coexistent cholangitis (autoimmune pancreato-cholangitis or AIPC), areas of pancreatitis and cholangitis are infiltrated by large numbers of $CD4^+$ $CD25^+T_{regs}$ [90]. The ratio of $Foxp3^+/CD4^+$ cells is higher in AIPC than in other autoimmune or non-autoimmune diseases, and infiltrating $T_{regs}$ may produce IL-10 and TGF-β which are highly expressed in AIPC [90]. Local IL-10 will promote B cell switching to $I_gG_4$-producing plasma cells, and TGF-β will activate pancreatic stellate cells (PSC) to myofibroblasts causing fibrosis. Interestingly, analysis of peripheral blood IL-10 and TGF-β in AIP patients revealed no difference from healthy controls or non-AIP chronic pancreatitis [91]. Other studies have analysed peripheral T cell counts in AIP patients and demonstrated that $T_h1$ cells predominate over $T_h2$ cells [70] with a marked increase in $CD4^+$ and $CD8^+$ T cells expressing $HLA\text{-}DR^+$ [70]; naïve $T_{regs}$ ($CD4^+$ $CD25^+$ $CD45RA^+$) are decreased while memory $T_{regs}$ ($CD4^+$ $CD25^+$ $CD45RA^-$) are elevated [91]. The increase of memory $T_{regs}$ may reflect the activation of $T_h0$ cells into effector and memory populations. However, it is difficult to reconcile the contrasting data on $T_h1/T_h2$ cytokine profiling in the pancreas [90] and in the peripheral blood [70] of AIP patients.

Circulating $CD4^+$ T cells expressing HLA-DR infiltrate pancreatic ductal epithelium in AIP [82, 83]. Although HLA-DR is mainly expressed by professional APCs, activated human T cells synthesise and express MHC class II molecules [92]. In vivo activated human T cells express MHC class II and co-stimulatory molecules and may be able to present peptide antigens to bystander T cells. Antigen presentation by MHC class II-expressing T cells provides downregulatory signals to antigen-responding $CD4^+$ T cells [92, 93]. This immunoregulatory role is emphasised by $HLA\text{-}DR^+$ $CD4^+$ $CD25^{hi}$ natural $T_{regs}$, which express the highest levels of Foxp3, rapidly induce strong suppression and exhibit low in vitro expansion capabilities [94, 95].

B cells may have a pro-fibrotic role in AIP. Peripheral blood B cells are recruited and activated due to repeated injury in sites of tissue fibrosis [96]. B cells secrete IL-4, IL-6 and IL-13 which cause paracrine activation of PSC [96–98] or induce macrophages to secrete TGF-β causing paracrine activation of PSC [99, 100]. The specific role of tissue $I_gG_4$ in AIP is uncertain, but it certainly does reflect the large number of B cells recruited to the pancreas and to extrapancreatic sites such as the salivary glands and liver [101].

The $T_h2$ cytokine IL-5 is expressed in tissue affected by AIP [90] and is an important stimulus to eosinophilic infiltration and activation [102]. The exact role played by eosinophils in AIP is uncertain, but they are capable of producing cytokines including IL-2, IL-3, IL-4, IL-5, IL-7, IL-13, IL-16, TNF-α, TGF-β and RANTES, as well as cationic proteins such as eosinophil cationic protein and reactive oxygen metabolites. As in AIP, profound fibrosis also occurs in eosinophilic pancreatitis where there is heavy eosinophilic infiltration of the pancreas [17]; eosinophilic pancreatitis may be an unusual variant form of AIP [103, 104]. Eosinophil-derived mediators may activate PSC similar to their effect on fibroblasts during fibrosis elsewhere [105–107].

## Rodent AIP

Spontaneous or induced rodent models of AIP have contributed to the understanding of the immune pathogenesis of AIP. Spontaneous experimental rodent models of AIP include the following (see also the complete list in Table 2.2):

(i) MRL/Mp mice spontaneously develop AIP after 22 weeks of age. Their pancreata are infiltrated by $CD4^+$ T cells and macrophages with destruction of acini that are replaced by adipose tissue [108]. Conplastic mouse strains containing the nuclear genome of MRL/MpJ mice and the mitochondrial genome of FVB/N mice (MRL/MpJ-$mt^{FVB/N}$) mice develop a more severe parenchymal destruction inflammatory infiltrate in the pancreas by 24 weeks of age compared with MRL/MpJ controls [109].

(ii) Mice homozygous for aly (alymphoplasia) mutation lack lymph nodes and Peyer's patches, show defects in humoral and cellular immunity and spontaneously develop AIP after 14 weeks of age. Pancreatic acinar cells are destroyed by infiltrating $CD4^+$ T cells and replaced by adipose tissue, while islet cells are completely spared [110].

(iii) Male Wistar Bonn Kobori (WBN/Kob) rats develop AIP spontaneously from 4 weeks of age marked by lymphocytic infiltration and acinar destruction. Fibrosis begins from 8 weeks of age and is accelerated with increased inflammatory cell infiltration from 12 weeks of age. The pancreas is infiltrated mainly by $CD8^+$ T cells expressing MHC I and II, serum $I_gG_{2b}$ levels are increased, peripheral blood $T_{regs}$ are reduced in count and extrapancreatic lesions exist [111].

(iv) NOD mice are prone to autoimmune diseases, but they do not spontaneously develop AIP. NOD mice with knockout of CD28 gene (NOD.CD28KO mice) show defective thymic development, maintenance of peripheral $T_{regs}$ and are predisposed to AIP. NOD.CD28KO mice transfused with islet-specific BDC2.5 $T_{regs}$ are protected from autoimmune islet injury but develop AIP from 8 weeks of age onwards. They show increasing infiltration of the pancreas by $CD4^+$ T cells, initially periductally then progressively spreading to result in atrophy of acinar cells and replacement by adipose tissue at 16 weeks. The inciting autoantigen was identified as α-amylase, and injecting mice with tolerance-inducing amylase-coupled splenic cells fixed with 1-ethyl-3-(3-dimethylaminopropyl)-carbodiimide (ECDI) has been shown to attenuate mononuclear cell infiltration and exocrine pancreatic injury [112].

(v) NOD mice lacking the tolerance-inducing autoimmune regulator (AIRE) gene show a shift in target autoantigen recognised by autoreactive T cells from islet-expressed antigen to acinar cell-expressed pancreas-

**Table 2.2** Summary of available rodent models of AIP

| Species | Mode | Autoantibody | Effector cell | Damage observed | Comment | Ref |
|---|---|---|---|---|---|---|
| AIRE KO mice | Spontaneous | Pancreas-specific protein disulfide isomerase (PDIp) | $CD4^+$ and $CD8^+$ T cells and B cells | Acinar destruction and fatty replacement | Polyclonal B cell activation occurs yielding $I_gM$, $I_gG_1$, $I_gG_2$ and $I_gG_4$ plasma cells | [88] |
| MRL/Mp mice | Spontaneous | Pancreatic secretory trypsin inhibitor (PSTI) | $CD4^+$ and macrophages | Acinar destruction and fatty replacement | Accelerated or worsened injury if treated with poly I:C or IFN- γ, respectively | [107–110] |
| MRL/MpJmt$^{FVB/N}$ mice | Spontaneous | Not specified | B cells and $CD8^+$ T cells | Acinar destruction, fibrosis, and fatty change | More severe parenchymal destruction than in MRL/MpJ controls at 24 weeks | [111] |
| aly/aly mice | Spontaneous | Not specified | $CD4^+$ T cells | Acinar destruction and fatty replacement | | [112] |
| WBN/Kob rats | Spontaneous | Not specified | $CD8^+$ mainly but also $CD4^+$ T cells | Acinar destruction and fibrosis | Peripheral blood Treg counts are reduced and extrapancreatic lesions exist | [113] |
| CD28-KO NOD mice | Spontaneous | Amylase | $CD4^+$ T cells | Acinar atrophy and fatty replacement | | [114] |
| HLA-DR*0405 transgenic Ab0 NOD mice | Spontaneous | Not specified | $CD4^+$ and $CD8^+$ T cells, B cells, and macrophages | Acinar destruction and fatty replacement | Also show acinar-to-ductal metaplasia | [115] |
| TGF-βR2$^{fspKO}$ mice | Spontaneous | Not specified | Macrophages and T cells | Acinar metaplasia | No significant fibrosis | [119] |
| Neonatally thymectomised BALB/c mice | Immunized with CA-II or LF antigens | Carbonic anhydrase II (CA-II) or Lactoferrin (LF) | $CD4^+$ T cells | Ductal and acinar cell apoptosis | | [116] |
| B6 mice | Infection with MuL V | Not specified | $CD4^+$ T cells, B cells and macrophages | Acinar destruction | ? Molecular mimicry | [117] |
| DA(RP) or Lewis rats | Adoptive transfer of amylase-specific T cells | Amylase | $CD4^+$ and $CD8^+$ T cells, macrophages, and dendritic cells | Ductal inflammation, acinar destruction and fibrosis | | [118] |

specific protein disulfide isomerase (PDIp) which protects AIRE-deficient NOD mice from autoimmune diabetes and induces spontaneous AIP [89]. Mice show pancreatic lymphoid cell infiltration starting at 2 weeks of age progressing to intense lymphocytic infiltration of acini that are completely destroyed and replaced with adipose tissue by 8–12 weeks after birth, leaving β cell islets and pancreatic ducts relatively well preserved [89].

(vi) HLA-DR*0405 transgenic Ab0 NOD develop spontaneous AIP by 18 weeks of age or earlier with periacinar leukocytic infiltration and destruction of acini, which are replaced by adipose tissue. HLA-DR*0405 transgenic Ab0 mice have near-normal $CD4^+$ T cell count and function, unlike Ab0 mice which are severely defective. These mice additionally show acinar-to-ductal metaplasia with loss of acinar zymogen granules and formation of ductular structures, but the islet cells are preserved [113].

(vii) C57BL/6 mice with conditional knockout of TGF-β type 2 receptor (TGF-βR2) in S100A4+ cells (TGF-$\beta R2^{fspKO}$ mice) show acinar metaplasia with infiltration by macrophages and T cells by 6 weeks of age, although islet cells are spared [114].

Induced models of AIP include the following:

(i) MLR/Mp mice treated with polyinosinic:polycytidylic acid (poly I:C) develop AIP earlier at 18 weeks [115, 116], and mice treated with IFN-γ show more prominent leukocyte infiltration and worsened histological injury [117]. Of note poly I:C-treated mice show elevated anti-PSTI but not anti-CA-II or anti-LF autoantibody titres and also elevated serum $I_gG_1$ and $I_gG_{2b}$ though not $I_gG_4$ [116].

(ii) Neonatally thymectomised BALB/c mice immunised with CA-II or LF antigens develop AIP with $CD4^+$ T cells infiltration of inflamed ductal or periductal areas and apoptotic ductal or acinar cells. Neonatally thymectomised mice lack peripheral $T_{regs}$ and are prone to autoimmunity. This was the first model to show AIP can be induced by treatment with autoantibodies and greatly strengthens their pathogenic role. Adoptive transfer of splenic T cell subsets from immunised to nude mice identified $CD4^+$ T cells as the effectors of immune damage in recipient mice. Insulitis was not induced by immunisation with CA-II or LF or by lymphocyte transfer [118].

(iii) Young B6 mice develop AIP 4 weeks after being infected with the LP-BM5 murine leukaemia retrovirus (MuLV) in addition to becoming profoundly immunodeficient, but islets are relatively preserved. Increasing leukocytic infiltration, initially seen around the pancreatic ducts with later involvement of the acini, causes acinar cell destruction peaking at 12 weeks after infection. A paucity of TUNEL-positive acinar cells suggests apoptosis is not the main mechanism of acinar cell death in this model, although lymphocytes undergo apoptosis, which may represent activation-induced cell death [119].

(iv) Adoptive transfer of amylase-specific activated $CD4^+$ T cell lines induces diffuse AIP in recipient DA(RP) rats, though less severe in Lewis rats. T cell lines specific for either CA-II or LF, however, did not induce AIP in DA(RP) rats [120].

Table 2.2 lists the various models of autoimmune pancreatitis so far described. Autoantigens thus so far identified in murine studies include pancreatic amylase [112, 120], CA-II and LF [118], PDIp [89] and PSTI [116].

## Canine AIP

A naturally occurring form of autoimmune chronic pancreatitis has been described in the English cocker spaniel (ECS) which develops pancreatic duct-centric immune damage with systemic manifestations, such as by keratoconjunctivitis sicca and autoimmune polyarthritis. Histology of the pancreas in affected dogs shows duct destruction associated with periductal and perivenular infiltration by T cells and progressive interlobular fibrosis [121]. Affected dogs often develop exocrine and endocrine insufficiency in end-stage disease, but neither serum nor tissue $I_gG$ subsets were measured in these studies. Autoimmune disease in ECS is associated with the dog leukocyte antigen system [122], but similar canine HLA association studies in AIP are lacking. German Shepherd dogs and rough-coated Collies also develop a distinct juvenile onset autoimmune-mediated atrophic lymphocytic pancreatitis with autoantibodies directed against acini. Their pancreata are infiltrated by lymphocytes and acini are destroyed causing exocrine insufficiency, but ductal epithelial cells are not targeted. Typically $CD8^+$ T cells predominate in areas of parenchymal destruction and destroyed acini of dogs are replaced by fat, but islets are relatively spared as seen in some rodent models of AIP, such as homozygous aly mice described in the preceding section [123, 124].

The burning question is to what extent these animal findings are relevant to, or can be transferred to, the human situation. There are likely to be significant insights from each species that could be applied to all. The dog has been suggested as a better model of pancreatic disease than rodents because the anatomy and function of the canine pancreas is more similar to humans [125], justifying very much further study to improve the management of AIP, not just in dogs but also in humans.

## TGF-B: Immunomodulator and Pro-fibrotic Factor in AIP

TGF-β signalling is essential for maintaining normal immune homeostasis of pancreatic acinar and ductal cells; indeed TGF-β1, TGF-β2 and TGF-β3 are highly pleiotropic cytokines that almost all cells secrete. Mice overexpressing a dominant-negative mutant form of TGF-β type 2 receptor under the influence of the pS2 promoter (which functionally inactivates TGF-β signalling selectively in pancreatic acinar and ductal cells) are more susceptible to developing autoimmune-mediated pancreatitis induced by caerulein injections [126]. Autoimmunity during pancreatitis in these mice is suggested by serum $I_gG$ and $I_gM$ autoantibodies targeting pancreatic acinar cells and ductal epithelial cells [126]. These transgenic mice show markedly increased MHC class II expression in the pancreatic acinar cells that enhances APC-T cell interactions during pancreatitis [126].

Adoptive transfer of TGF-βR2-deficient dendritic cells (DC) from TGF-$\beta R2^{fspKO}$ mice induced AIP in syngeneic wild-type mice in vivo and caused enhanced T cell activation during in vitro assays using ovalbumin antigen, likely due to enhanced maturation of DCs in response to antigen [120].

TGF-β is crucial for transforming PSC into proliferating myofibroblasts [127, 128] and is expressed alongside its receptor in AIP tissue. In pancreatic tissue specimens from patients affected by AIP, macrophages express the TGF-β1 propeptide called latency-associated peptide (LAP) [9]; pancreatic ductal cells and infiltrating mononuclear cells express TGF-β1 itself [129], while myofibroblasts and ductal cells express TGF-βR2 [9]. TGF-β and other pro-fibrotic cytokines including PDGF-B transform PSC into myofibroblasts causing intense periductal fibrosis [9].

## Potential Triggers of Disease

### Effect of Immunological Genotype on AIP

The occurrence and outcome of AIP is associated with genetic factors within and outside the major histocompatibility complex (MHC). Polypeptide chains encoded by MHC I genes are HLA-A, HLA-B, HLA-C, HLA-E, HLA-G and HLA-F (all belong to human leukocyte antigen or HLA class I), and those encoded by MHC II genes are HLA-DR, HLA-DQ and HLA-DP (all HLA class II). DR and DQ subregion genes are closely linked and usually inherited together such that DR and DQ alleles form stable haplotypes in the population; α and β denote functional genes, while ψ denotes non-functional genes. A diagrammatic representation of potential triggers of AIP is given in the summary (Fig. 2.4).

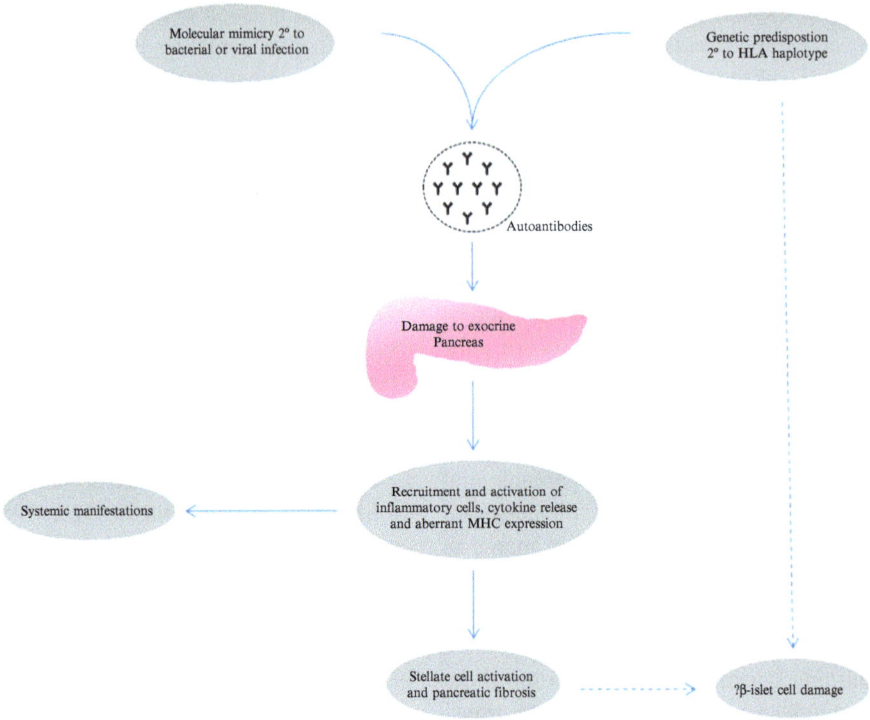


**Fig. 2.4** *Overview of mechanisms leading to injury in AIP*. Triggers, such as molecular mimicry and genetic susceptibility, lead to the expression of autoantigenic epitopes and subsequently the production of autoantibodies that target the exocrine pancreas. Pancreatic injury generates a cytokine milieu that recruits inflammatory cells which become activated to secrete cytokines and cause further damage. Pro-fibrotic cytokines activate pancreatic stellate cells leading to fibrosis. Activated immune cells and cytokines entering the circulating blood may partly account for the systematic manifestations of AIP. β-islet cells may be damaged by surrounding fibrosis, but it is recognised that AIP and autoimmune diabetes share susceptibility haplotypes

Molecular genotyping of 40 Japanese patients with AIP showed that HLA haplotype DRβ1*0405-DQβ1*0401 is associated with AIP [130], and this was confirmed in a more recent study of 15 Japanese patients with AIP [78]. Another study of 43 Japanese patients with AIP showed that in addition to the haplotype HLA-DRβ1*0405-DQβ1*0401 of HLA class II, there also exists a susceptibility region that includes the C3-2-11 microsatellite located between HLA-A and HLA-E genes in the HLA class I region [131]. However, no mutual association was found between HLA-DRB1*0405-DQB1*0401 and the C3-2-11 microsatellite region suggesting these are two distinct genetic susceptibility factors for AIP. Susceptibility conferred by HLA-DR*0405 in man is reproduced in HLA-DR*0405 transgenic Ab0 NOD mice that develop spontaneous AIP closely mimicking human disease [113]. The association of AIP and the DRB1*0405 allele may be explained by linkage disequilibrium with promoter polymorphisms in nuclear factor kappa light polypeptide gene enhancer in B cells inhibitor-like 1 (NFκBI-L1), which may represent a true susceptibility allele as it has crucial roles in inflammation and immunity [131]. The HLA-DRB1*0405-DQB1*0401 haplotype is also linked with autoimmune type 1 diabetes in Japanese patients [132].

Susceptibility MHC alleles were not found in a study of 40 Korean patients with AIP, but it was demonstrated that the HLA DQB1*0302 allele showed a significant association with the relapse of AIP [133], and amino acid sequencing identified a single-nucleotide substitution of aspartic acid to non-aspartic acid at position 57 of the DQβ1 residue [133]. HLA susceptibility haplotypes may alter antigen presentation to T cells, enhancing responses following antigen recognition and promoting development of autoimmunity.

Polymorphisms of alleles 110G and 110A/A of Fc-receptor-like 3 (FCRL3) gene, which belongs to the Fc-receptor-like family of genes that bear homology with classical Fcγ receptor genes, have also shown association with AIP in a study of 59 Japanese patients [134]. Although independently associated with AIP, no association was found between FCRL3-110 alleles and the HLA DRB1*0405-DQB1*0401 haplotype [134]. FCRL3 gene is located on chromosome 1q21 and encodes a glycoprotein of unknown function, but is suspected to play a role in immune regulation as it contains intracellular domain tyrosine-based activation and inhibition motifs [135]. The majority of FCRL3 is expressed in germinal-centre centrocytes that are the precursors of B cells. An effect on B cell development may explain the positive correlation between the number of polymorphisms of FCRL3 susceptibility alleles and serum $I_gG_4$ concentrations in patients with AIP [134]. FCRL3 is expressed on B cells, and single-nucleotide polymorphisms (SNP) within the FCRL3 gene are associated with susceptibility to rheumatoid arthritis, autoimmune thyroiditis and systemic lupus erythematosus, possibly linked to altered binding affinity of the transcription factor NF-κB [136]. FCRL3 may actually be a true susceptibility gene for AIP as it causes $T_{reg}$ dysfunction that promotes loss of self-tolerance and onset of autoimmunity [137].

Genes encoding non-MHC proteins such as cytokines may also affect susceptibility to AIP. There is a lower relative risk of disease resulting from these non-MHC genes compared with the disease-associated MHC haplotypes. CTLA-4 is a key negative regulator of the T cell immune response. The G/G genotype of a CTLA-4 SNP at position +6230 increased susceptibility to AIP (OR 2.48) in a study of 59 Japanese patients with AIP [138]. The +6230A/A genotype was found to be associated with AIP resistance (OR 0.49) but was associated with an enhanced risk of relapse, as was the +49A/A genotype (OR 5.45 and 12.66, respectively) [138]. Serum soluble CTLA-4 levels were found to be significantly higher in patients with AIP but showed no correlation with +6230 alleles [138]. CTLA-4 49A polymorphisms and the -318C/+49A/CT60G haplotype increased susceptibility to AIP in Taiwanese patients [139]. CTLA-4 polymorphisms may induce susceptibility to AIP by causing loss of self-tolerance. Adenine to guanine polymorphism at position +49 of exon 1 of CTLA-4 (CTLA4 +49A/G) is also associated with increased susceptibility to autoimmune thyroiditis and type 1 diabetes [140].

Polymorphisms of TLR4 [141] and the TNF-α promoter gene [131] were shown to have no association with susceptibility to AIP in Japanese patients. Polymorphism of the TNF-α promoter -863A, however, was found to be associated with extrapancreatic disease including nephritis, lymphadenopathy, thyroiditis and hepatitis in Taiwanese patients with AIP [139].

## Molecular Mimicry

Molecular mimicry, a mechanism by which pathogens can induce autoimmune disease, is the development of cross-reactivity to a self-peptide that may arise during the immune response to a foreign peptide. An allogeneic peptide-MHC complex may resemble a self-peptide-MHC complex, which can lead to cross-reactivity by lymphocytes. Although the cross-reactivity of lymphocytes with an array of antigens allows response to diverse pathogens, cross-reactivity with self-antigens is inappropriate and breaks down immune tolerance. AIP may arise from protracted or repeated exposure to indigenous etiologic agents that can break self-tolerance, by activating $CD4^+$ T cells because of incomplete specificity, or the regulation of specificity, of T cell antigen receptors, leading to expansion of cytotoxic T cells and antigen-sensitised plasma cells that produce autoantibodies.

*Helicobacter pylori* (*H. pylori*) is strongly associated with peptic ulceration and is suggested to be a pathogenic trigger of AIP [142]. Gastric peptic ulcers infiltrated by abundant $I_gG_4$-bearing plasma cells occur more frequently in patients with AIP compared to non-diseased controls or patients with non-autoimmune CP [143, 144], and it has recently been proposed that AIP-related gastritis is added to the list of $I_gG_4$-related sclerosing diseases [145]. In considering the potential role of *H. pylori* as a trigger of molecular mimicry, it must be acknowledged that AIP-related gastric ulcers also occur in the absence of *H. pylori* [144, 145].

The role of *H. pylori* in causing AIP by molecular mimicry is supported by the significant homology that exists between human carbonic anhydrase type II and an important *H. pylori* survival enzyme called α-carbonic anhydrase (α-CA), with the binding motif of the AIP susceptibility allele HLA DRB1*0405 also being present in the homologous segment [146]. This suggests that *H. pylori* may trigger AIP in genetically predisposed individuals [146]. Direct bacterial infection of the pancreas by *H. pylori* as part of molecular mimicry is unlikely because *H. pylori* DNA is not detectable in the pancreas of patients with AIP [147].

Screening of serum specimens from 35 AIP patients identified a peptide called AIP1-7 bearing sequence homology to the *H. pylori* peptide plasminogen-binding protein (PBP) and also to the pancreatic acinar enzyme ubiquitin-protein ligase E3 component n-recognin 2 (UBR2) [52]. Anti-PBP antibodies were detected in nearly all screened patients, raising the possibility that molecular mimicry due to homology of URB2 with PBP drives acinar damage [52].

Mice treated with avirulent *Escherichia coli* for 8 weeks develop delayed onset AIP with lymphoplasmacytic infiltration and anti-CA, anti-LF and antinuclear autoantibodies. The authors of the aforementioned study speculated that host self-antigen(s) may act as molecular mimics of *Escherichia coli*, stimulating host immune response in this model [148]. Gastric *Helicobacter* species (not pylori) are also detected in most dogs [149] and may drive molecular mimicry during AIP in dogs.

## Action of Corticosteroids in AIP

The clinical symptoms of AIP are readily relieved by steroid therapy in the majority of patients [50]. Corticosteroids significantly lower the relapse of AIP [150], as achieved by other immunosuppressants such as azathioprine and mycophenolate [151].

Corticosteroids inhibit antigen-specific antibodies, but the relative amounts of total $I_gG_4$ in human peripheral blood mononuclear cells can increase after steroid therapy [152]. The differential effect of corticosteroids on circulating specific and total $I_g$ isotype formation is due to suppression of antigen-specific lymphocyte responses that does not reduce total $I_gG_4$ production. The number of pancreatic $I_gG_4^+$ plasma cells, however, is reduced by corticosteroids [153]. Such therapy also significantly decreases serum immune complex concentrations in AIP patients, most likely by inhibiting the classic complement pathway, as mannose-binding lectin levels are unaffected by corticosteroid therapy [56]. Corticosteroids may also reduce antigen presentation to lymphocytes in AIP, as this therapy significantly decreases the number of peripheral myeloid and $CD123^+$ plasmacytoid DC [91].

Although corticosteroids enhance differentiation of $T_{regs}$ [154], the number of peripheral $CD4^+CD25^{hi}$ $T_{regs}$ in AIP patients treated with corticosteroids remains unaffected, but this may be related to the dosage used [91]. In vitro assays show corticosteroids reduce expression of ICAM-1 and E-selectin on human umbilical vein endothelial cells stimulated with LPS, suggesting corticosteroids attenuate immune cell recruitment during inflammation [155].

Corticosteroids support pancreatic function by correcting CFTR localization to the apical membrane of pancreatic duct cells, restoring $HCO_3^-$ secretion, and by promoting the regeneration of acinar cells, improving digestive enzyme secretion [153]. While the above effects of corticosteroids are advantageous, there are many well-known disadvantages, including a lack of effect on some areas of fibrotic tissue injury damage and major side effects.

The search for greater understanding of the pathogenesis of AIP will help inform the development of new therapies, which can sensibly draw upon novel approaches under development for other autoimmune diseases. To maximise the potential for progress, the pancreatic community should be ready to adopt developments from both within and outside, whether in basic or clinical research. Advances are likely to occur faster if committed centres collaborate, including with industry, to explore applications of new molecules and trial new treatments.

## Learning Points

1. Autoimmune pancreatitis (AIP) is typically recognised as a distinct form of chronic pancreatitis with key features of diffuse lymphoplasmacytic infiltration and chronic inflammatory sclerosis of the pancreas associated with hypergammaglobulinaemia.
2. The two predominant patterns of AIP are lymphoplasmacytic sclerosing pancreatitis (LPSP or type 1) with elevated tissue and serum expression of $I_gG4$ and idiopathic duct-centric pancreatitis (IDCP or type 2) with granulocyte epithelial lesions.
3. Both acinar and ductal cells are the targets of autoantibodies in AIP; islets are most likely attacked in more advanced disease through epitope spreading. Polyclonal lymphocyte populations suggest numerous antigenic epitopes are targeted.
4. $I_gG_4$ may be induced by IL-4, IL-13, IL-10 or TGF-β and may serve an anti-inflammatory role because of its ability to undergo Fab-arm exchange.
5. Pancreatic stellate cells may be transformed into myofibroblasts by the important regulatory cytokine TGF-β family or by IL-4, IL-6 and IL-13 produced by $T_{regs}$ and B cells or by mediators secreted by infiltrating eosinophils.
6. Autoantigens identified in patients with AIP include lactoferrin, carbonic anhydrase types II and IV, SPINK-1 (PSTI), α-Fodrin, amylase α-2A and anti-HSP 10; those in rodents with AIP include lactoferrin, carbonic anhydrase type II, PSTI, amylase and PDIp. Pancreatic digestive enzymes have been identified as important autoantigens that may provide the basis for more sensitive and specific diagnostic tests.
7. Fibrosis usually occurs following exocrine damage in man; however, some rodents and dogs show replacement of destroyed parenchyma with adipose tissue.
8. Individual genotypes can increase susceptibility to AIP (HLA-DRβ1*0405-DQβ1*0401, C3-2-11 microsatellite, FCRL3 and CTLA-4 gene polymorphisms), relapse of AIP (HLA DQB1*0302, CTLA-4 polymorphism) or resistance to AIP (+6230A/A genotype of CTLA4).
9. Homology between carbonic anhydrase type II and α-carbonic anhydrase as well as between URB2 and PBP of humans and *H. pylori*, respectively, implicates *H. pylori* as a pathogen that may trigger AIP through molecular mimicry.
10. Steroid therapy inhibits antigen-specific antibodies, classic complement pathway activation and dendritic cells. Increasing understanding of AIP will assist efforts to develop new and improved therapies, more likely to accelerate through collaboration between committed centres and with industry.

## References


1. Sutton R. Autoimmune pancreatitis – also a Western disease. Gut. 2005;54(5):581–3.
2. Park DH, Kim MH, Chari ST. Recent advances in autoimmune pancreatitis. Gut. 2009;58(12):1680–9.
3. Mihaljevic AL, et al. Histopathological features of autoimmune pancreatitis. Minerva Gastroenterol Dietol. 2008;54(4):365–74.
4. Kamisawa T, et al. Autoimmune pancreatitis and IgG4-related sclerosing disease. Nat Rev Gastroenterol Hepatol. 2010;7(7):401–9.
5. Goldfine ID, Williams JA. Receptors for insulin and CCK in the acinar pancreas: relationship to hormone action. Int Rev Cytol. 1983;85:1–38.
6. Sunamura M, et al. Pancreatic microcirculation in acute pancreatitis. J Hepatobiliary Pancreat Surg. 1998;5(1):62–8.

7. Navas V, O'Morchoe PJ, O'Morchoe CC. Lymphatic system of the rat pancreas. Lymphology. 1995;28(1):4–20.
8. O'Morchoe CC. Lymphatic system of the pancreas. Microsc Res Tech. 1997;37(5–6):456–77.
9. Detlefsen S, et al. Autoimmune pancreatitis: expression and cellular source of profibrotic cytokines and their receptors. Am J Surg Pathol. 2008;32(7):986–95.
10. Notohara K, et al. Idiopathic chronic pancreatitis with periductal lymphoplasmacytic infiltration: clinicopathologic features of 35 cases. Am J Surg Pathol. 2003;27(8):1119–27.
11. Weber SM, et al. Lymphoplasmacytic sclerosing pancreatitis: inflammatory mimic of pancreatic carcinoma. J Gastrointest Surg. 2003;7(1):129–37; discussion 137–9.
12. Zamboni G, et al. Histopathological features of diagnostic and clinical relevance in autoimmune pancreatitis: a study on 53 resection specimens and 9 biopsy specimens. Virchows Arch. 2004;445(6):552–63.
13. Kloppel G. Chronic pancreatitis, pseudotumors and other tumor-like lesions. Mod Pathol. 2007;20 Suppl 1:S113–31.
14. Wang WL, et al. Autoimmune pancreatitis-related cholecystitis: a morphologically and immunologically distinctive form of lymphoplasmacytic sclerosing cholecystitis. Histopathology. 2009;54(7):829–36.
15. Nakanuma Y. A novel approach to biliary tract pathology based on similarities to pancreatic counterparts: is the biliary tract an incomplete pancreas? Pathol Int. 2010;60(6):419–29.
16. Wang Q, et al. Eosinophilia associated with chronic pancreatitis. Pancreas. 2009;38(2):149–53.
17. Abraham SC, et al. Eosinophilic pancreatitis and increased eosinophils in the pancreas. Am J Surg Pathol. 2003;27(3):334–42.
18. Sah RP, et al. Eosinophilia and allergic disorders in autoimmune pancreatitis. Am J Gastroenterol. 2010;105(11):2485–91.
19. Sasahira N, et al. Inflammatory pseudotumor of the liver and peripheral eosinophilia in autoimmune pancreatitis. World J Gastroenterol. 2005;11(6):922–5.
20. Okazaki K. Autoimmune pancreatitis: etiology, pathogenesis, clinical findings and treatment. The Japanese experience. JOP. 2005;6(1 Suppl):89–96.
21. Farris III AB, Lauwers GY, Deshpande V. Autoimmune pancreatitis-related diabetes: quantitative analysis of endocrine islet cells and inflammatory infiltrate. Virchows Arch. 2010;457(3):329–36.
22. Ito T, et al. Evaluation of pancreatic endocrine and exocrine function in patients with autoimmune pancreatitis. Pancreas. 2007;34(2):254–9.
23. Tanaka S, et al. Evidence of primary beta-cell destruction by T-cells and beta-cell differentiation from pancreatic ductal cells in diabetes associated with active autoimmune chronic pancreatitis. Diabetes Care. 2001;24(9):1661–7.
24. Tessem JS, et al. Critical roles for macrophages in islet angiogenesis and maintenance during pancreatic degeneration. Diabetes. 2008;57(6):1605–17.
25. Delves PJ, Roitt IM. The immune system. First of two parts. N Engl J Med. 2000;343(1):37–49.
26. Medzhitov R, Janeway Jr C. The Toll receptor family and microbial recognition. Trends Microbiol. 2000;8(10):452–6.
27. Hoebe K, Janssen E, Beutler B. The interface between innate and adaptive immunity. Nat Immunol. 2004;5(10):971–4.
28. Bluestone JA. Is CTLA-4 a master switch for peripheral T cell tolerance? J Immunol. 1997;158(5):1989–93.
29. Quandt D, et al. A new role of CTLA-4 on B cells in thymus-dependent immune responses in vivo. J Immunol. 2007;179(11):7316–24.
30. Liang B, Mamula MJ. Molecular mimicry and the role of B lymphocytes in the processing of autoantigens. Cell Mol Life Sci. 2000;57(4):561–8.
31. Tarlinton D. Germinal centers: form and function. Curr Opin Immunol. 1998;10(3):245–51.
32. Mosmann TR, Sad S. The expanding universe of T-cell subsets: Th1, Th2 and more. Immunol Today. 1996;17(3):138–46.
33. Korn T, et al. IL-17 and Th17 cells. Annu Rev Immunol. 2009;27:485–517.
34. Cua DJ, Tato CM. Innate IL-17-producing cells: the sentinels of the immune system. Nat Rev Immunol. 2010;10(7):479–89.
35. Hsu HC, et al. Interleukin 17-producing T helper cells and interleukin 17 orchestrate autoreactive germinal center development in autoimmune BXD2 mice. Nat Immunol. 2008;9(2):166–75.
36. Konforte D, Simard N, Paige CJ. IL-21: an executor of B cell fate. J Immunol. 2009;182(4):1781–7.
37. Sakaguchi S, et al. FOXP3+ regulatory T cells in the human immune system. Nat Rev Immunol. 2010;10(7):490–500.
38. Baecher-Allan C, Hafler DA. Human regulatory T cells and their role in autoimmune disease. Immunol Rev. 2006;212:203–16.
39. Chaplin DD. Overview of the immune response. J Allergy Clin Immunol. 2010;125(2 Suppl 2):S3–23.
40. Goodnow CC, et al. Cellular and genetic mechanisms of self tolerance and autoimmunity. Nature. 2005;435(7042):590–7.
41. Cappione III A, et al. Germinal center exclusion of autoreactive B cells is defective in human systemic lupus erythematosus. J Clin Invest. 2005;115(11):3205–16.
42. Kilmon MA, et al. Macrophages prevent the differentiation of autoreactive B cells by secreting CD40 ligand and interleukin-6. Blood. 2007;110(5):1595–602.
43. Tiller T, et al. Autoreactivity in human IgG+ memory B cells. Immunity. 2007;26(2):205–13.

44. Shlomchik MJ. Sites and stages of autoreactive B cell activation and regulation. Immunity. 2008;28(1):18–28.
45. Aloisi F, Pujol-Borrell R. Lymphoid neogenesis in chronic inflammatory diseases. Nat Rev Immunol. 2006;6(3):205–17.
46. Bour-Jordan H, et al. Constitutive expression of B7-1 on B cells uncovers autoimmunity toward the B cell compartment in the nonobese diabetic mouse. J Immunol. 2007;179(2):1004–12.
47. Hu CY, et al. Treatment with CD20-specific antibody prevents and reverses autoimmune diabetes in mice. J Clin Invest. 2007;117(12):3857–67.
48. Edwards JC, et al. Efficacy of B-cell-targeted therapy with rituximab in patients with rheumatoid arthritis. N Engl J Med. 2004;350(25):2572–81.
49. Fillatreau S, Gray D, Anderton SM. Not always the bad guys: B cells as regulators of autoimmune pathology. Nat Rev Immunol. 2008;8(5):391–7.
50. Chari ST, et al. Diagnosis of autoimmune pancreatitis: the Mayo Clinic experience. Clin Gastroenterol Hepatol. 2006;4(8):1010–16. quiz 934.
51. Kojima M, et al. Autoimmune pancreatitis: frequency, IgG4 expression, and clonality of T and B cells. Am J Surg Pathol. 2007;31(4):521–8.
52. Frulloni L, et al. Identification of a novel antibody associated with autoimmune pancreatitis. N Engl J Med. 2009;361(22):2135–42.
53. French MA, Harrison G. Serum IgG subclass concentrations in healthy adults: a study using monoclonal antisera. Clin Exp Immunol. 1984;56(2):473–5.
54. Esposito I, et al. Autoimmune pancreatocholangitis, non-autoimmune pancreatitis and primary sclerosing cholangitis: a comparative morphological and immunological analysis. PLoS One. 2008;3(7):e2539.
55. Oliveira DB. Membranous nephropathy: an IgG4-mediated disease. Lancet. 1998;351(9103):670–1.
56. Muraki T, et al. Autoimmune pancreatitis and complement activation system. Pancreas. 2006;32(1):16–21.
57. Kawa S, et al. A novel immunoglobulin-immunoglobulin interaction in autoimmunity. PLoS One. 2008;3(2):e1637.
58. Song TJ, et al. The combined measurement of total serum IgG and IgG4 may increase diagnostic sensitivity for autoimmune pancreatitis without sacrificing specificity, compared with IgG4 alone. Am J Gastroenterol. 2010;105(7):1655–60.
59. Lundgren M, et al. Interleukin 4 induces synthesis of IgE and IgG4 in human B cells. Eur J Immunol. 1989;19(7):1311–15.
60. Punnonen J, et al. Interleukin 13 induces interleukin 4-independent IgG4 and IgE synthesis and CD23 expression by human B cells. Proc Natl Acad Sci USA. 1993;90(8):3730–4.
61. Meiler F, et al. Distinct regulation of IgE, IgG4 and IgA by T regulatory cells and toll-like receptors. Allergy. 2008;63(11):1455–63.
62. Satoguina JS, et al. Tr1 and naturally occurring regulatory T cells induce IgG4 in B cells through GITR/GITR-L interaction, IL-10 and TGF-beta. Eur J Immunol. 2008;38(11):3101–13.
63. van der Neut KM, et al. Anti-inflammatory activity of human IgG4 antibodies by dynamic Fab arm exchange. Science. 2007;317(5844):1554–7.
64. Aalberse RC, et al. Immunoglobulin G4: an odd antibody. Clin Exp Allergy. 2009;39(4):469–77.
65. Holland M, et al. Anti-neutrophil cytoplasm antibody IgG subclasses in Wegener's granulomatosis: a possible pathogenic role for the IgG4 subclass. Clin Exp Immunol. 2004;138(1):183–92.
66. Mihai S, et al. IgG4 autoantibodies induce dermal-epidermal separation. J Cell Mol Med. 2007;11(5):1117–28.
67. Puig-Divi V, et al. Induction of chronic pancreatic disease by trinitrobenzene sulfonic acid infusion into rat pancreatic ducts. Pancreas. 1996;13(4):417–24.
68. Aoki S, et al. Immunohistochemical study of autoimmune pancreatitis using anti-IgG4 antibody and patients' sera. Histopathology. 2005;47(2):147–58.
69. Kino-Ohsaki J, et al. Serum antibodies to carbonic anhydrase I and II in patients with idiopathic chronic pancreatitis and Sjogren's syndrome. Gastroenterology. 1996;110(5):1579–86.
70. Okazaki K, et al. Autoimmune-related pancreatitis is associated with autoantibodies and a Th1/Th2-type cellular immune response. Gastroenterology. 2000;118(3):573–81.
71. Aparisi L, et al. Antibodies to carbonic anhydrase and IgG4 levels in idiopathic chronic pancreatitis: relevance for diagnosis of autoimmune pancreatitis. Gut. 2005;54(5):703–9.
72. Nishimori I, et al. Serum antibodies to carbonic anhydrase IV in patients with autoimmune pancreatitis. Gut. 2005;54(2):274–81.
73. Asada M, et al. Identification of a novel autoantibody against pancreatic secretory trypsin inhibitor in patients with autoimmune pancreatitis. Pancreas. 2006;33(1):20–6.
74. Andoh A, et al. Elevated serum anti-carbonic anhydrase II antibodies in patients with ulcerative colitis. Int J Mol Med. 2002;9(5):499–502.
75. Muratori L, et al. Antilactoferrin antibodies in autoimmune liver disease. Clin Exp Immunol. 2001;124(3):470–3.
76. Horiuchi A, et al. Does a lack of reactivity to alpha-fodrin indicate the existence of primary autoimmune pancreatitis? Am J Gastroenterol. 2002;97(5):1275–7.
77. Haneji N, et al. Identification of alpha-fodrin as a candidate autoantigen in primary Sjogren's syndrome. Science. 1997;276(5312):604–7.
78. Endo T, et al. Amylase alpha-2A autoantibodies: novel marker of autoimmune pancreatitis and fulminant type 1 diabetes. Diabetes. 2009;58(3):732–7.
79. Takizawa S, et al. HSP 10 is a new autoantigen in both autoimmune pancreatitis and fulminant type 1

diabetes. Biochem Biophys Res Commun. 2009;386(1):192–6.
80. Löhr JM, et al. Autoantibodies against the exocrine pancreas in autoimmune pancreatitis: gene and protein expression profiling and immunoassays identify pancreatic enzymes as a major target of the inflammatory process. Am J Gastroenterol. 2010;105(9):2060–71.
81. Ectors N, et al. Non-alcoholic duct destructive chronic pancreatitis. Gut. 1997;41(2):263–8.
82. Uchida K, et al. Clinical analysis of autoimmune-related pancreatitis. Am J Gastroenterol. 2000;95(10):2788–94.
83. Kamisawa T, et al. Close relationship between autoimmune pancreatitis and multifocal fibrosclerosis. Gut. 2003;52(5):683–7.
84. Jalleh RP, et al. Expression of major histocompatibility antigens in human chronic pancreatitis. Gut. 1993;34(10):1452–7.
85. Cavallini G, et al. Autoimmunity and chronic pancreatitis. Gut. 1995;36(5):799–800.
86. Bovo P, et al. HLA molecule expression on chronic pancreatitis specimens: is there a role for autoimmunity? A preliminary study. Pancreas. 1987;2(3):350–6.
87. Bedossa P, et al. Lymphocyte subsets and HLA-DR expression in normal pancreas and chronic pancreatitis. Pancreas. 1990;5(4):415–20.
88. Williams PE. Lymphoid tissues and organs. In: Williams PE, editor. Fundamental immunology. Philadelphia: Lippincott Williams & Wilkins; 2008. p. 27–55.
89. Niki S, et al. Alteration of intra-pancreatic target-organ specificity by abrogation of Aire in NOD mice. J Clin Invest. 2006;116(5):1292–301.
90. Zen Y, et al. Th2 and regulatory immune reactions are increased in immunoglobin G4-related sclerosing pancreatitis and cholangitis. Hepatology. 2007;45(6):1538–46.
91. Miyoshi H, et al. Circulating naive and CD4+CD25high regulatory T cells in patients with autoimmune pancreatitis. Pancreas. 2008;36(2):133–40.
92. Holling TM, Schooten E, van Den Elsen PJ. Function and regulation of MHC class II molecules in T-lymphocytes: of mice and men. Hum Immunol. 2004;65(4):282–90.
93. Costantino CM, Ploegh HL, Hafler DA. Cathepsin S regulates class II MHC processing in human CD4+ HLA-DR+ T cells. J Immunol. 2009;183(2):945–52.
94. Baecher-Allan C, Wolf E, Hafler DA. MHC class II expression identifies functionally distinct human regulatory T cells. J Immunol. 2006;176(8):4622–31.
95. Swiatek-de Lange M, et al. Comment on "MHC class II expression identifies functionally distinct human regulatory T cells". J Immunol. 2008;180(6):3625; author reply 3626.
96. Novobrantseva TI, et al. Attenuated liver fibrosis in the absence of B cells. J Clin Invest. 2005;115(11):3072–82.
97. Harris DP, et al. Reciprocal regulation of polarized cytokine production by effector B and T cells. Nat Immunol. 2000;1(6):475–82.
98. Chiaramonte MG, et al. An IL-13 inhibitor blocks the development of hepatic fibrosis during a T-helper type 2-dominated inflammatory response. J Clin Invest. 1999;104(6):777–85.
99. Lee CG, et al. Interleukin-13 induces tissue fibrosis by selectively stimulating and activating transforming growth factor beta(1). J Exp Med. 2001;194(6):809–21.
100. Fichtner-Feigl S, et al. IL-13 signaling through the IL-13alpha2 receptor is involved in induction of TGF-beta1 production and fibrosis. Nat Med. 2006;12(1):99–106.
101. Ohara H, et al. Systemic extrapancreatic lesions associated with autoimmune pancreatitis. J Gastroenterol. 2007;42 Suppl 18:15–21.
102. Simon D, Simon HU. Eosinophilic disorders. J Allergy Clin Immunol. 2007;119(6):1291–300; quiz 1301–2.
103. Detlefsen S, et al. Diagnosis of autoimmune pancreatitis by core needle biopsy: application of six microscopic criteria. Virchows Arch. 2009;454(5):531–9.
104. Iwamuro M, et al. Eosinophilic cholangitis with initial clinical features indistinguishable from IgG4-related cholangitis. Intern Med. 2009;48(13):1143–7.
105. Furuta GT, et al. Eosinophil granule-derived major basic protein induces IL-8 expression in human intestinal myofibroblasts. Clin Exp Immunol. 2000;122(1):35–40.
106. Huaux F, et al. Eosinophils and T lymphocytes possess distinct roles in bleomycin-induced lung injury and fibrosis. J Immunol. 2003;171(10):5470–81.
107. Zagai U, et al. Eosinophil cationic protein stimulates migration of human lung fibroblasts in vitro. Scand J Immunol. 2009;69(4):381–6.
108. Kanno H, et al. Spontaneous development of pancreatitis in the MRL/Mp strain of mice in autoimmune mechanism. Clin Exp Immunol. 1992;89(1):68–73.
109. Yu X, et al. The mtDNA nt7778 G/T polymorphism affects autoimmune diseases and reproductive performance in the mouse. Hum Mol Genet. 2009;18(24):4689–98.
110. Tsubata R, et al. Autoimmune disease of exocrine organs in immunodeficient alymphoplasia mice: a spontaneous model for Sjogren's syndrome. Eur J Immunol. 1996;26(11):2742–8.
111. Sakaguchi Y, et al. The Wistar Bonn Kobori rat, a unique animal model for autoimmune pancreatitis with extrapancreatic exocrinopathy. Clin Exp Immunol. 2008;152(1):1–12.
112. Meagher C, et al. Spontaneous development of a pancreatic exocrine disease in CD28-deficient NOD mice. J Immunol. 2008;180(12):7793–803.
113. Freitag TL, et al. Human risk allele HLA-DRB1*0405 predisposes class II transgenic Ab0

NOD mice to autoimmune pancreatitis. Gastroenterology. 2010;139(1):281–91.
114. Boomershine CS, et al. Autoimmune pancreatitis results from loss of TGFbeta signalling in S100A4-positive dendritic cells. Gut. 2009;58(9):1267–74.
115. Qu WM, et al. A novel autoimmune pancreatitis model in MRL mice treated with polyinosinic:polycytidylic acid. Clin Exp Immunol. 2002;129(1):27–34.
116. Asada M, et al. Analysis of humoral immune response in experimental autoimmune pancreatitis in mice. Pancreas. 2010;39(2):224–31.
117. Fitzner B, et al. Interferon-gamma treatment accelerates and aggravates autoimmune pancreatitis in the MRL/Mp-mouse. Pancreatology. 2009;9(3):233–9.
118. Uchida K, et al. Experimental immune-mediated pancreatitis in neonatally thymectomized mice immunized with carbonic anhydrase II and lactoferrin. Lab Invest. 2002;82(4):411–24.
119. Watanabe S, et al. Kinetic analysis of the development of pancreatic lesions in mice infected with a murine retrovirus. Clin Immunol. 2003;109(2):212–23.
120. Davidson TS, Longnecker DS, Hickey WF. An experimental model of autoimmune pancreatitis in the rat. Am J Pathol. 2005;166(3):729–36.
121. Watson PJ, et al. Prevalence and breed distribution of chronic pancreatitis at post-mortem examination in first-opinion dogs. J Small Anim Pract. 2007;48(11):609–18.
122. Day MJ. Inheritance of serum autoantibody, reduced serum IgA and autoimmune disease in a canine breeding colony. Vet Immunol Immunopathol. 1996;53(3–4):207–19.
123. Wiberg ME, et al. Cellular and humoral immune responses in atrophic lymphocytic pancreatitis in German shepherd dogs and rough-coated collies. Vet Immunol Immunopathol. 2000;76(1–2):103–15.
124. Wiberg ME. Pancreatic acinar atrophy in German shepherd dogs and rough-coated collies. Etiopathogenesis, diagnosis and treatment. A review. Vet Q. 2004;26(2):61–75.
125. Case RM. Is the rat pancreas an appropriate model of the human pancreas? Pancreatology. 2006;6(3):180–90.
126. Hahm KB, et al. Loss of TGF-beta signaling contributes to autoimmune pancreatitis. J Clin Invest. 2000;105(8):1057–65.
127. Kordes C, et al. Differential and synergistic effects of platelet-derived growth factor-BB and transforming growth factor-beta1 on activated pancreatic stellate cells. Pancreas. 2005;31(2):156–67.
128. Blaine SA, et al. Epidermal growth factor receptor regulates pancreatic fibrosis. Am J Physiol Gastrointest Liver Physiol. 2009;297(3):G434–41.
129. Choi EK, et al. Differences in pancreatic immunohistochemical staining profiles of TGF-beta1, MMP-2, and TIMP-2 between autoimmune and alcoholic chronic pancreatitis. Pancreas. 2009;38(7):739–45.
130. Kawa S, et al. HLA DRB10405-DQB10401 haplotype is associated with autoimmune pancreatitis in the Japanese population. Gastroenterology. 2002;122(5):1264–9.
131. Ota M, et al. Two critical genes (HLA-DRB1 and ABCF1)in the HLA region are associated with the susceptibility to autoimmune pancreatitis. Immunogenetics. 2007;59(1):45–52.
132. Kawabata Y, et al. Asian-specific HLA haplotypes reveal heterogeneity of the contribution of HLA-DR and -DQ haplotypes to susceptibility to type 1 diabetes. Diabetes. 2002;51(2):545–51.
133. Park OJ, et al. The association of osteoprotegerin gene polymorphisms with periodontitis. Oral Dis. 2008;14(5):440–4.
134. Umemura T, et al. Genetic association of Fc receptor-like 3 polymorphisms with autoimmune pancreatitis in Japanese patients. Gut. 2006;55(9):1367–8.
135. Ravetch JV, Lanier LL. Immune inhibitory receptors. Science. 2000;290(5489):84–9.
136. Chistiakov DA, Chistiakov AP. Is FCRL3 a new general autoimmunity gene? Hum Immunol. 2007;68(5):375–83.
137. Swainson LA, et al. Expression of the autoimmune susceptibility gene FcRL3 on human regulatory T cells is associated with dysfunction and high levels of programmed cell death-1. J Immunol. 2010;184(7):3639–47.
138. Umemura T, et al. Association of autoimmune pancreatitis with cytotoxic T-lymphocyte antigen 4 gene polymorphisms in Japanese patients. Am J Gastroenterol. 2008;103(3):588–94.
139. Chang MC, et al. T-cell regulatory gene CTLA-4 polymorphism/haplotype association with autoimmune pancreatitis. Clin Chem. 2007;53(9):1700–5.
140. Ueda H, et al. Association of the T-cell regulatory gene CTLA4 with susceptibility to autoimmune disease. Nature. 2003;423(6939):506–11.
141. Umemura T, et al. Association analysis of Toll-like receptor 4 polymorphisms with autoimmune pancreatitis. Hum Immunol. 2009;70(9):742–6.
142. Kountouras J, Zavos C, Chatzopoulos D. A concept on the role of *Helicobacter pylori* infection in autoimmune pancreatitis. J Cell Mol Med. 2005;9(1):196–207.
143. Shinji A, et al. Autoimmune pancreatitis is closely associated with gastric ulcer presenting with abundant IgG4-bearing plasma cell infiltration. Gastrointest Endosc. 2004;59(4):506–11.
144. Chang MC, et al. Autoimmune pancreatitis associated with high prevalence of gastric ulcer independent of *Helicobacter pylori* infection status. Pancreas. 2009;38(4):442–6.
145. Uehara T, et al. Chronic gastritis in the setting of autoimmune pancreatitis. Am J Surg Pathol. 2010;34(9):1241–9.
146. Guarneri F, Guarneri C, Benvenga S. *Helicobacter pylori* and autoimmune pancreatitis: role of carbonic anhydrase via molecular mimicry? J Cell Mol Med. 2005;9(3):741–4.
147. Jesnowski R, et al. *Helicobacter pylori* in autoimmune pancreatitis and pancreatic carcinoma. Pancreatology. 2010;10(4):462–6.

148. Haruta I, et al. A mouse model of autoimmune pancreatitis with salivary gland involvement triggered by innate immunity via persistent exposure to avirulent bacteria. Lab Invest. 2010;90(12):1757–69.
149. Happonen I, et al. Detection and effects of helicobacters in healthy dogs and dogs with signs of gastritis. J Am Vet Med Assoc. 1998;213(12):1767–74.
150. Hirano K, et al. Long-term prognosis of autoimmune pancreatitis with and without corticosteroid treatment. Gut. 2007;56(12):1719–24.
151. Ghazale A, Chari ST. Optimising corticosteroid treatment for autoimmune pancreatitis. Gut. 2007;56(12):1650–2.
152. Akdis CA, et al. Glucocorticoids inhibit human antigen-specific and enhance total IgE and IgG4 production due to differential effects on T and B cells in vitro. Eur J Immunol. 1997;27(9):2351–7.
153. Ko SB, et al. Corticosteroids correct aberrant CFTR localization in the duct and regenerate acinar cells in autoimmune pancreatitis. Gastroenterology. 2010;138(5):1988–96.
154. Karagiannidis C, et al. Glucocorticoids upregulate FOXP3 expression and regulatory T cells in asthma. J Allergy Clin Immunol. 2004;114(6):1425–33.
155. Cronstein BN, et al. A mechanism for the antiinflammatory effects of corticosteroids: the glucocorticoid receptor regulates leukocyte adhesion to endothelial cells and expression of endothelial-leukocyte adhesion molecule 1 and intercellular adhesion molecule 1. Proc Natl Acad Sci USA. 1992;89(21):9991–5.

# Overview of Types 1 and 2

# 3

Tooru Shimosegawa

## Definition of Type 1 and Type 2 AIP

Type 1 autoimmune pancreatitis (AIP) is defined as a pancreatitis with unique morphological features of diffuse or segmental/focal enlargement of the pancreas and narrowing of short segment or entire length of the MPD, serologically the elevation of serum IgG4, histologically lymphoplasmacytic sclerosing pancreatitis (LPSP), and an association of various extrapancreatic lesions.

Type 2 AIP is defined by the histological findings of idiopathic duct-centric pancreatitis (IDCP) or granulocytic epithelial lesions (GELs). Type 2 AIP shows imaging findings and response to steroids similar to type 1 AIP but lacks serological biomarker and is occasionally complicated with inflammatory bowel disease (IBD).

## Clinical Features

The clinical and pathological features of AIP are summarized below, and they are compared between type 1 and type 2 AIP (Table 3.1).

T. Shimosegawa, M.D. (✉)
Department of Gastroenterology,
Hohoku University Hospital, 1-1 Seiryo-machi,
Aoba-ku, Sendai, Miyagi, Japan
e-mail: tshimosegawa@int3.med.tohoku.ac.jp

1. Symptoms
   As the initial symptoms, type 1 AIP patients have obstructive jaundice in 33–59 %, abdominal pain in 32 %, back pain in 15 %, weight loss in 15 %, and appetite loss and general fatigue in about 10 % each. Fifteen percent of patients are asymptomatic [1]. Abdominal pain is usually absent or mild to moderate if present, and severe pain like acute pancreatitis is rare. Since AIP develops frequently in elderly males with painless obstructive jaundice, mild abdominal pain, or nonspecific symptoms such as weight loss and appetite loss, differentiation between AIP and pancreatobiliary malignant tumors is very important [2]. Type 2 AIP patients are more likely to show more severe pain resembling acute pancreatitis than type 1 AIP (46.2 % vs. 11.1 %) [3].
2. Imaging
   Imaging findings of type 1 and type 2 AIP are essentially similar, although pancreatic swelling is more frequently diffuse type in type 1 compared with type 2 AIP [3].
   (a) *Ultrasound (US), Endoscopic US (EUS), and Intraductal US (IDUS)*
   The US imaging of typical AIP is diffuse enlargement of the pancreas showing a homogenously hypoechoic pattern, occasionally scattered with tiny bright spots. The imaging is called "sausage-like" [1, 4, 5] (Fig. 3.1a, b). In cases of segmental/focal enlargement, the US

M.J. Levy and S.T. Chari (eds.), *Autoimmune (IgG4-related) Pancreatitis and Cholangitis*,
DOI 10.1007/978-1-4419-6430-4_3, © Springer Science+Business Media New York 2013

**Table 3.1** Comparison of clinical features between type 1 and type 2 AIP

| | | Type 1 | Type 2 |
|---|---|---|---|
| Age | | 50–70 y.o. | 20–40 y.o. |
| Presentation | | M>F | M=F |
| Imaging | CT/MRI | Diffuse/segmental/focal enlargement of the pancreas | Mass forming>diffuse enlargement |
| | ERP | Irregular narrowing of the MPD (diffuse/segmental/focal) | Irregular narrowing/obstruction of the MPD |
| | PET | Pancreas/extrapancreatic lesions | Pancreas |
| Serology | | IgG4, IgG, ANA, RF | – |
| Histology | | LPSP | IDCP/GELs |
| OOI | | Sclerosing cholangitis<br>Sclerosing sialadenitis<br>Retroperitoneal fibrosis<br>Tubulointerstitial nephritis | UC<br>Crohn's disease |
| Therapy | | PSL | PSL |

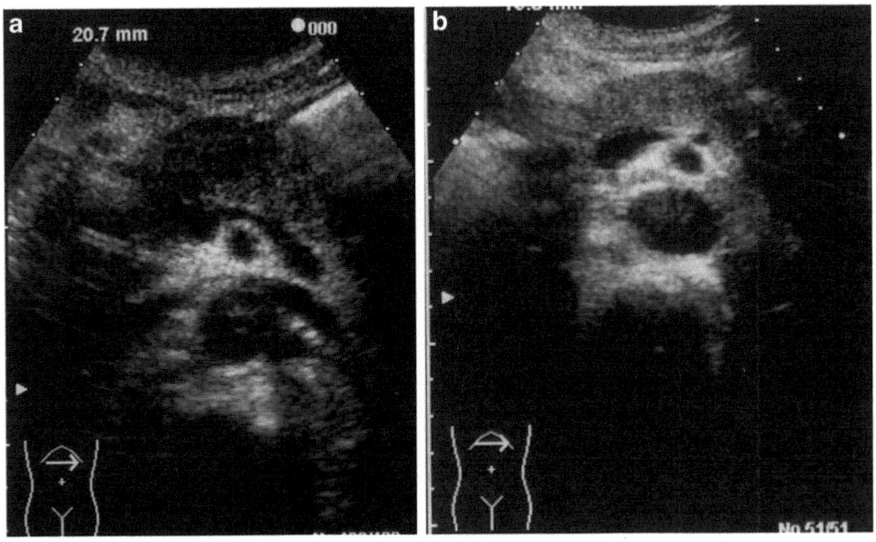


**Fig. 3.1** US imaging of the pancreas in a patient with AIP. The swollen pancreas before treatment (**a**) showed "sausage-like" appearance with homogeneously low-echoic pattern. Diffuse enlargement of the pancreas was improved remarkably in response to steroid treatment (**b**)

imaging may show a relatively clearly margined hypoechoic lesion that is sometimes difficult to differentiate from pancreatic cancer (PCa) [5]. The EUS findings of AIP are essentially the same, although the involved area can be seen more clearly [5].

US is useful to detect wall thickening of the biliary tract, the finding characteristic for sclerosing cholangitis, an extrapancreatic lesion seen in approximately 60 % of AIP patients. The wall thickening is detected chiefly in the common bile duct, occasionally spreading to the gallbladder and even to the intrahepatic bile ducts [6]. Examination by the IDUS reveals thickening of the inner hypoechoic zone of the bile duct wall, with the outer hyperechoic zone being preserved [7] (Fig. 3.2a–d).

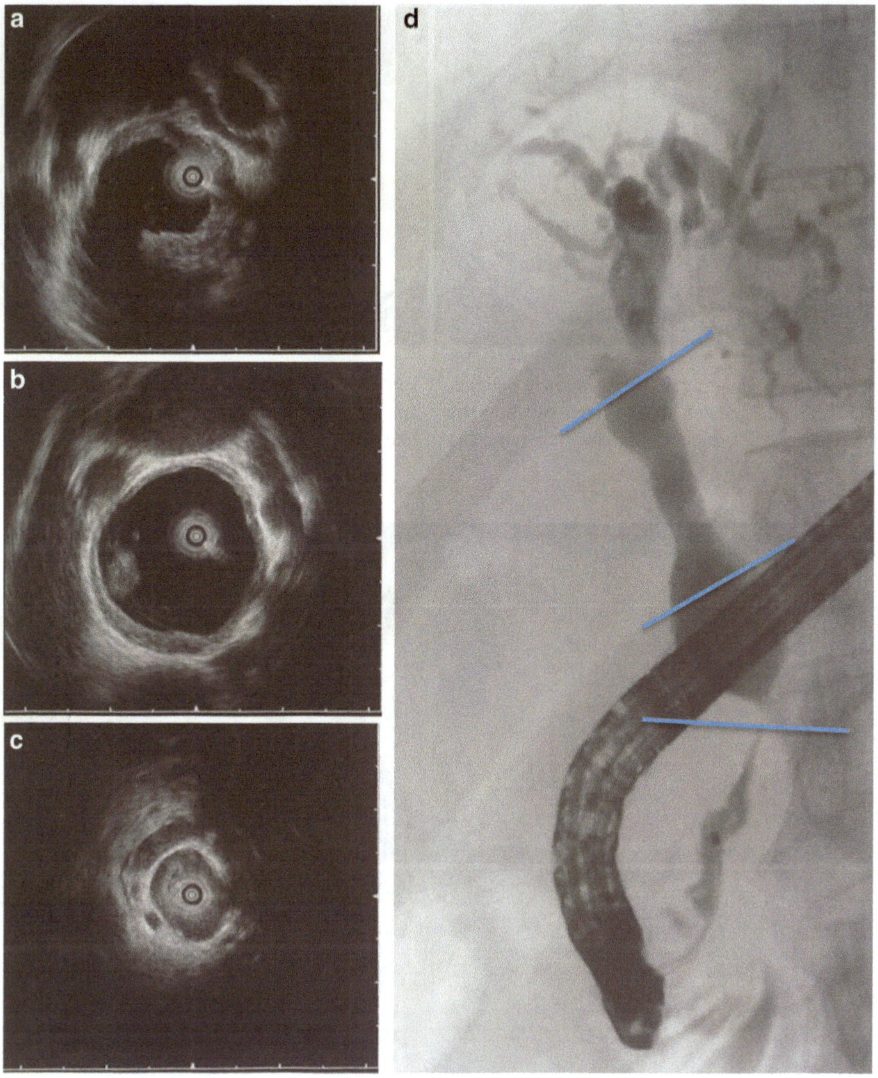


**Fig. 3.2** IDUS findings of sclerosing cholangitis complicated to AIP. The respective IDUS imaging in the left panels (**a**–**c**) corresponds to the line markers on the cholangiogram in the right (**d**)

(b) *Computed Tomography (CT) and Magnetic Resonance Imaging (MRI)*
The CT finding of AIP is characterized by the delayed enhancement of the swollen pancreas on dynamic CT [8] (Fig. 3.3a, b). Irrespective of diffuse or segmental/focal enlargement, the involved area shows slightly low density compared with the uninvolved area in early imaging and increases the density in delayed phases. A very unique finding of AIP is a low-density marginal zone in the periphery of the pancreas called "capsule-like rim" which may indicate fibro-inflammatory changes of peripancreatic area [8] (Fig. 3.3a).

In the MRI, the involved area of the pancreas typically shows signals lower than the liver in T1-weighted imaging. The signal intensity in T2-weighted imaging is variable depending on the fibrosis [8] (Fig. 3.4a–d). The characteristic finding

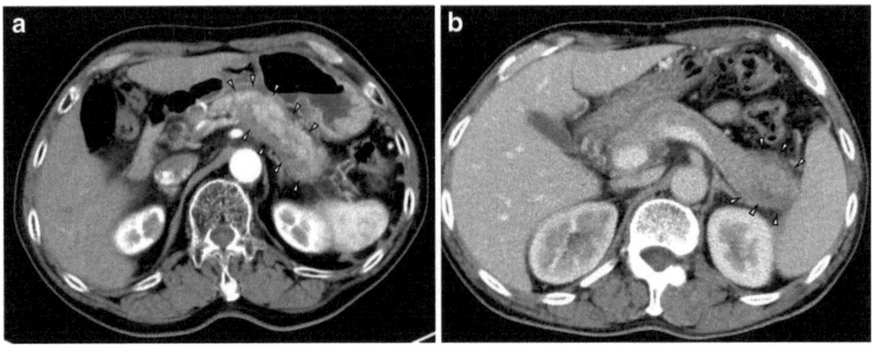


**Fig. 3.3** Dynamic CT imaging of the pancreas in patients with AIP. Diffuse enlargement (**a**) and focal swelling (**b**) of the pancreas in AIP patients. The swollen pancreas shows a low-density rim-like structure (*arrowheads* in **a** and **b**) in the periphery of the pancreas called "capsule-like rim"

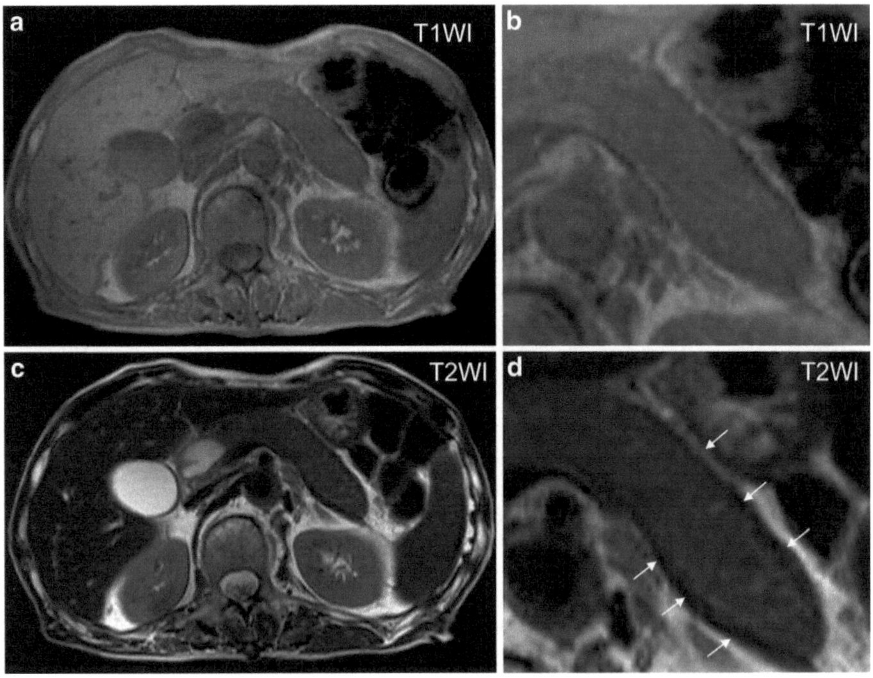


**Fig. 3.4** MR imaging of the pancreas in a patient with AIP. The T1-weighted imaging (**a, b**) shows the swollen pancreas with slightly low signal intensity compared with the liver. "Capsule-like rim" is clearly seen in the T2-weighted imaging as marginal low signal area in the periphery of the pancreas (d, *arrows*)

of AIP on dynamic MRI is a delayed enhancement of the involved area. The "capsule-like rim" can be shown in T2-weighted images as a low signal structure which is enhanced in a delayed manner [8] (Fig. 3.4c, d). At present, MRCP is considered to have insufficient resolution for the visualization of MPD narrowing in AIP.

(c) *Endoscopic Retrograde Cholangiopancreatography (ERCP)*
One of the most characteristic findings of AIP is the diffuse or segmental/focal, irregular narrowing of the MPD

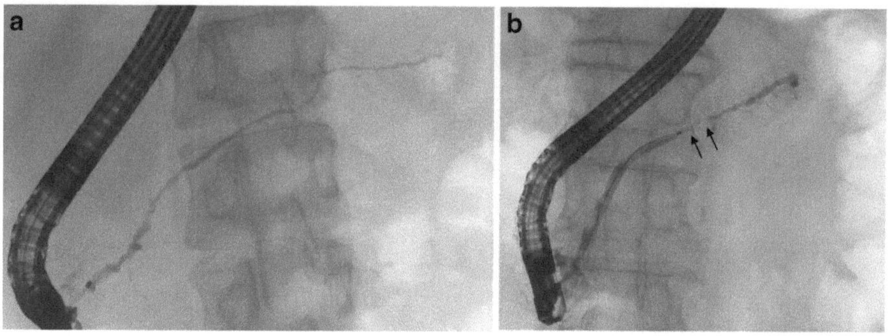


**Fig. 3.5** ERP imaging of diffuse-type and localized-type AIP. The main pancreatic duct (MPD) shows diffuse narrowing with irregular wall (**a**). The localized type shows MPD narrowing in a short segment in the pancreas body (*arrows*), but the upstream MPD does not show remarkable dilatation (**b**)

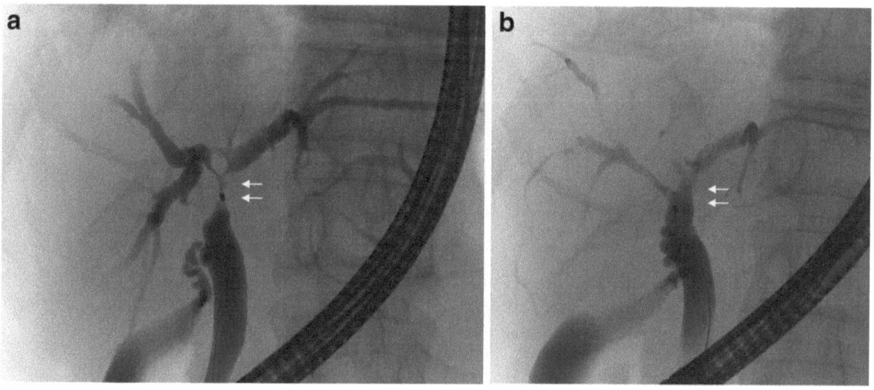


**Fig. 3.6** Bile duct stricture at the liver hilum due to sclerosing cholangitis complicated to AIP. Severe stricture at the hepatic hilum before treatment with PSL (*white arrows* in **a**) was remarkably ameliorated in response to steroid treatment (*white arrows* in **b**)

on pancreatogram. Typically, the duct narrowing spans more than 1/3 of the entire pancreatic duct or occurs as multiple segmental narrowing [9–11] (Fig. 3.5a). Characteristically, even in the case of short-segment narrowing, the upstream MPD usually does not show remarkable dilatation, an important sign to differentiate AIP from PCa [12] (Fig. 3.5b). Up to 80 % of AIP patients show biliary stenosis in any site of the extra or intrahepatic biliary tract, most frequently occurring in the lower part of the common bile duct [13]. The hilar biliary duct lesions in AIP patients are occasionally difficult to differentiate from bile duct carcinoma [12, 13] (Fig. 3.6a, b).

(d) *[$^{18}$F]Fluorodeoxyglucose Positron Emission Tomography (FDG-PET)*
In AIP patients, FDG is taken up strongly in the involved area of the pancreas, which disappears quickly in response to steroid treatment [14]. Although the FDG-PET is unable to differentiate AIP from PCa, it is helpful to detect the systemic distribution of extrapancreatic lesions of AIP [15, 16] (Fig. 3.7a, b).

3. Serology
Type 1 AIP is characterized by the elevation of serum IgG4. According to the original report by Hamano H et al., serum IgG4 alone

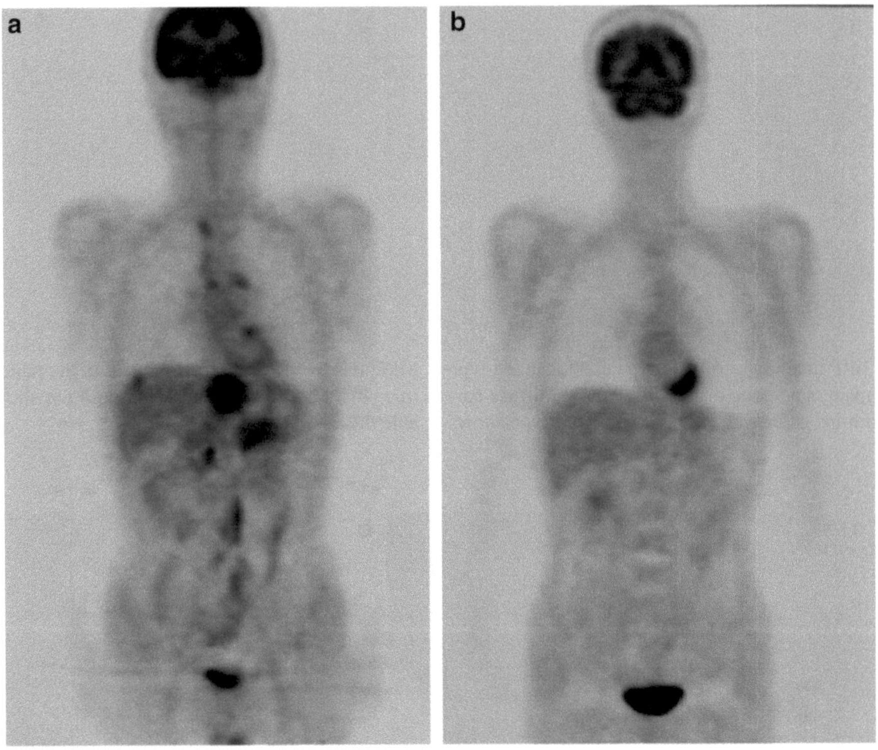


**Fig. 3.7** Whole-body FDG-PET imaging of a patient with AIP. FDG was taken up to the body and tail of the swollen pancreas, the large pseudotumor of the liver, the pulmonary hilar lymph nodes, and to the salivary glands (**a**). They disappeared shortly after the steroid treatment (**b**)

is an excellent marker with high accuracy (97 %), sensitivity (95 %), and specificity (97 %) for the differentiation of AIP from PCa [17]. However, Ghazale A et al. reported that 13 out of 135 PCa patients (10 %) showed slight elevation of serum IgG4 and called attention to overconfidence on IgG4 as it is not a disease-specific marker [18]. Other than IgG4, serum γ-globulin and IgG can be used for the evaluation of disease activity, response to steroids, and prediction of recurrence.

Various antibodies appear in the sera of type 1 AIP patients. Representatives include anti-lactoferrin antibody (ALF), anti-carbonic anhydrase II antibody (CA-II), anti-nuclear antibody (ANA), anti-pancreatic secretory trypsin inhibitor (PSTI) antibody, and rheumatoid factor (RF) with the respective frequency for the appearance of 75 %, 55 %, 60 %, 30.8 %, and 20–30 % [19, 20]. In differentiation from PCa, the sensitivity, specificity, and accuracy of ANA are 58 %, 79 %, and 67 %, respectively, while those of RF are 23 %, 94 %, and 54 %, respectively [19]. Recently, Frulloni L et al. suggested the involvement of *H. pylori* infection in the pathogenesis of AIP, because reportedly plasminogen-binding protein (PBP) of *H. pylori* could have been detected in 95 % of AIP patients [21].

It should be noted that anti-SSA/Ro and anti-SSB/La antibodies, well-known markers of Sjögren's syndrome, are rarely seen in AIP patients. Anti-mitochondrial antibody (AMA), a marker of primary biliary cirrhosis (PBC), is also rarely detected [19]. One fourth of AIP patients show a decrease in thyroid function, and 34 % and 17 % of them have positive anti-thyroglobulin and anti-

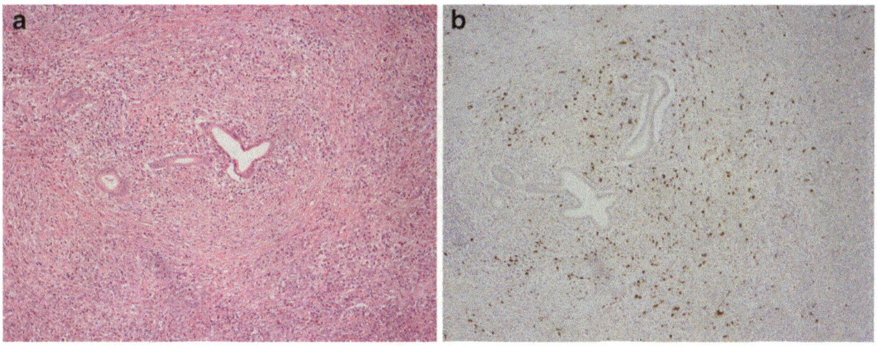


**Fig. 3.8** LPSP. (**a**) The pancreas tissue section stained by hematoxylin-eosin (H-E) shows characteristic findings of lymphoplasmacytic sclerosing pancreatitis (LPSP), "storiform fibrosis," and massive infiltration of plasma cells and lymphocytes. (**b**) Immunohistochemistry for IgG4 on the adjacent section to (**a**) demonstrates the presence of numerous IgG4-positive plasma cells

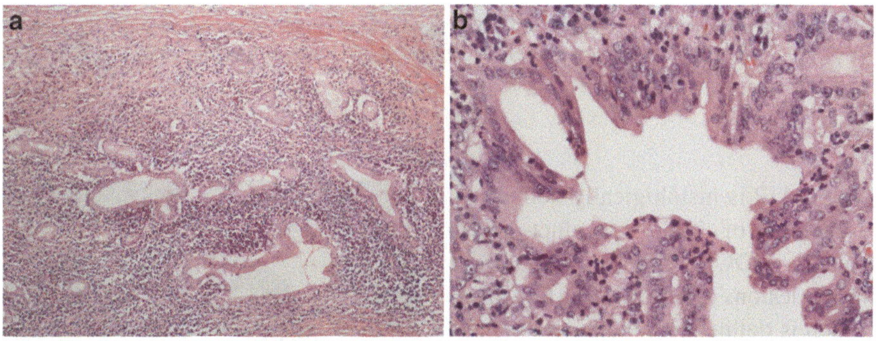


**Fig. 3.9** IDCP. The pancreas tissue section stained by hematoxylin-eosin (H-E) shows characteristic findings of idiopathic duct-centric pancreatitis (IDCP) which is characterized by a massive infiltration of inflammatory cells (including neutrophils) around medium- and small-size ducts (**a**). A magnified view (**b**) shows the infiltration of numerous neutrophils into the duct epithelium and the destruction of epithelial lining

thyroid peroxidase (TPO) antibodies, respectively [22].

At present, there is no known serum biomarker specific to type 2 AIP [23]. Conversely, type 2 AIP is suspected in the patients who show imaging findings suggestive of AIP but show negative results for serum IgG4 and other organ involvement (OOI) which are characteristic features of type 1 AIP.

4. Histology
Type 1 AIP is defined histologically as lymphoplasmacytic sclerosing pancreatitis (LPSP) [24] (Fig. 3.8a, b). The diagnosis can be made solely with the histological finding of LPSP when large specimens are obtained for evaluation. The finding is characterized by dense and unique fibrosis called "storiform fibrosis" which is associated with massive infiltration of lymphocytes and plasma cells and obliterative phlebitis [25] (Fig. 3.8a). These changes are prominent around the medium- to small-size ducts. Immunohistochemistry can clearly demonstrate that plasma cells seen in the lesion are largely positive for IgG4 [26, 27] (Fig. 3.8b). However, caution is required for IgG4-positive plasma cells, because they are not specific to AIP but can be seen occasionally in the lesion of PCa or alcoholic CP [26, 27].

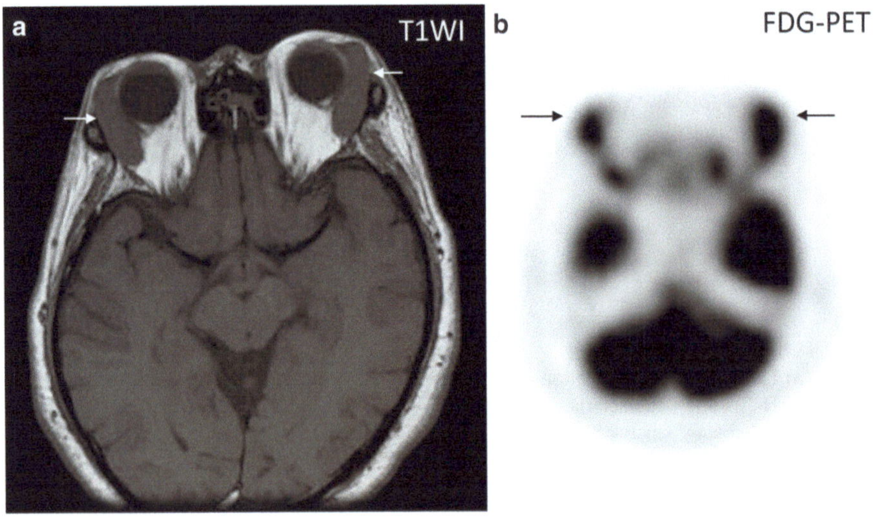


**Fig. 3.10** Lachrymal gland adenitis. MRI T1W1 imaging (**a**) shows bilateral enlargement of the lachrymal glands (*white arrows*). FDG-PET (**b**) demonstrates densely accumulated FDG in these glands (*black arrows*)

Type 2 AIP is histologically defined by the presence of idiopathic duct-centric pancreatitis (IDCP) [28] or granulocytic epithelial lesions (GELs) [29] (Fig. 3.9a, b), which is defined as inflammatory infiltrates seen densely in the lobules than in interlobular fibrotic areas, accompanied by numerous neutrophils and destruction of duct epithelium (Fig. 3.9a). Klöppel G defined "GELs" as focal disruption and destruction of the duct epithelium resulting from invasion of mainly granulocytes [30] (Fig. 3.9b). GELs are typically seen in medium- to small-caliber ducts.

5. Other Organ Involvement (OOI)
It is well known that type 1 AIP is frequently associated with various extrapancreatic lesions, such as adenitis of lachrymal (Fig. 3.10a, b), submandibular and/or parotid glands [31], pulmonary hilar lymph node swelling [32] (Fig. 3.11), sclerosing cholangitis [33] (Fig. 3.6a, b), retroperitoneal fibrosis [34] (Fig. 3.12), renal involvement [35] (Fig. 3.13a, b), and interstitial pneumonitis [36] (Fig. 3.14a, b). Other lesions reported so far include hypophysitis [37] (Fig. 3.15), chronic thyroiditis [22], pseudotumor of the liver [38, 39], gastric ulcer [40], prostatitis [41], Schönlein-Henoch purpura, and autoimmune thrombocytopenia [42]. Typical sialadenitis is recognized as bilateral, symmetrical, hard, and painless swelling of submandibular

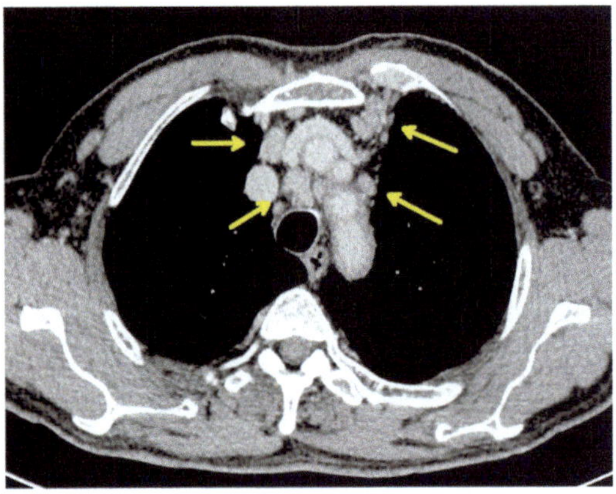

**Fig. 3.11** Pulmonary hilar lymph node swelling. CT imaging depicts enlargement of multiple lymph nodes (*yellow arrows*) around the pulmonary hilum

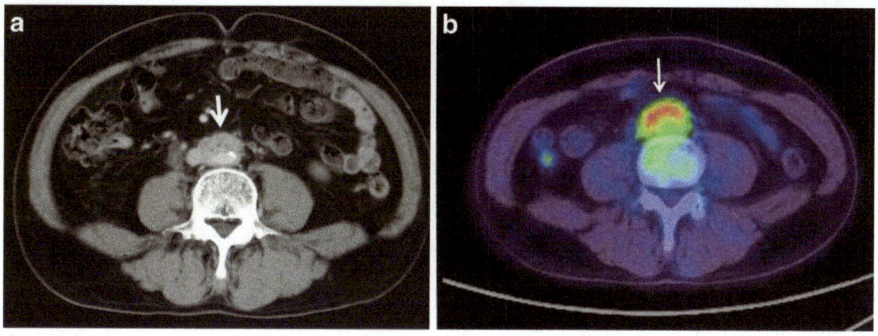

**Fig. 3.12** Retroperitoneal fibrosis. The CT imaging shows a soft tissue mass at the ventral side of abdominal aorta (*white arrow* in **a**), which is strongly labeled by FDG on PET scan (*white arrows* in **b**)

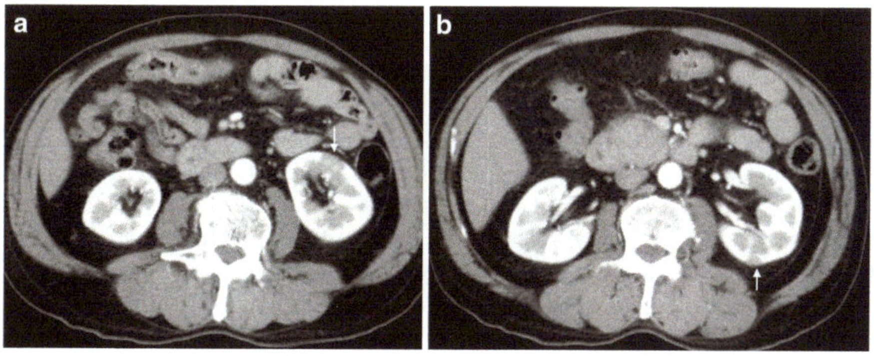

**Fig. 3.13** Renal involvement. Renal involvements can be observed as multiple low-density band-like (*white arrow* in **a**) and wedge-like (*white arrow* in **b**) structures in the renal cortex

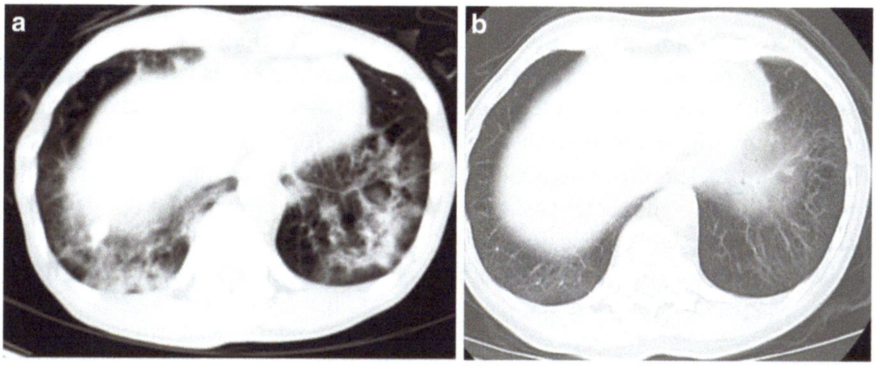

**Fig. 3.14** CT imaging of interstitial pneumonitis seen in a patient with AIP. The pulmonary lesions in the periphery of the lung (**a**) almost completely disappeared after steroid treatment (**b**)

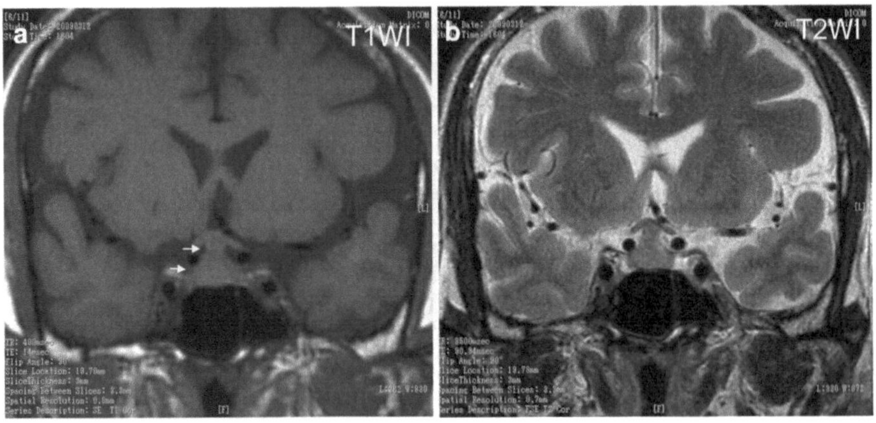


**Fig. 3.15** Hypophyseal involvement. This patient developed suddenly bitemporal hemianopsia and diabetes insipidus shortly after discontinuation of steroid maintenance therapy for AIP. The MRI imaging shows swelling of the stalk and the gland of hypophysis

and/or lachrymal glands, with mild sicca symptom and negative anti-SSA/Ro and anti-SSB/La antibodies, features compatible with Mikulicz disease or Küttner tumor [43, 44]. In addition, sclerosing cholangitis complicated to AIP (SC-AIP) shows the morphology distinct from primary sclerosing cholangitis (PSC) on cholangiogram [45, 46]. Since the similar inflammatory changes seen in the pancreas often occur in the major duodenal papilla, its biopsy can be used as a diagnostic adjunct for type 1 AIP [47]. Steroids are effective for extrapancreatic lesions as well and improvement can be achieved in a short time after the beginning of treatment [14–16].

Kamisawa et al. proposed the concept of "IgG4-related sclerosing disease" in which pancreatitis is a manifestation of systemic disease [48, 49]. The word "sclerosing" comes from similarity in the distribution of involved organs and the pathological features to multifocal fibrosclerosis [50]. Because some extrapancreatic lesions lack or show less fibrous tissues, the term "IgG4-related disease" is now accepted for the disease entity [51]. Currently type 1 AIP is considered to be a pancreatic manifestation of the systemic "IgG4-related disease" [51].

It is reported that type 2 AIP patients do not develop various extrapancreatic lesions which are characteristically seen in the type 1 AIP patients, but up to 30 % of them are complicated with inflammatory bowel diseases (IBDs) such as ulcerative colitis (UC) and Crohn's disease synchronously or heterochronously [52].

## Diagnosis

1. Diagnostic Criteria
Since Japan Pancreas Society (JPS) first proposed the diagnostic criteria of AIP in 2002 [53], various criteria have been proposed from many countries, such as the Korean diagnostic criteria by Asan Medical Center [54] and by Korean Pancreas-Biliary Association (KPBA) [55], the HISORt criteria

by Mayo Clinic [56], the revised Japanese criteria by JPS [2], and so on. The reasons why multiple criteria were created in a short period may be the rapid understanding of this disease, the alteration of disease concept in a short period (such as the recognition of IgG4 as a serum marker and the association of various extrapancreatic lesions), the difference in the diagnostic approaches to this disease (ERCP-oriented or histology-oriented), and the appearance of another type different from the originally defined AIP (type 2). The first attempt to integrate different criteria was made by Japanese and Korean experts, resulting in successful compilation of the Asian criteria published in 2008 [57]. However, different diagnostic approaches to AIP between Japan/Korea (ERCP-oriented) and Western countries (histology-oriented) and growing attention to another type AIP hampered the integration of the Asian criteria [57] and the HISORt criteria [56]. Experts from Eastern and Western countries gathered and exchanged hot discussions from various points of view on AIP at the Satellite symposium of the joint conference of the 40th annual meeting of APA and JPS in 2009, which was summarized as the "Honolulu consensus" later [58]. Based on the consensus, a draft of diagnostic criteria was made and discussed by experts from various countries at the joint conference of the 14th IAP meeting and the 41st JPS annual meeting in Fukuoka in 2010, and, based on the agreement and after the brush up, it was finally reported as the International Consensus Diagnostic Criteria for AIP (ICDC) in 2011 [59]. The ICDC is the latest criteria for AIP, which can be used worldwide.

2. Diagnosis of AIP

   At present, the ICDC are the sole criteria that can make separate diagnoses of type 1 and type 2 AIP [59]. In addition, the ICDC are designed to reach the diagnosis of AIP by various diagnostic approaches irrespective of the practice patterns in different countries. Although it is mentioned that the ICDC can be tailored for use in individual institutions depending on local expertise [59], the comparison of clinical and pathological features of AIP and search for the most suitable treatment should be discussed beyond countries based on the ICDC.

3. ICDC

   To accomplish the goal that the consensus diagnostic criteria should be used worldwide irrespective of practical patterns in different countries, the ICDC were designed to make the diagnosis by a combination of 6 factors, namely, parenchymal imaging (P), ductal imaging (D), serology (S), other organ involvement (OOI), histology of the pancreas (H), and response to steroid (Rt) [59] (Tables 3.2, 3.3, 3.4, 3.5, and 3.6). In order to add more flexibility in the diagnostic measures, the respective five factors (P, D, S, OOI, H) have Level 1 and Level 2 findings according to the grade of specificity to AIP (Tables 3.2 and 3.3). The diagnostic procedures would be initiated by the parenchymal (P) imaging (CT or MRI) suggestive of AIP, which was followed by different diagnostic flows depending on whether the P finding was typical or indeterminate/atypical [59]. According to the ICDC, the diagnosis of "definitive" or "probable" is made for type 1 and type 2 AIP depending on the reliability of the diagnosis (Tables 3.4 and 3.5). Patients who show pancreatic imaging compatible with AIP but have no other factors suggestive of AIP can be diagnosed with AIP-not otherwise specified (AIP-NOS) if they respond to steroid treatment (Table 3.6).

**Table 3.2** Factors and Findings of ICDC for type 1 AIP

| Factor | Level 1 finding | Level 2 finding |
|---|---|---|
| **P** Parenchymal imaging | **Typical:**<br>Diffuse enlargement with delayed enhancement (sometimes associated with rim like enhancement) | **Indeterminate** (including atypical*):<br>Segmental/focal enlargement with delayed enhancement |
| **D** Ductal imaging (ERP) | Long (>1/3 length of the main pancreatic duct) or multiple strictures without marked upstream dilatation | Segmental/focal narrowing without marked upstream<br>Dilatation (duct size < 5 mm) |
| **S** Serology | **IgG4:**<br>> 2 X upper limit of normal value | **IgG4:**<br>1 – 2 X upper limit of normal value |
| **OOI** Other Organ Involvement | **a or b:** | **a or b:** |
| | **a. Histology of extrapancreatic organs:**<br>**Any 3 of the following**<br>(1) Marked lymphoplasmacytic infiltration with fibrosis and without<br>(2) Storiform fibrosis<br>(3) Obliterative phlebitis<br>(4) Abundant (> 10 cells/hpf) IgG4-positive cells | **a. Histology of extrapancreatic organs including endoscopic biopsies of bile duct:**<br>**Both of the following**<br>(1) Marked lymphoplasmacytic infiltration with fibrosis and without granulocytic infiltration<br>(2) Abundnat (> 10 cells/hpf) IgG4-positive cells |
| | **b. Typical radiological evidence: at least one of the following**<br>(1) Segmental/multiple proximal (hilar/intrahepatic) or proximal and distal bile duct stricture<br>(2) Retroperitoneal fibrosis | **b. Physical or radiological evidence: At lease one of the following**<br>(1) Symmetrically enlarged salivary/lachrymal glands<br>(2) Radiologic evidence of renal involvement described in association with AIP |
| **H** Histology of the pancreas | **LPSP** (core biopsy/resection)<br>**At least 3 of the following**<br>(1) Periductal lymphoplasmacytic infiltrate without granulocytic Infiltration<br>(2) Storiform fibrosis<br>(3) Obliterative phlebitis<br>(4) Abundant (> 10 cells/hpf) IgG4-positive cells | **LPSP** (core biopsy)<br>**Any 2 of the following**<br>(1) Periductal lymphoplasmacytic infiltrate without granulocytic infiltration<br>(2) Storiform fibrosis<br>(3) Obliterative phlebitis<br>(4) Abundant (> 10 cells/hpf) IgG4-positive cells |
| **Rt**# Response to steroid | Rapid (< 2 wk) radiologically demonstrable resolution or marked improvement in pancreatic or extra-pancreatic manifestations | |

# Rt should be used with these cavieats:

a. Rt should be exercised only after negative work-up for cancer including EUS-FNA.

b. General feeling of well being, resolution of mild symptoms (e.g., arthralgia, dyspepsia) and reduction in serum IgG4 levels are not included in "response".

c. In patients with clinical pancreatitis at presentation, spontaneous improvement in pancreatic swelling may occur with resolution of pancreatitis and "response" to steroids should be interpreted with caution.

d. Currently recognized spectrum of presentation of type 1 AIP does not include idiopathic recurrent pancreatitis or typical painfu chronic pancreatitis. Diagnosis of AIP in this setting is to be made by definitive histology rather than by response to steroid therapy.

* Atypical: Some AIP cases may show low-density mass, pancreatic ductal dilatation, or distal atrophy. Such atypical imaging findings in patients with obstructive jaundice and/or pancreatic mass are highly suggestive of pancreatic cancer. Such patients should be managed as pancreatic cancer unless there is strong collateral evidence for AIP, and thorough workup for cancer is negative.

**Table 3.3** Factors and Findings of ICDC for type 2 AIP

| Factor | Level 1 finding | Level 2 finding |
|---|---|---|
| **P** Parenchymal imaging | **Typical:**<br>Diffuse enlargement with delayed enhancement (sometimes associated with rim like enhancement) | **Indeterminate** (including atypical*):<br>Segmental/focal enlargement with delayed enhancement |
| **D** Ductal imaging (ERP) | Long (>1/3 length of the main pancreatic duct) or multiple strictures without marked upstream dilatation | Segmental/focal narrowing without marked upstream<br>Dilatation (duct size < 5 mm) |
| **OOI** Other Organ Involvement | | **IBD**<br>Clinically diagnosed inflammatory bowel disease |
| **H** Histology of the pancreas | IDCP :<br>Both of the following<br>(1) Granulocytic infiltration of duct wall (GEL) with or without granulocytic acinar inflammation<br>(2) Absent or scant (0 – 10 cells/hpf) IgG4-positive cells | Both of the following<br>(1) Granulocytic and lymphoplasmacytic acinar infiltrate<br>(2) Absent or scant (0 – 10 cells/hpf) IgG4-positive cells |
| **Rt**# Response to steroid | Rapid (< 2 wk) radiologically demonstrable resolution or marked improvement in pancreatic or extra-pancreatic manifestations | |

# Rt should be used with these cavieats:

a. Rt should be exercised only after negative work-up for cancer including EUS-FNA.

b. General feeling of well being, resolution of mild symptoms (e.g., arthralgia, dyspepsia) and reduction in serum IgG4 levels are not included in "response".

c. In patients with clinical pancreatitis at presentation, spontaneous improvement in pancreatic swelling may occur with resolution of pancreatitis and "response" to steroids should be interpreted with caution.

d. Currently recognized spectrum of presentation of type 1 AIP does not include idiopathic recurrent pancreatitis or typical painfu chronic pancreatitis. Diagnosis of AIP in this setting is to be made by definitive histology rather than by response to steroid therapy.

* Atypical: Some AIP cases may show low-density mass, pancreatic ductal dilatation, or distal atrophy. Such atypical imaging findings in patients with obstructive jaundice and/or pancreatic mass are highly suggestive of pancreatic cancer. Such patients should be managed as pancreatic cancer unless there is strong collateral evidence for AIP, and thorough workup for cancer is negative.

**Table 3.4** Diagnosis of Definitive/Probable type 1 AIP (see Table 3.2)

| Diagnosis | Factor | Imaging (P) | Collateral Evidence |
|---|---|---|---|
| Definitive type 1 AIP | Histology | Typical /indeterminate | Histologically confirmed LPSP (Level 1 H) |
| | Imaging | Typical<br>Indeterminate | Any non-D Level 1 or Level 2 finding<br>Two or more from Level 1 findings (+ Level 2 D *) |
| | Response to steroid | Indeterminate | Level 1 S or OOI + Rt<br>Or<br>Level 1 D + Level 2 S or OOI or H + Rt |
| Probable type 1 AIP | | Indeterminate | Level 2 S or OOI or H + Rt |

* Level 2 D is counted as Level 1 in this setting.

**Table 3.5** Diagnosis of Definitive/Probable type 2 AIP (see Table 3.3)

| Diagnosis | Imaging (P) | Collateral Evidence |
|---|---|---|
| Definitive type 2 AIP | Typical /indeterminate | Histologically confirmed IDCP (Level 1 H)<br>Clinical IBD and Level 2 H + Rt |
| Probable type 2 AIP | Typical /indeterminate | Clinical IBD and Level 2 H + Rt |

**Table 3.6** Diagnosis of AIP Not Otherwise Specified (AIP-NOS) (see Table 3.2 or 3.3)

| Diagnosis | Imaging (P) | Collateral Evidence |
|---|---|---|
| AIP-NOS | Typical /indeterminate | Clinical 1 D or Level 2 D + Rt |

## Treatment

1. Achievement of Remission
According to a survey on 563 AIP patients in Japan, the remission rate by steroid treatment was 98 % [60], a value which was significantly higher than without steroids (74 %), endorsing oral prednisolone (PLS) as a standard therapy for AIP. The Japanese guidelines for the treatment of AIP [61] recommend the biliary drainage for jaundice associated with AIP and the control of blood glucose for DM before steroid use (Fig. 3.16). The guidelines recommend oral PSL for patients who have symptoms such as jaundice, biliary stenosis, and abdominal pain, but strictly prohibit a facile use of steroids before cautious rule out of pancreatobiliary cancer. The recommended initial dose of PSL is 0.6 mg/kg/day. After administration of the initial dose for 2–4 weeks, it is to be reduced gradually (by 5 mg every 1–2 weeks) depending on the improvement of clinical manifestations, blood test results, and imaging findings to the maintenance dose roughly within 2–3 months. Because radiological improvement appears around 1–2 weeks after the start of steroid therapy [61], morphological and serological evaluations should be followed 2 weeks after the start of steroids. As poor responses suggest the possibility of PCa and other malignant diseases, reevaluation should be carried out promptly.
2. Maintenance Therapy
The important issue in the treatment of AIP is how to inhibit the frequently occurring relapses. AIP is reported to recur in 18–32 % cases under steroid maintenance and in 53 % cases after cessation of steroids [62, 63]. Japanese experts recommended steroid maintenance therapy after remission in order to prevent relapse [1, 60]. On the other hand, Chari ST of Mayo Clinic recommended early discontinuation of steroids and restart of oral PSL when AIP recurred. Their protocol consists of PSL at a dose of 40 mg/day for 4 weeks as the initial treatment, followed by a reduction by 5 mg every week and a withdrawal within 11 weeks [56] (Fig. 3.17).
Recently Kamisawa T et al. retrospectively analyzed the treatment of 563 AIP patients in 17 centers in Japan [60]. The results showed that the relapse rate on maintenance therapy was 23 %, whereas it increased to significantly higher 34 % after the discontinuation of steroids. Relapses occurred within 1 year after the withdrawal of steroids in 56 % cases and within 3 years in 92 % cases. The PSL doses at the time of relapse were 10 mg/day in 16 % cases, 7.5 mg/day in 11 %, 5 mg/day in 46 %, and 2.5 mg/day in 13 %. Even if AIP recurred, patients responded well to restart or dose-up of PSL. However, it is still controversial whether the maintenance therapy with PSL really contributes to the prognosis in the light of unfavorable side effects.
Type 2 AIP reportedly responds very well to steroids as type 1 AIP does. Sah RP et al. showed that the patients with histologically confirmed type 2 AIP responded well to the steroid treatment and none of them developed recurrence during the follow-up period of 9–108 months [3]. None or less frequent relapse is considered to form another important clinical feature that distinguishes type 2 from type 1 AIP.
3. Other Medicine
The use of immune-modulating medicine for patients with steroid resistant AIP has been reported chiefly from Western countries. The medicine so far reported includes azathioprine [64, 65], a combination of PSL and azathioprine [66], mycophenolate mofetil [67], cytoxan [67], and 6-mercaptopurine [68]. In addition to these drugs, there are several recent reports on the successful use of rituximab for the treatment of patients with AIP or IgG4-related sclerosing cholangitis (IgG4-SC), who were refractory to steroids and/or other immune-modulating drugs [68–70]. Because rituximab exerts its effects through the depletion of B-lymphocytes, B cell activity may play important role in the pathogenesis of AIP.

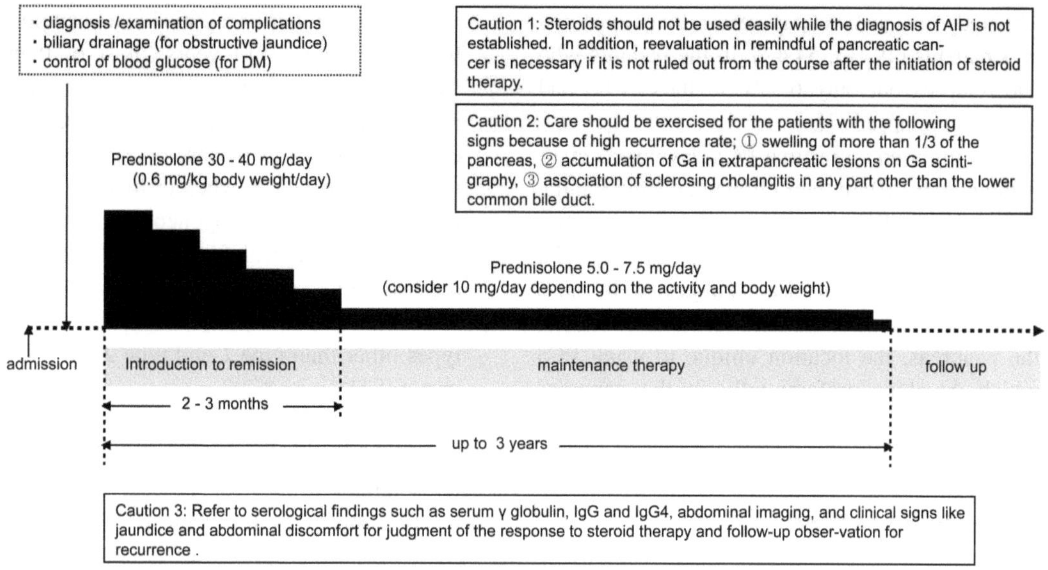


**Fig. 3.16** A schematic drawing of the steroid regimen for AIP recommended by Japanese experts

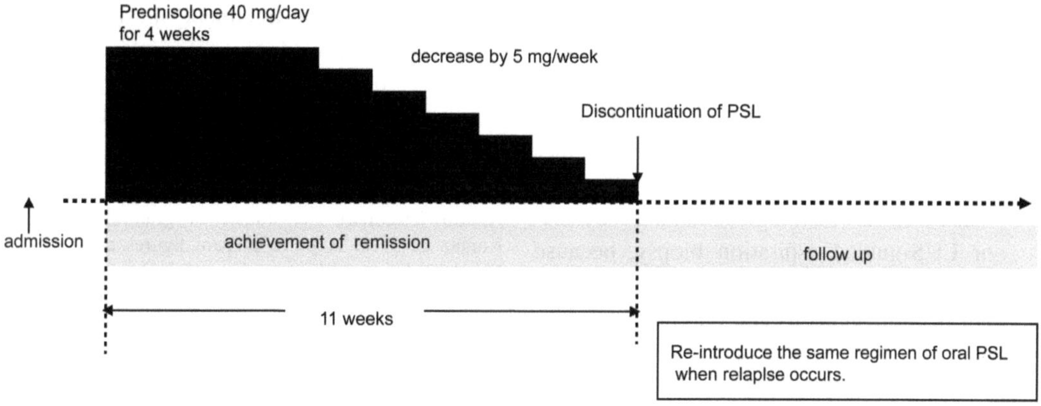


**Fig. 3.17** A schematic drawing of the steroid regimen for AIP recommended by Mayo Clinic

## Prognosis

According to a recent follow-up study of 78 patients with type 1 and 19 patients with type 2 AIP for the median period of 58 and 89 months, respectively, the long-term survival of AIP patients was not significantly different from that of the demographically similar US population [3]. In addition, there was no difference in the survival between type 1 and type 2 AIP patients. Although the study suggested that neither type of AIP affects the long-term survival, some earlier reports demonstrated the development of pancreatic atrophy and pancreatic stones in 30–40 % and 6.5–25 % of AIP patients, respectively [71–73]. The stone formation seemed to be related to the occurrence of relapses. Takayama M et al. reported the prognosis of 42 cases of AIP who had been followed for median periods of 54.5 months.

The study revealed that pancreatic stones appeared in 8 patients (19 %), 54.4 % in the patients who had relapses but only 6.5 % in those who had never had relapse [73].

It is reported so far that PCa developed in 11 patients with AIP in their clinical course: 5 at the diagnosis of AIP and 6 at around 3–5 years after the initiation of steroid therapy [74–76]. The unique localization of PCa is suggested, because 9 of these 11 cases had PCa in the body or tail of the pancreas, the location unique to usual PCa which develops preferentially in the pancreas head [74].

## Issues to Be Settled

1. How to Obtain High-Quality Tissue Specimens
   Currently, the diagnosis of type 2 AIP is solely based on the pathological findings of IDCP/GELs, which holds true even by the ICDC. Even in the diagnosis of type 1 AIP, histological evaluation would be decisive when the case lacks characteristic features like elevation of serum IgG4 or typical other organ involvement. However, it is difficult to make a correct histological diagnosis by US- or EUS-guided aspiration biopsy, because pathological changes in the pancreas may not be homogeneous and may not be evaluated precisely in small specimens. Indeed, a recent report from Korea demonstrated that transabdominal US-guided pancreatic core biopsy could give correct diagnosis only in 26 % of the AIP patients examined [77]. Some experts recommended the use of 19-gauge Trucut needles to obtain large samples [78], but there are limitations for the use due to a fear for complications or difficulty in insertion of such thick needles into the targeted lesions [79]. Therefore, it is strongly desired to develop devices that enable to obtain high-quality tissue specimens safely and with high certainty.
2. Establishment of Clinical and Pathological Features of AIP in the World
   Although AIP has attracted attention since the original report in 1995 [80] and an increasing number of reports have been published in the past 17 years, most of them came from limited countries in the world. It is expected that a spread of the ICDC may clarify whether this disease distributes more widely in the world, whether this disease is homogeneous or heterogeneous in the clinical and pathological features, whether this disease shows racially or geographically different characteristics, and whether unique types other than type 1 and type 2 AIP exist or not [81].
3. Best Treatment for Quality of Life (QOL)
   There is no clear evidence whether long-term administration of PSL at low doses really suppresses the relapse of AIP and improves the prognosis of patients or not. There is no evidence whether other immune-modulating drugs are more effective and safer than steroids and could improve the QOL of patients [82]. To establish the best regimen for the treatment of AIP, prospective randomized clinical trials and long-term follow-up for the effectiveness are required under a cooperation of multiple countries.

**Acknowledgment** The author is grateful to Atushi Kanno for great helps to prepare figures and to Kenji Notohara for providing the beautiful pictures of IDCP/GELs (Fig. 3.9). This manuscript is made with a support in part by the Research Committee of Intractable Pancreatic Diseases provided by the Ministry of Health, Labour, and Welfare of Japan.

## References

1. Okazaki K, Kawa S, Kamisawa T, Ito T, Inui K, Irie H, Irisawa A, Kubo K, Notohara K, Hasebe O, Fujinaga Y, Ohara H, Tanaka S, Nishino T, Nishimori I, Nishiyama T, Suda K, Shiratori K, Shimosegawa T, Tanaka M. Japanese clinical guidelines for autoimmune pancreatitis. Pancreas. 2009;38:849–66.
2. Okazaki K, Kawa S, Kamisawa T, Naruse S, Tanaka S, Nishimori I, Ohara H, Ito T, Kiriyama S, Inui K, Shimosegawa T, Koizumi M, Suda K, Shiratori K, Yamaguchi K, Yamaguchi T, Sugiyama M, Otsuki M. Clinical diagnostic criteria of autoimmune pancreatitis: revised proposal. J Gastroenterol. 2006;41: 626–31.
3. Sah RP, Chari ST, Pannala R, Sugumar A, Clain JE, Levy MJ, Pearson RK, Smyrk TC, Petersen BT, Topazian MD, Takahash N, Farnell MB, Vege SS. Differences in clinical profile and relapse rate of type

1 versus type 2 autoimmune pancreatitis. Gastroenterology. 2010;139:140–8.
4. Kawa S, Hamano H. Clinical features of autoimmune pancreatitis. J Gastroenterol. 2007;42(Suppl XVIII):9–14.
5. Sahani DV, Kalva SP, Farrell J, Maher MM, Saini S, Mueller PR, Lauwers GY, Fernandez CD, Warshaw AL, Simeone JF. Autoimmune pancreatitis: imaging features. Radiology. 2004;233:345–52.
6. Kamisawa T, Tu Y, Nakajima H, Egawa N, Tsuruta K, Okamoto A, Horiguchi S. Sclerosing cholecystitis associated with autoimmune pancreatitis. World J Gastroenterol. 2006;12:3736–9.
7. Hyodo N, Hyodo T. Ultrasonographic evaluation in patients with autoimmune-related pancreatitis. J Gastroenterol. 2003;38:1155–61.
8. Irie H, Honda H, Baba S, Kuroiwa T, Yoshimitsu K, Tajima T, Jimi M, Sumii T, Masuda K. Autoimmune pancreatitis: CT and MR characteristics. Am J Roentgenol. 1998;170:1323–7.
9. Ito T, Nakano I, Koyanagi S, Miyahara T, Migita Y, Ogoshi K, Sakai H, Matsunaga S, Yasuda O, Sumii T, Nawata H. Autoimmune pancreatitis as a new clinical entity. Three cases of autoimmune pancreatitis with effective steroid therapy. Dig Dis Sci. 1997;42:1458–68.
10. Wakabayashi T, Motoo Y, Kojima Y, Makino H, Sawabu N. Chronic pancreatitis with diffuse irregular narrowing of the main pancreatic duct. Dig Dis Sci. 1998;43:2415–25.
11. Horiuchi A, Kawa S, Hamano H, Hayama M, Ota H, Kiyosawa K. ERCP features in 27 patients with autoimmune pancreatitis. Gastrointest Endosc. 2002;55:494–9.
12. Kamisawa T, Tu Y, Egawa N, Nakajima H, Tsuruta K, Okamoto A. Involvement of pancreatic and bile ducts in autoimmune pancreatitis. World J Gastroenterol. 2006;12:612–4.
13. Hirano K, Shiratori Y, Komatsu Y, Yamamoto N, Sasahira N, Toda N, Isayama H, Tada M, Tsujino T, Nakata R, Kawase T, Katamoto T, Kawabe T, Omata M. Involvement of the biliary system in autoimmune pancreatitis: a follow-up study. Clin Gastroenterol Hepatol. 2003;1:453–64.
14. Higashi T, Saga T, Nakamoto Y, Ishimori T, Fujimoto K, Doi R, Imamura M, Konishi J. Diagnosis of pancreatic cancer using fluorine-18 fluorodeoxyglucose positron emission tomography (FDG-PET) – usefulness and limitations in "clinical reality". Ann Nucl Med. 2003;17:261–79.
15. Ozaki Y, Oguchi K, Hamano H, Arakura N, Muraki T, Kiyosawa K, Momose M, Kadoya M, Miyata K, Aizawa T, Kawa S. Differentiation of autoimmune pancreatitis from suspected pancreatic cancer by fluorine-18 fluorodeoxyglucose positron emission tomography. J Gastroenterol. 2008;43:144–51.
16. Sato M, Okumura T, Shioyama Y, Imura J. Extrapancreatic F-18 FDG accumulation in autoimmune pancreatitis. Ann Nucl Med. 2008;22:215–9.
17. Hamano H, Kawa S, Horiuchi A, Unno H, Furuya N, Akamatsu T, Fukushima M, Nikaido T, Nakayama K, Usuda N, Kiyosawa K. High serum IgG4 concentrations in patients with sclerosing pancreatitis. N Engl J Med. 2001;344:732–8.
18. Ghazale A, Chari ST, Smyrk TC, Levy MJ, Topazian MD, Takahashi N, Clain JE, Pearson RK, Pelaez-Luna M, Petersen BT, Vege SS, Farnell MB. Value of serum IgG4 in the diagnosis of autoimmune pancreatitis and in distinguishing it from pancreatic cancer. Am J Gastroenterol. 2007;102:1646–53.
19. Okazaki K, Uchida K, Ohana M, Nakase H, Uose S, Inai M, Matsushima Y, Katamura K, Ohmori K, Chiba T. Autoimmune-related pancreatitis is associated with autoantibodies and a Th1/Th2-type cellular immune response. Gastroenterology. 2000;118:573–81.
20. Asada M, Nishio A, Uchida K, Kido M, Ueno S, Uza N, Kiriya K, Inoue S, Kitamura H, Ohashi S, Tamaki H, Fukui T, Matsuura M, Kawasaki K, Nishi T, Watanabe N, Nakase H, Chiba T, Okazaki K. Identification of a novel autoantibody against pancreatic secretory trypsin inhibitor in patients with autoimmune pancreatitis. Pancreas. 2006;33:20–6.
21. Frulloni L, Lunardi C, Simone R, Dolcino M, Scattolini C, Falconi M, Benini L, Vantini I, Corrocher R, Puccetti A. Identification of a novel antibody associated with autoimmune pancreatitis. N Engl J Med. 2009;361:2135–42.
22. Komatsu K, Hamano H, Ochi Y, Takayama M, Muraki T, Yoshizawa K, Sakurai A, Ota M, Kawa S. High prevalence of hypothyroidism in patients with autoimmune pancreatitis. Dig Dis Sci. 2005;50:1052–7.
23. Sugumar A, Klöppel G, Chari ST. Autoimmune pancreatitis: pathologic subtypes and their implications for its diagnosis. Am J Gastroenterol. 2009;104:2308–10.
24. Kawaguchi K, Koike M, Tsuruta K, Okamoto A, Tabata I, Fujita N. Lymphoplasmacytic sclerosing pancreatitis with cholangitis. Hum Pathol. 1991;22:387–95.
25. Suda K, Takase M, Fukumura Y, Ogura K, Ueda A, Matsuda T, Suzuki F. Histopathologic characteristics of autoimmune pancreatitis based on comparison with chronic pancreatitis. Pancreas. 2005;30:355–8.
26. Kojima M, Sipos B, Klapper W, Frahm O, Knuth HC, Yanagisawa A, Zamboni G, Morohoshi T, Klöppel G. Autoimmune pancreatitis: frequency, IgG4 expression, and clonality of T and B cells. Am J Surg Pathol. 2007;31:521–8.
27. Zhang L, Notohara K, Levy MJ, Chari ST, Smyrk TC. IgG4-positive plasma cell infiltration in the diagnosis of autoimmune pancreatitis. Mod Pathol. 2007;20:23–8.
28. Notohara K, Burgart LJ, Yadav D, Chari S, Smyrk TC. Idiopathic chronic pancreatitis with periductal lymphoplasmacytic infiltration. Clinicopathologic features of 35 cases. Am J Surg Pathol. 2003;27:1119–27.
29. Zamboni G, Lüttges J, Capelli P, Frulloni L, Cavallini G, Pederzoli P, Leins A, Longnecker D, Klöppel G. Histopathological features of diagnostic and clinical

relevance in autoimmune pancreatitis: a study on 53 resection specimens and biopsy specimens. Virchows Arch. 2004;445:552–63.
30. Klöppel G, Detlefsen S, Chari ST, Longnecker DS, Zamboni G. Autoimmune pancreatitis: the clinico-pathological characteristics of the subtype with granulocytic epithelial lesions. J Gastroenterol. 2010;45: 787–93.
31. Kamisawa T, Funata N, Hayashi Y, Tsuruta K, Okamoto A, Amemiya K, Egawa N, Nakajima H. Close relationship between autoimmune pancreatitis and multifocal fibrosclerosis. Gut. 2003;52:683–7.
32. Saegusa H, Momose M, Kawa S, Hamano H, Ochi Y, Takayama M, Kiyosawa K, Kadoya M. Hilar and pancreatic gallium-67 accumulation is characteristic feature of autoimmune pancreatitis. Pancreas. 2003;27:20–5.
33. Nakazawa T, Ohara H, Yamada T, Ando H, Sano H, Kajino S, Hashimoto T, Nakamura S, Ando T, Nomura T, Joh T, Itoh M. Atypical primary sclerosing cholangitis cases associated with unusual pancreatitis. Hepatogastroenterology. 2001;48:625–30.
34. Hamano H, Kawa S, Ochi Y, Unno H, Shiba N, Wajiki M, Nakazawa K, Shimojo H, Kiyosawa K. Hydronephrosis associated with retroperitoneal fibrosis and sclerosing pancreatitis. Lancet. 2002;359: 1403–4.
35. Takeda S, Haratake J, Kasai T, Takaeda C, Takazakura E. IgG4-associated idiopathic tubulointerstitial nephritis complicating autoimmune pancreatitis. Nephrol Dial Transplant. 2004;19:474–6.
36. Taniguchi T, Ko M, Seko S, Nishida O, Inoue F, Kobayashi H, Saiga T, Okamoto M, Fukuse T. Interstitial pneumonia associated with autoimmune pancreatitis. Gut. 2003;52:683–7.
37. Taniguchi T, Hamasaki A, Okamoto M. A case of suspected lymphocytic hypophysitis and organizing pneumonia during maintenance therapy for autoimmune pancreatitis associated with autoimmune thrombocytopenia. Endocr J. 2006;53:563–6.
38. Kanno A, Satoh K, Kimura K, Masamune A, Asakura T, Unno M, Matsuno S, Moriya T, Shimosegawa T. Autoimmune pancreatitis with hepatic inflammatory pseudotumor. Pancreas. 2005;31:420–3.
39. Zen Y, Harada K, Sasaki M, Sato Y, Tsuneyama K, Haratake J, Kurumaya H, Katayanagi K, Masuda S, Niwa H, Morimoto H, Miwa A, Uchiyama A, Portmann BC, Nakanuma Y. IgG4-realted sclerosing cholangitis with and without hepatic inflammatory pseudotumor, and sclerosing pancreatitis-associated sclerosing cholangitis. Am J Surg Pathol. 2004;28:1193–203.
40. Kamisawa T, Egawa N, Nakajima H, Tsuruta K, Okamoto A, Hayashi Y, Funata N. Gastrointestinal findings in patients with autoimmune pancreatitis. Endoscopy. 2005;37:1127–30.
41. Yoshimura Y, Takeda S, Ieki Y, Takazakura E, Koizumi H, Takagawa K. IgG4-associated prostatitis complicating autoimmune pancreatitis. Intern Med. 2006;45:897–901.
42. Ohara H, Nakazawa T, Sano H, Ando T, Okamoto T, Takada H, Hayashi K, Kitajima Y, Nakao H, Joh T. Systemic extrapancreatic lesions associated with autoimmune pancreatitis. Pancreas. 2005;31:232–7.
43. Yamamoto M, Ohara M, Suzuki C, Naishiro Y, Yamamoto H, Takahashi H, Imai K. Elevated IgG4 concentrations in serum of patients with Mikulicz's disease. Scand J Rheumatol. 2004;33:432–3.
44. Yamamoto M, Harada S, Ohara M, Suzuki C, Naishiro Y, Yamamoto H, Takahashi H, Imai K. Clinical and pathological differences between Mikulicz's disease and Sjögren syndrome. Rheumatology. 2005;44:227–34.
45. Nakazawa T, Ohara H, Sano H, Aoki S, Kobayashi S, Okamoto T, Imai H, Nomura T, Joh T, Itoh M. Cholangiography can discriminate sclerosing cholangitis with autoimmune pancreatitis from primary sclerosing cholangitis. Gastrointest Endosc. 2004;60:937–44.
46. Nakazawa T, Ohara H, Sano H, Ando T, Aoki S, Kobayashi S, Okamoto T, Nomura T, Joh T, Itoh M. Clinical differences between primary sclerosing cholangitis and sclerosing cholangitis with autoimmune pancreatitis. Pancreas. 2005;30:20–5.
47. Kamisawa T, Tu Y, Egawa N, Tsuruta K, Okamoto A. A new diagnostic endoscopic tool for autoimmune pancreatitis. Gastrointest Endosc. 2008;68:358–61.
48. Kamisawa T, Funata N, Hayashi Y, Eishi Y, Koike M, Tsuruta K, Okamoto A, Egawa N, Nakajima H. A new clinicopathological entity of IgG4-related autoimmune disease. J Gastroenterol. 2003;38:982–4.
49. Kamisawa T, Nakajima H, Egawa N, Funata N, Tsuruta K, Okamoto A. IgG4-related sclerosing disease incorporating sclerosing pancreatitis, cholangitis, sialadenitis and retroperitoneal fibrosis with lymphadenopathy. Pancreatology. 2006;6:132–7.
50. Kamisawa T, Funata N, Hayashi Y, Eishi Y, Koike M, Tsuruta K, Okamoto A, Egawa N, Nakajima H. Close relationship between autoimmune pancreatitis and multifocal fibrosclerosis. Gut. 2003;52:683–7.
51. Stone JH, Zen Y, Deshpande V. IgG4-related disease. N Engl J Med. 2012;366:539–51.
52. Sugumar A, Smyrk TC, Takahashi N, Levy MJ, Chari ST. Lymphoplasmacytic sclerosing pancreatitis (LPSP) and idiopathic duct centric pancreatitis (IDCP) are distinct clinical forms of autoimmune pancreatitis (AIP). Pancreas. 2008;37:497.
53. Members of the Criteria Committee for Autoimmune Pancreatitis of the Japan Pancreas Society. Diagnostic criteria for autoimmune pancreatitis by the Japan Pancreas Society (2002) (in Japanese with English abstract). Suizo. 2002;17:585–7.
54. Kim K-P, Kim M-H, Kim JC, Lee SS, Seo DW, Lee SK. Diagnostic criteria for autoimmune chronic pancreatitis revisited. World J Gastroenterol. 2006;12: 2487–96.
55. Choi EK, Kim M-H, Kim JC, Han J, Seo DW, Lee SS, Lee SK. The Japanese diagnostic criteria for autoimmune chronic pancreatitis: Is it completely satisfactory? Pancreas. 2006;33:13–9.
56. Chari ST, Smyrk TC, Levy MJ, Topazian MD, Takahashi N, Zhang L, Clain JE, Pearson RK, Petersen BT, Vege SS, Farnell MB. Diagnosis of auto-

immune pancreatitis: the Mayo Clinic experience. Clin Gastroenterol Hepatol. 2006;4:1010–6.
57. Otsuki M, Chung JB, Okazaki K, Kim M-H, Kamisawa T, Kawa S, Park SW, Shimosegawa T, Lee K, Ito T, Nishimori I, Notohara K, Naruse S, Ko SBH, Ko SBH, Kihara Y, The Research Committee of Intractable Pancreatic Diseases provided by the Ministry of Health, Labour and Welfare of Japan and the Korean Society of Pancreatobiliary Diseases. Asian diagnostic criteria for autoimmune pancreatitis: consensus of the Japan-Korea symposium on autoimmune pancreatitis. J Gastroenterol. 2008;43:403–8.
58. Chari ST, Kloeppel G, Zhang L, Notohara K, Lerch MM, Shimosegawa T, The Autoimmune Pancreatitis International Cooperative Study Group (APICS). Histopathologic and clinical subtypes of autoimmune pancreatitis: the Honolulu consensus document. Pancreas. 2010;39:549–54.
59. Shimosegawa T, Chari ST, Frulloni L, Kamisawa T, Kawa S, Mino-Kenudson M, Kim M-H, Klöppel G, Lerch MM, Löhr M, Notohoara K, Okazaki K, Schneider A, Zhang L. International consensus diagnostic criteria for autoimmune pancreatitis. Guidelines of the International Association of Pancreatology. Pancreas. 2011;40:352–8.
60. Kamisawa T, Shimosegawa T, Okazaki K, Nishino T, Watanabe H, Kanno A, Okumura F, Nishikawa T, Kobayashi K, Ichiya T, Takatori H, Yamakita K, Kubota K, Hamano H, Okamura K, Hirano K, Ito T, Ko SBH, Omata M. Standard steroid treatment for autoimmune pancreatitis. Gut. 2009;58:1504–7.
61. Ito T, Nishimori I, Inoue N, Kawabe K, Gibo J, Arita Y, Okazaki K, Takayanagi R, Otsuki M. Treatment for autoimmune pancreatitis: consensus on the treatment for patients with autoimmune pancreatitis in Japan. J Gastroenterol. 2007;42(Suppl XVIII):50–8.
62. Hirano K, Tada M, Isayama H, Yagioka H, Sasaki T, Kogure H, Nakai Y, Sasahira N, Tsujino T, Yoshida H, Kawabe T, Omata M. Long-term prognosis of autoimmune pancreatitis with and without corticosteroid treatment. Gut. 2007;56:1719–24.
63. Kamisawa T, Okamoto A, Wakabayashi T, Watanabe H, Sawabu N. Appropriate steroid therapy for autoimmune pancreatitis based on long-term outcome. Scand J Gastroenterol. 2008;43:609–13.
64. Church NI, Pereira S, Deheragoda MG, Sandanayake N, Amin Z, Lees WR, Gillams A, Rodriguez-Justo M, Novelli M, Seward EW, Hatfield ARW, Webster GJM. Autoimmune pancreatitis: clinical and radiological features and objective response to steroid therapy in a UK series. Am J Gastroenterol. 2007;102:2417–25.
65. Sandanayake NS, Church NI, Chapman MH, Johnson GJ, Dhar DK, Amin Z, Deheragoda MG, Novelli M, Winstanley A, Rodrizuez-Justo M, Hatfield ARW, Pereira SP, Webster GJM. Presentation and management of post-treatment relapse in autoimmune pancreatitis/immunoglobulin G4-associated cholangitis. Clin Gastroenterol Hepatol. 2009;7:1089–96.
66. Raina A, Yadav D, Krasinskas AM, McGrath KM, Khalid A, Sanders M, Witcomb DC, Slivka A. Evaluation and management of autoimmune pancreatitis: experience at a large US center. Am J Gastroenterol. 2009;104:2295–306.
67. Ghazale A, Chari ST, Zhang L, Smyrk TC, Takahashi N, Levy MJ, Topazian MD, Clain JE, Pearson RK, Petersen BT, Vege SS, Lindor K, Farnell MB. Immunoglobulin G4-associate cholangitis: clinical profile and response to therapy. Gastroenterology. 2008;134:706–15.
68. Topazian M, Witzig TE, Smyrk TC, Pulido JS, Levy MJ, Kamath PS, Chari ST. Rituximab therapy for refractory biliary strictures in immunoglobulin G4-associated cholangitis. Clin Gastroenterol Hepatol. 2008;6:364–6.
69. Rueda JC, Duarte-Rey C, Casas N. Successful treatment of relapsing autoimmune pancreatitis in primary Sjögren's syndrome with rituximab: report of a case and review of the literature. Rheumatol Int. 2009;29:1481–5.
70. Khosroshahi A, Bloch DB, Deshpande V, Stone JH. Rituximab therapy leads to rapid decline of serum IgG4 levels and prompt clinical improvement in IgG4-realted systemic disease. Arthritis Rheum. 2010;62:1755–62.
71. Kamisawa T, Yoshiike M, Egawa N, Nakajima H, Tsuruta K, Okamoto A. Treating patients with autoimmune pancreatitis: results from a long-term follow-up study. Pancreatology. 2005;5:234–8.
72. Nishino T, Toki F, Oyama H, Shimizu K, Shiratori K. Long-term outcome of autoimmune pancreatitis after oral prednisolone therapy. Intern Med. 2006;45:497–501.
73. Takayama M, Hamano H, Ochi Y, Saegusa H, Komatsu K, Muraki T, Arakura N, Imai Y, Hasebe O, Kawa S. Recurrent attacks of autoimmune pancreatitis result in pancreatic stone formation. Am J Gastroenterol. 2004;99:932–7.
74. Iida H, Kubota K, Mawatari H, Yoneda M, Goto A, Abe Y, Inamori M, Kobayashi N, Kirikoshi H, Saito S, Nakajima A. A case of autoimmune pancreatitis developed pancreatic tail cancer. (Japanese and English abstract) Suizo. 2008;23:608–14.
75. Inoue H, Miyatani H, Sawada Y, Yoshida Y. A case of pancreas cancer with autoimmune pancreatitis. Pancreas. 2006;33:208–9.
76. Ghazale A, Chari S. Is autoimmune pancreatitis a risk factor for pancreatic cancer. Pancreas. 2007;35:376.
77. Bang S-J, Kim M-H, Kim DH, Lee TY, Kwon S, Oh H-C, Kim JY, Hwang CY, Lee SS, Seo DW, Kee SK, Song DE, Jang SJ. Is pancreatic core biopsy sufficient to diagnose autoimmune chronic pancreatitis? Pancreas. 2008;36:84–9.
78. Levy MJ, Reddy RP, Wiersema MJ, Smyrk TC, Clain JE, Harewood GC, Pearson RK, Rajan E, Topazian MD, Yusuf TE, Chari ST, Peterson BT. EUS-guided trucut biopsy in establishing autoimmune pancreatitis as the cause of obstructive jaundice. Gastrointest Endosc. 2005;61:467–72.

79. DeWitt J, McGreevy K, LeBlanc J, McHenry L, Cummings O, Sherman S. EUS-guided Trucut biopsy of suspected nonfocal chronic pancreatitis. Gastrointest Endosc. 2005;62:76–84.
80. Yoshida K, Toki F, Takeuchi T, Watanabe S-I, Shiratori K, Hayashi N. Chronic pancreatitis caused by an autoimmune abnormality. Proposal of the concept of autoimmune pancreatitis. Dig Dis Sci. 1995;40:1561–8.
81. Kamisawa T, Chari ST, Giday SA, Kim M-H, Chang JB, Lee KT, Werner J, Bergmann F, Lerch MM, Mayerle J, Pickartz T, Lohr M, Schneider A, Frulloni L, Webster GJM, Reddy ND, Liao W-C, Wang H-P, Okazaki K, Shimosegawa T, Kloeppel G, Go VLW. Clinical profile of autoimmune pancreatitis and its histological subtypes. An international multicenter survey. Pancreas. 2011;40: 809–14.
82. Hart PA, Topazian MD, Witzig TE, Clain JE, Gleeson FC, Klebig RR, Levy MJ, Pearson RK, Petersen BT, Smyrk TC, Sugumar A, Takahashi N, Vege SS, Chari ST. Treatment of relapsing autoimmune pancreatitis with immunomodulators and rituximab: the Mayo Clinic experience. Gut. 2012;0:1–8. doi:10.1136/gutjnl-2012-302886.

# Histologic Features

# 4

Günter Klöppel and Thomas C. Smyrk

## Introduction

To the pathologist, chronic pancreatitis is a combination of inflammation, fibrosis, and loss of acinar tissue, accompanied by secondary changes in ducts and islets. Long thought to be nondescript and nonspecific, there are in fact histologic clues to various etiologic possibilities, including alcoholic chronic pancreatitis, hereditary pancreatitis, paraduodenal pancreatitis, obstructive chronic pancreatitis, and autoimmune pancreatitis [1]. Recent work further suggests that the term "autoimmune pancreatitis" encompasses at least two entities, one related to a systemic IgG4 disease process referred to as $IgG_4$-related disease ($IgG_4$-RD) and one not, and that histology can generally separate the two. The two entities are provisionally termed autoimmune pancreatitis, type 1 and type 2 [2].

G. Klöppel, MD
Department of Pathology, University Hospital, University of Kiel, Ismaningersts 22, Munich, Bavaria 81675, Germany
e-mail: guenter.kloeppel@alumni.uni-kiel.de

T.C. Smyrk, MD (✉)
Department of Pathology, Mayo Clinic, 200 1st ST., SW, Rochester, MN 55905, USA
e-mail: smyrk.thomas@mayo.edu

## Histopathology of Type 1 AIP

Type 1 AIP is the pancreatic manifestation of $IgG_4$-RD. It is characterized by periductal lymphoplasmacytic inflammation, phlebitis, and fibrosis, almost always accompanied by increased numbers of IgG4-positive plasma cells (Fig. 4.1) [3]. The distribution within the pancreas is usually diffuse, but can be localized, mimicking neoplasm. Even when the pancreas is diffusely involved by imaging and gross examination, histology reveals focal parenchymal sparing in the majority of resected organs [4].

The periductal inflammation involves medium-sized ducts. It is dominated by lymphocytes, but substantial numbers of plasma cells are also present (Fig. 4.2). Duct epithelium is intact and does not show reactive or hyperplastic changes. At times, the periductal inflammation is accompanied by a collar of dense fibrous tissue (Fig. 4.3). Occasional lymphoid aggregates, some with germinal centers, accompany the periductal inflammation. Eosinophils may be seen, sometimes in large numbers [5], but neutrophils are not a feature of type 1 AIP.

Inflammation and fibrosis are the parenchymal changes characteristic of type 1 AIP (Fig. 4.4). A fibroinflammatory process encroaches on and overruns lobules. The fibrosing process forms short fascicles of collagen arranged in a swirled, cartwheel pattern. Adding to the distinctive appearance is the fact that the storiform fibrosis is almost

M.J. Levy and S.T. Chari (eds.), *Autoimmune (IgG4-related) Pancreatitis and Cholangitis*, DOI 10.1007/978-1-4419-6430-4_4, © Springer Science+Business Media New York 2013

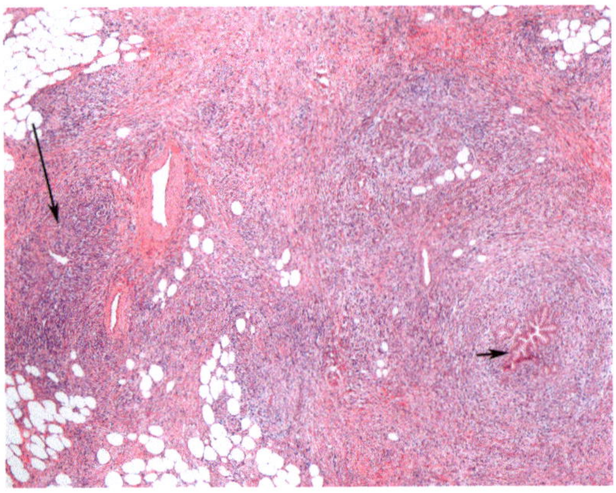

**Fig. 4.1** Type 1 AIP. This low-power view shows phlebitis (*long arrow*) and a medium-sized duct with inflammation (*short arrow*). Fibrosis and inflammation occupy the center of the field

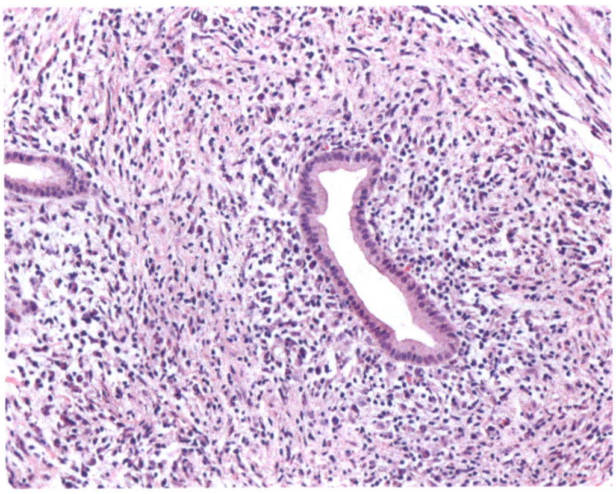

**Fig. 4.2** Dense periductal lymphoplasmacytic inflammation. The epithelium is not inflamed and appears undamaged

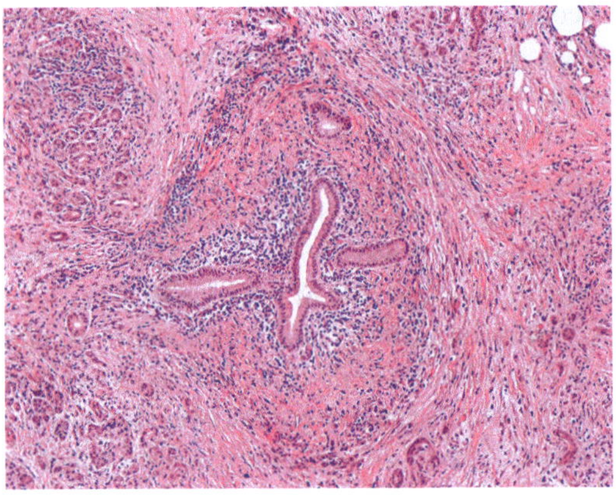

**Fig. 4.3** The periductal inflammation is accompanied by a collar of fibrous tissue

always accompanied by dense lymphoplasmacytic inflammation. Eosinophils may be seen, but, just as in the periductal infiltrate, the presence of neutrophils suggests a diagnosis other than type 1 AIP. The infiltrate typically spills into peripancreatic soft tissue, where one very commonly sees lymphoid aggregates and perineural inflammation (Fig. 4.5). Lymphoid aggregates are also present in the parenchyma, but are not a prominent feature.

The lymphoplasmacytic infiltrate of type 1 AIP involves vein walls. This is always a striking finding in the resected pancreas, where one can locate large muscular arteries at low power and contrast the usual absence of inflammation there to the dense lymphoplasmacytic infiltrate that compresses and often obliterates the lumen of the adjacent vein (Fig. 4.6). Rarely, the artery may also have some lymphoplasmacytic inflammation, but neutrophils are not present in either vein or artery, and there is no fibrin or nuclear dust.

As the pancreatic form of systemic IgG4-related disease, type 1 AIP typically has increased numbers of IgG4-positive plasma cells (Fig. 4.7). Various definitions for "increased" have been proposed, with any particular cutoff value necessarily reflecting a trade-off between sensitivity and specificity [6–8]. A recent consensus statement has chosen to utilize different cutoff values depending on the nature of the specimen, requiring more than 50 positive cells per high power field to support the diagnosis in resection specimens, but only 10 per high power field in needle biopsies [3].

In some organ systems, the IgG4 to IgG ratio may be more specific for the diagnosis of type 1 AIP [9], particularly those such as lung, that tend to have a very rich plasma cell infiltrate [10, 11]. Those who find the IgG4/IgG ratio useful suggest that 40 % is the best cutoff value [12]. In the pancreas, we feel that IgG4 counts alone, combined with appropriate histology, are sufficient to make an accurate diagnosis.

It is important to note that increased numbers of IgG4-positive plasma cells are not specific for the diagnosis of type 1 AIP. Other situations in which the pancreas can have increased IgG4 include type 2 AIP (discussed below), primary

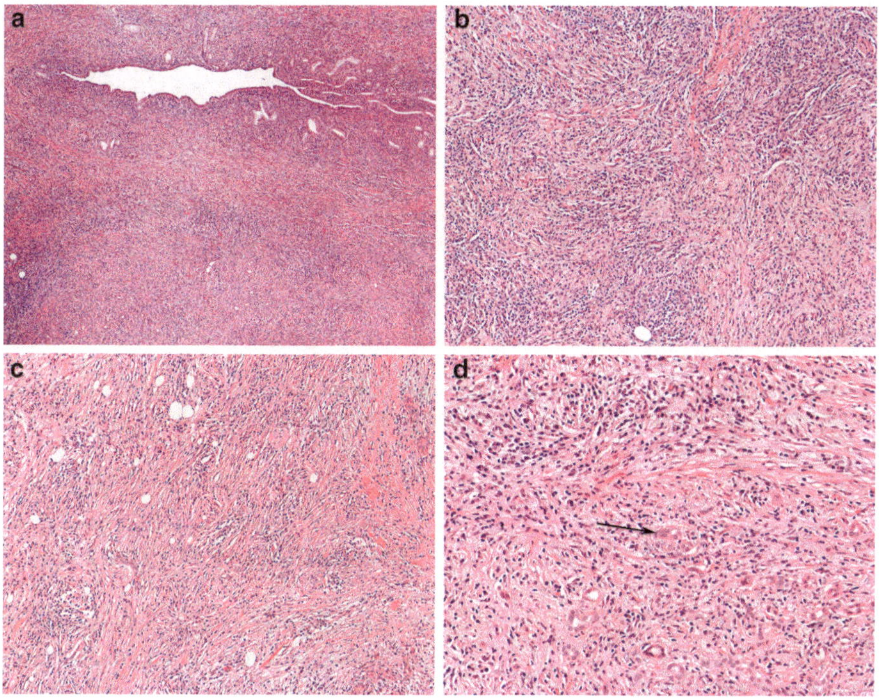

**Fig. 4.4** (**a**) A preserved duct occupies the *top* half of the field. In the *lower* half, pancreatic lobules have been replaced by a fibroinflammatory process. (**b**) Swirling fascicles of collagen, accompanied by lymphoplasmacytic inflammation. (**c**) Another example of storiform fibrosis, this one with slightly less inflammation. (**d**) The fibroinflammatory process is both interlobular (*top*) and intralobular (*bottom*). A few attenuated acini survive (*arrow*). There are no neutrophils

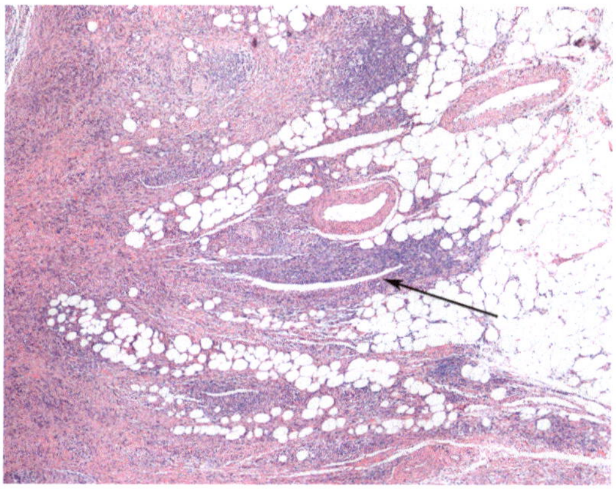

**Fig. 4.5** Lymphoid follicles extend into peripancreatic parenchyma in type 1 AIP. A peripancreatic vein is involved by phlebitis (*arrow*)

sclerosing cholangitis, adenocarcinoma, and malignant lymphoma. Conversely, the *absence* of tissue IgG4 does not necessarily rule out type 1 AIP. This is an unusual event (two patients in our experience), but rare patients can have compelling clinical and morphologic changes of IgG4-related disease without detectable tissue IgG4, suggesting that IgG4 is a characteristic but not necessary marker for this idiopathic condition.

## Needle Biopsy and Fine Needle Aspiration in Type 1 AIP

Increasing recognition of systemic IgG4-related disease has made pancreatoduodenectomy specimens less common in recent years, although van Heerde et al. still found a prevalence of AIP of 2.6 % among patients undergoing this operation at a Dutch tertiary care center between 2000 and 2009 [13]. Large-caliber (19-gauge) trucut biopsy (TCB) obtained via endoscopic ultrasound can provide diagnostic histology. In some TCB specimens, all three of the supportive criteria (periductal inflammation, storiform fibrosis, phlebitis)

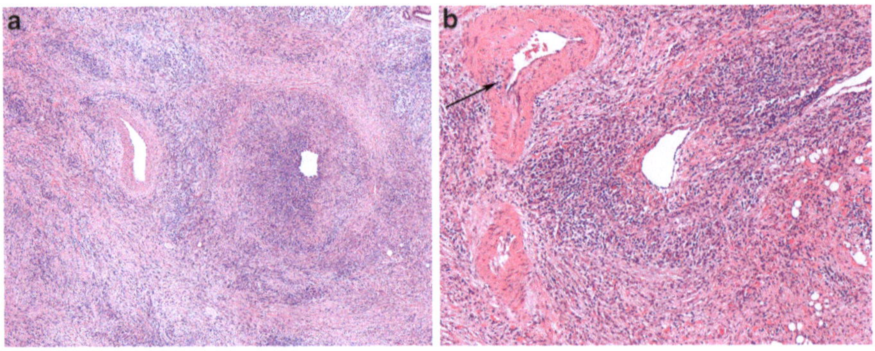


**Fig. 4.6** Obliterative phlebitis. (**a**) Mononuclear inflammatory cells infiltrate the vein wall, leaving the adjacent muscular artery untouched. (**b**) Another vein encased in a fibroinflammatory process. Note the focal arteritis (*arrow*)

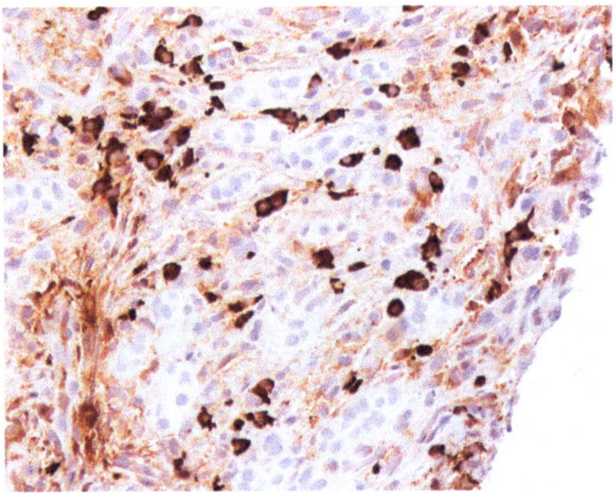

**Fig. 4.7** Increased numbers of IgG4-positive plasma cells in type 1 AIP

can be found. Given the importance of phlebitis to the diagnosis, some authors have recommended the use of special stains to highlight blood vessel walls [14]. In practice, the presence of two criteria plus increased numbers of IgG4-positive plasma cells (more than 10 per high power field) is sufficient to provide strong support for a diagnosis of type 1 AIP (Fig. 4.8). Fine needle aspiration (FNA) is more problematic: while some authors have been able to use the tissue fragments garnered during such a procedure to identify storiform fibrosis and increased IgG4 [15], others warn than fine needle aspiration is often interpreted as "atypical," increasing the likelihood of unnecessary surgery [16].

## Histopathology of Type 2 AIP

The pancreas of patients with type 2 AIP is often only focally involved. The region that seems to be most often affected is the pancreatic head including the pancreatic portion of the distal bile duct. As in type 1 AIP, the outstanding histologic feature is a periductal lymphoplasmacytic infiltrate usually affecting some or all of the medium-sized ducts (Fig. 4.9). As in type 1, the inflammation is often accompanied by periductal fibrosis, which may narrow the affected duct. In contrast to type 1, the epithelium in type 2 is inflamed and damaged. This is the so-called granulocytic epithelial lesion (GEL), a change that is specific to type 2 AIP [17]. This lesion is characterized by focal disruption and destruction of the duct epithelium due to the invasion of neutrophilic granulocytes (Fig. 4.9). The number of GELs and their severity differs from patient to patient. The lymphoplasmacytic infiltrate may extend from the periductal area to the acinar tissue, but here too neutrophils are an almost invariable component (Fig. 4.10). Perilobular fibrosis, occasionally of the storiform type, can be seen, as can phlebitis, but they are usually less pronounced than that in type 1 AIP (Fig. 4.11). Another sometimes helpful criterion for the diagnosis of type 2 AIP is that IgG4-positive plasma cells are absent or present only in small numbers (<10 cells/HPF) [7, 18].

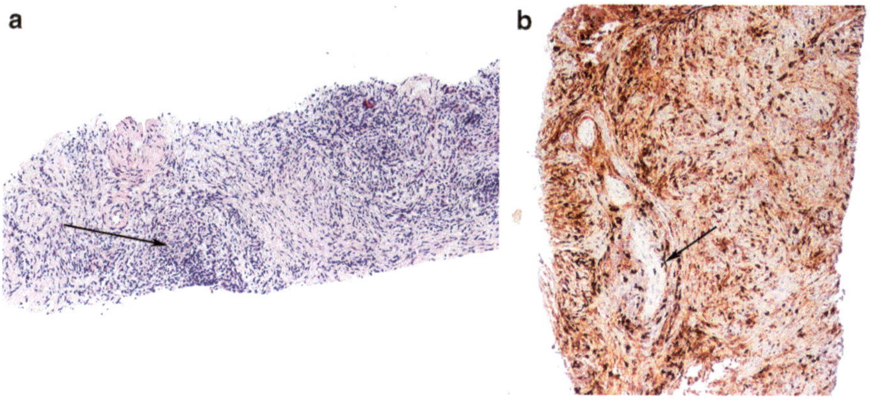


**Fig. 4.8** (**a**) Lymphoplasmacytic inflammation, storiform fibrosis, and phlebitis (*arrow*) in a needle biopsy of AIP type1. (**b**) IgG4-positive plasma cells in a needle biopsy. Some of the positive cells are perineural (*arrow*)

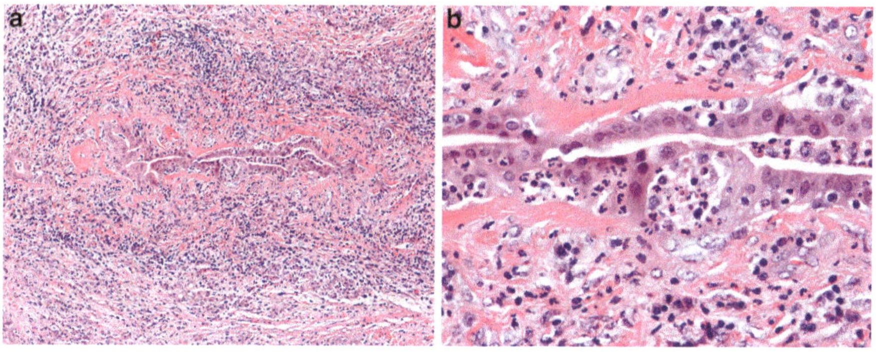


**Fig. 4.9** Duct changes in type 2 AIP. (**a**) The periductal inflammation and fibrosis are similar to type 1 AIP. (**b**) Neutrophils infiltrate and damage duct epithelium, the granulocytic epithelial lesion (GEL) of type 2 AIP

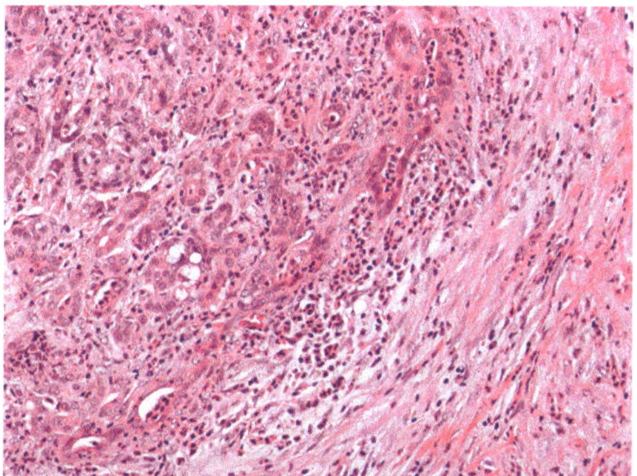

**Fig. 4.10** Neutrophils at the periphery of, and partly infiltrating, a pancreatic lobule in type 2 AIP

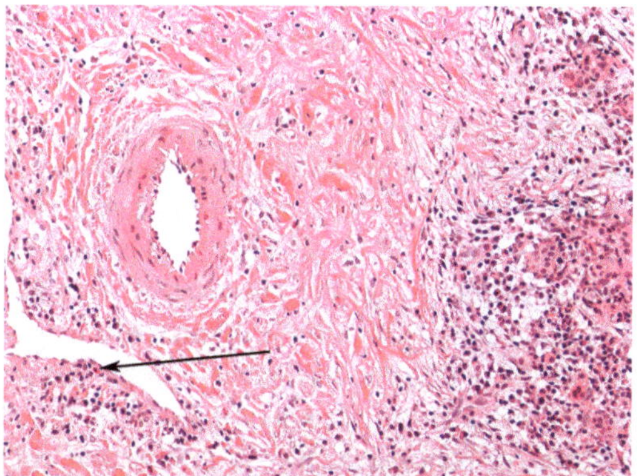

**Fig. 4.11** Sparse phlebitis in type 2 AIP (*arrow*). Note the lobular neutrophils on the *right*

## Large-Caliber TCB in Type 2 AIP

It can be difficult to establish a diagnosis of type 2 AIP on clinical grounds alone, since this condition lacks both the elevated serum IgG4 and the presence of other organ involvement that contribute to a diagnosis of type 1 AIP. Thus, TCB can be a critical part of the workup. A biopsy with periductal lymphoplasmacytic inflammation, sparse to no tissue IgG4, and perhaps a bit of storiform fibrosis can be considered suggestive of type 2 AIP in the right clinical setting. A GEL in a pancreatic biopsy from a patient suspected of having AIP is diagnostic for type 2 AIP [18]. Neutrophils in pancreatic acini are also characteristic of type 2 AIP and can increase one's confidence in the diagnosis.

## Differential Diagnosis of Type 2 AIP Versus Type 1 AIP

Macroscopically, type 1 AIP and 2 are indistinguishable. In many cases, they present as a tumorous mass in the head of the pancreas mimicking ductal adenocarcinoma [17, 19]. The inflammatory infiltration of the pancreas head and the wall of the extrahepatic bile duct leads to narrowing of the distal bile duct and the main pancreatic duct. Both types of AIP share the absence of pseudocysts and, in most cases, calculi [2, 17].

The histopathology of the two types of AIP differs in the following features: type 2 AIP is characterized by the presence of GELs, which are absent in type 1 AIP [2, 17]. Neutrophils are also commonly seen in the pancreatic lobule in type 2, but are not a feature of type 1. Type 2 AIP typically has few or no IgG4- positive plasma cells, which contrasts with the presence of abundant (>10 cells/hpf) IgG4-positive plasma cells in type 1 AIP. Other features that are not specific but are usually more pronounced in type 1 AIP are (1) an intense lymphoplasmacytic infiltration not only around ducts but also in the acinar tissue; (2) a swirling (storiform) fibrosis centered around ducts and extending into the lobules; and (3) a vasculitis with lymphoplasmacytic infiltration surrounding and obliterating the veins (phlebitis) and, to a lesser extent, also the arteries (arteritis). Immunohistochemistry for CD3-, CD4-, and CD8-positive lymphocytes, CD79a-positive plasma cells, and CD68-positive macrophages often reveals a higher number of the abovementioned cells in AIP type1 than 2 [7, 20].

## Extrapancreatic Disease in Type 2 AIP

Patients with type 2 AIP usually do not show the immune-mediated diseases that are observed in a subset of type 1 AIP, summarized under the term IgG4-related sclerosing disease [21, 22]. Instead, they sometimes suffer from chronic inflammatory bowel disease [17] (Kamisawa et al. 2011). Moreover, these patients mostly fail to exhibit elevated IgG4 serum levels and increased IgG4-positive plasma cells.

## Epidemiology of Type 2 AIP

The two groups of AIP patients differ in their clinical features such as gender and mean age. Type 2 AIP is associated with an equal gender distribution and a mean age (45–48 years) that is considerably lower than that of type 1 AIP patients, which peaks between 60 and 65 years [2, 17, 22].

It is interesting to note that the relative frequency of the two AIP types in Europe and the USA seems to differ from that in East Asia. While in Europe each subtype can be expected in about 40–60 % of the cases (in biopsy series they amount to 38 % and 45 %, respectively), the type 2 AIP seems to be rare in East Asia [23].

## Clinical Features and Laboratory Data of Type 2 Versus Type 1 AIP

Clinically, both types of AIP patients are indistinguishable. Many patients complain of abdominal pain, although the frequency and intensity of pain attacks tend to be lower than in type 1

AIP patients than in type 2 AIP patients [22]. Other frequent symptoms are jaundice and loss of weight. Corticosteroid treatment resolves strictures of the extrahepatic bile ducts and main pancreatic duct, as well as the pancreatic mass and focal lesions in the lungs, kidneys, and retroperitoneal inflammatory pseudotumors. This can be the case after only 1–2 weeks of steroid therapy [22, 24, 25].

Long-term follow-up in patients with AIP after pancreatic resection revealed that recurrence of the disease may be observed in type 1 AIP, while this seems to be not the case or only very rare in type 2 AIP [17, 26, 27].

Among the autoantibodies that may be detected are antibodies against antigens from the pancreatic ducts and acini such as lactoferrin, carbonic anhydrase type II, and SPINK1 and trypsinogen [28, 29]. Other autoantibodies associated with AIP are antinuclear antibody, rheumatoid factor, and anti-smooth muscle antibody.

## Pathogenesis

The pathogenesis of AIP is still not known, but several findings, common to both types of AIP, are suggestive of an immune-related etiopathogenesis. These include the general histopathological features of both AIP types, their frequent association with immune-related disorders such as the IgG4-systemic diseases on the one hand and the idiopathic inflammatory bowel diseases on the other, and the response to steroid treatment. Whether the demonstrated circulating autoantibodies against carboanhydrase II, lactoferrin, and nuclear and smooth muscle antigens as well as SPINK1 are found in the same frequency in type 1 AIP as in type 2 AIP is so far not known.

A clear difference between type 1 AIP and 2 concerns the presence or absence of abundant IgG4-positive plasma cells in the pancreatic tissue, a finding that seems to correlate with either elevated or normal IgG4 serum levels in the respective patients. Recently it was found that renal tissue from AIP patients with tubulointerstitial nephritis contained granular deposits at the tubular basement membranes, that were positive for IgG4 and complement C3, and occasionally IgG1, IgG2, and IgG3 [30]. In a similar study on pancreatic tissue and bile duct tissue of six GEL-negative AIP patients, using double immunofluorescence microscopy, deposits of IgG, IgG4, and C3c (but not C1q, IgA, and IgM) were identified that colocalized with basement membrane-associated collagen IV of ducts and acini [31]. On the basis of these findings, it may be hypothesized that IgG4 could play a role in the deposition of immune complexes at pancreatic structures that seem to be the target of the fibroinflammatory process characterizing AIP. In order to clarify whether this hypothesis is only valid in IgG4-positive patients with type 1 AIP, a patient was included in the study whose clinical features were indistinguishable from those of the other six patients of the series but who showed a type 2 AIP with very low numbers of IgG4-positive plasma cells in the pancreatic tissue. This patient failed to show any IgG4-positive deposits at the basement membranes of the ducts and acini but remained positive for C3c and IgG. If this thus far unique finding is confirmed in future studies, it would imply that in type 2 AIP the pathomechanisms leading to the changes in the ducts and acini and the fibrosis are independent of the effects of IgG4. This then raises the question as to whether the increased number of IgG4 plasma cells, the high IgG4 serum levels, and the tissue depositions of IgG4 play a primary and active role in the pathogenesis of AIP or are rather secondary phenomena.

## Autoimmune Pancreatitis as a Pre- or Paraneoplastic Condition

There are rare reports of pancreatic ductal adenocarcinoma discovered in association with AIP [32, 33]. Thus far, the three documented cases have been in patients with type 1 AIP [33]. Others have proposed the intriguing idea that type 1 AIP might be a paraneoplastic inflammatory condition, reacting to clonal proliferations that are often eradicated, but sometimes develop into malignancies. This is currently no published data to support this idea.

## References


1. Kloppel G. Chronic pancreatitis, pseudotumors and other tumor-like lesions. Mod Pathol. 2007;20 Suppl 1:S113–31.
2. Chari ST, Kloeppel G, Zhang L, et al. Histopathologic and clinical subtypes of autoimmune pancreatitis: the Honolulu consensus document. Pancreas. 2010;39: 549–54.
3. Deshpande V, Zen Y, Chan JK, et al. Consensus statement on the pathology of IgG4-related disease. Mod Pathol. 2012;25(9):1181–92.
4. Chandan VS, Iacobuzio-Donahue C, Abraham SC. Patchy distribution of pathologic abnormalities in autoimmune pancreatitis: implications for preoperative diagnosis. Am J Surg Pathol. 2008;32:1762–9.
5. Abraham SC, Leach S, Yeo CJ, et al. Eosinophilic pancreatitis and increased eosinophils in the pancreas. Am J Surg Pathol. 2003;27:334–42.
6. Kamisawa T, Funata N, Hayashi Y, et al. A new clinicopathological entity of IgG4-related autoimmune disease. J Gastroenterol. 2003;38:982–4.
7. Zhang L, Notohara K, Levy MJ, et al. IgG4-positive plasma cell infiltration in the diagnosis of autoimmune pancreatitis. Mod Pathol. 2007;20:23–8.
8. Dhall D, Suriawinata AA, Tang LH, et al. Use of immunohistochemistry for IgG4 in the distinction of autoimmune pancreatitis from peritumoral pancreatitis. Hum Pathol. 2010;41:643–52.
9. Zen Y, Nakanuma Y. IgG4-related disease: a cross-sectional study of 114 cases. Am J Surg Pathol. 2010;34:1812–9.
10. Shrestha B, Sekiguchi H, Colby TV, et al. Distinctive pulmonary histopathology with increased IgG4-positive plasma cells in patients with autoimmune pancreatitis: report of 6 and 12 cases with similar histopathology. Am J Surg Pathol. 2009;33:1450–62.
11. Zen Y, Inoue D, Kitao A, et al. IgG4-related lung and pleural disease: a clinicopathologic study of 21 cases. Am J Surg Pathol. 2009;33:1886–93.
12. Cheuk W, Chan JK. IgG4-related sclerosing disease: a critical appraisal of an evolving clinicopathologic entity. Adv Anat Pathol. 2010;17:303–32.
13. van Heerde MJ, Biermann K, Zondervan PE, et al. Prevalence of autoimmune pancreatitis and other benign disorders in pancreatoduodenectomy for presumed malignancy of the pancreatic head. Dig Dis Sci. 2012;57(9):2458–65.
14. Chu KE, Papouchado BG, Lane Z, et al. The role of Movat pentachrome stain and immunoglobulin G4 immunostaining in the diagnosis of autoimmune pancreatitis. Mod Pathol. 2009;22:351–8.
15. Deshpande V, Mino-Kenudson M, Brugge WR, et al. Endoscopic ultrasound guided fine needle aspiration biopsy of autoimmune pancreatitis: diagnostic criteria and pitfalls. Am J Surg Pathol. 2005;29:1464–71.
16. Holmes BJ, Hruban RH, Wolfgang CL, et al. Fine needle aspirate of autoimmune pancreatitis (lymphoplasmacytic sclerosing pancreatitis): cytomorphologic characteristics and clinical correlates. Acta Cytol. 2012;56: 228–32.
17. Zamboni GLJ, Capelli P. Histopathological features of diagnostic and clinical relevance in autoimmune pancreatitis: a study of 53 resection specimens and 9 biopsy specimens. Virchows Arch. 2004;445: 552–63.
18. Detlefsen S, Mohr Drewes A, Vyberg M, et al. Diagnosis of autoimmune pancreatitis by core needle biopsy: application of six microscopic criteria. Virchows Arch. 2009;454:531–9.
19. Notohara K, Burgart LJ, Yadav D, et al. Idiopathic chronic pancreatitis with periductal lymphoplasmacytic infiltration: clinicopathologic features of 35 cases. Am J Surg Pathol. 2003;27:1119–27.
20. Kojima M, Sipos B, Klapper W, et al. Autoimmune pancreatitis: frequency, IgG4 expression, and clonality of T and B cells. Am J Surg Pathol. 2007;31:521–8.
21. Kamisawa T, Okamoto A. Autoimmune pancreatitis: proposal of IgG4-related sclerosing disease. J Gastroenterol. 2006;41:613–25.
22. Kamisawa T, Chari ST, Giday SA, et al. Clinical profile of autoimmune pancreatitis and its histological subtypes: an international multicenter survey. Pancreas. 2011;40:809–14.
23. Kloppel G, Detlefsen S, Chari ST, et al. Autoimmune pancreatitis: the clinicopathological characteristics of the subtype with granulocytic epithelial lesions. J Gastroenterol. 2010;45:787–93.
24. Ito T, Nishimori I, Inoue N, et al. Treatment for autoimmune pancreatitis: consensus on the treatment for patients with autoimmune pancreatitis in Japan. J Gastroenterol. 2007;42 Suppl 18:50–8.
25. Saito T, Tanaka S, Yoshida H, et al. A case of autoimmune pancreatitis responding to steroid therapy. Evidence of histologic recovery. Pancreatology. 2002;2:550–6.
26. Chari ST, Murray JA. Autoimmune pancreatitis, Part II: the relapse. Gastroenterology. 2008;134:625–8.
27. Detlefsen S, Zamboni G, Frulloni L, et al. Clinical features and relapse rates after surgery in type 1 autoimmune pancreatitis differ from type 2: a study of 114 surgically treated European patients. Pancreatology. 2012;12:276–83.
28. Taniguchi T, Okazaki K, Okamoto M, et al. High prevalence of autoantibodies against carbonic anhydrase II and lactoferrin in type 1 diabetes: concept of autoimmune exocrinopathy and endocrinopathy of the pancreas. Pancreas. 2003;27:26–30.
29. Lohr JM, Faissner R, Koczan D, et al. Autoantibodies against the exocrine pancreas in autoimmune pancreatitis: gene and protein expression profiling and immunoassays identify pancreatic enzymes as a major target of the inflammatory process. Am J Gastroenterol. 2010;105:2060–71.

30. Deshpande V, Chicano S, Finkelberg D, et al. Autoimmune pancreatitis: a systemic immune complex mediated disease. Am J Surg Pathol. 2006;30:1537–45.
31. Detlefsen S, Brasen JH, Zamboni G, et al. Deposition of complement C3c, immunoglobulin (Ig)G4 and IgG at the basement membrane of pancreatic ducts and acini in autoimmune pancreatitis. Histopathology. 2010;57:825–35.
32. Inoue H, Miyatani H, Sawada Y, et al. A case of pancreas cancer with autoimmune pancreatitis. Pancreas. 2006;33:208–9.
33. Witkiewicz AK, Kennedy EP, Kennyon L, et al. Synchronous autoimmune pancreatitis and infiltrating pancreatic ductal adenocarcinoma: case report and review of the literature. Hum Pathol. 2008;39: 1548–51.

# CT and MRI Features

# 5

Naoki Takahashi and Dushyant V. Sahani

## Introduction

Patients with autoimmune pancreatitis (AIP) commonly present with vague abdominal pain, jaundice, or weight loss, and contrast-enhanced computed tomography (CT) is often the first imaging study obtained. Radiological evaluation is crucial in making the correct diagnosis. Differentiating AIP from pancreatic cancer is the main goal to avoid unnecessary surgery or invasive intervention. One should be aware of various pancreatic and extrapancreatic manifestations of AIP in order to facilitate diagnosis.

## Pancreatic Morphological Changes

Diffuse parenchymal enlargement of the pancreas is a characteristic feature of AIP seen in 24–73 % of patients (Figs. 5.1a, b, and 5.2) [1–5]. The pancreatic border becomes featureless with effacement of the lobular contour of the pancreas [2]. The pancreatic tail may become foreshortened [6]. On CT, the pancreas shows delayed enhancement during the late phase of contrast enhancement [1, 7]. On magnetic resonance imaging (MRI), the pancreas is diffusely hypointense on T1-weighted images, slightly hyperintense on T2-weighted images, and shows heterogeneous and diminished enhancement during the early phase with delayed increased enhancement during the late phase of contrast enhancement [1, 2, 8].

Focal, mass-like enlargement of the pancreas is seen in 18–40 % of patients with AIP (Fig. 5.3) [2, 4, 5, 9]. Any portion of the pancreas can be involved, although involvement of the pancreatic head is more common [5, 10]. On CT, the enlarged segment of the pancreas typically demonstrates iso-attenuation compared to the non-enlarged segment of pancreatic parenchyma [2]. In a small number of cases, the focally enlarged segment is low attenuation compared to the uninvolved pancreatic parenchyma and may be indistinguishable from pancreatic cancer [2, 4, 9, 11]. The demarcation between the normal parenchyma tends to be sharp in such cases [11]. Atrophy of the pancreas upstream to the focally involved area is uncommon in patients with AIP in contrast to patients with pancreatic carcinoma. The pancreas may also appear as an area of segmental low density without mass-like enlargement. Multifocal pancreatic involvement is rare, but occasionally multiple low-attenuation lesions may be seen [12]. When the pancreas is focally enlarged, the normal appearing segment should be carefully examined, as the apparent normal

N. Takahashi, M.D.
Department of Radiology, Mayo Clinic,
200 First Street SW, Rochester, MN 55905, USA
e-mail: takahashi.naoki@mayo.edu

D.V. Sahani, M.D. (✉)
Department of Radiology, Massachusetts General Hospital (ADK, DS), 55 Fruit Street, Boston, MA 02114, USA
e-mail: dsahani@partners.org

M.J. Levy and S.T. Chari (eds.), *Autoimmune (IgG4-related) Pancreatitis and Cholangitis*,
DOI 10.1007/978-1-4419-6430-4_5, © Springer Science+Business Media New York 2013

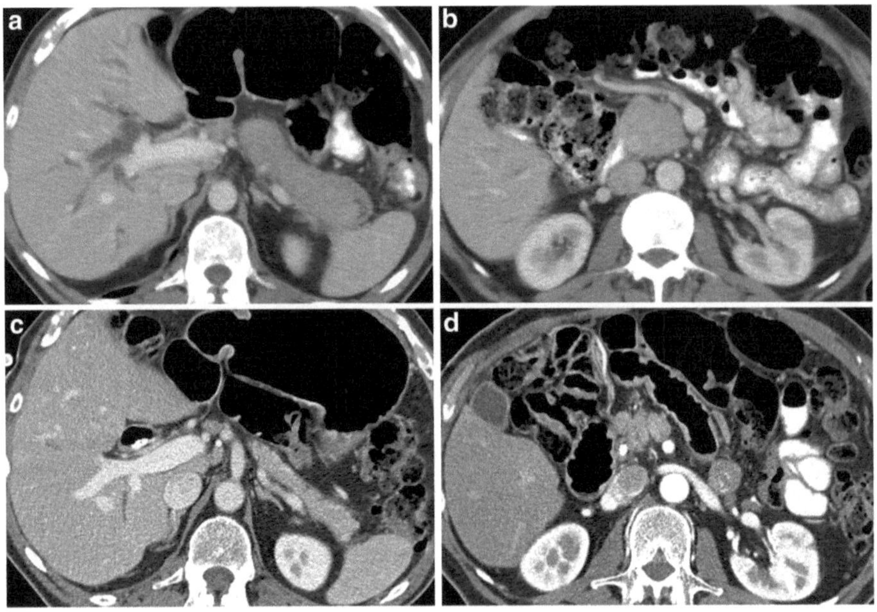


**Fig. 5.1** (**a**–**d**) A 68-year-old male with autoimmune pancreatitis. (**a**, **b**) Contrast-enhanced CT shows diffuse enlargement of the pancreas. Capsule-like rim is present around the tail of the pancreas. Enhancement of intrapancreatic portion of the bile duct is suggestive of biliary involvement. Note the intrahepatic biliary dilation. (**c**, **d**) Contrast-enhanced CT obtained after steroid treatment shows diffuse atrophy of the pancreas

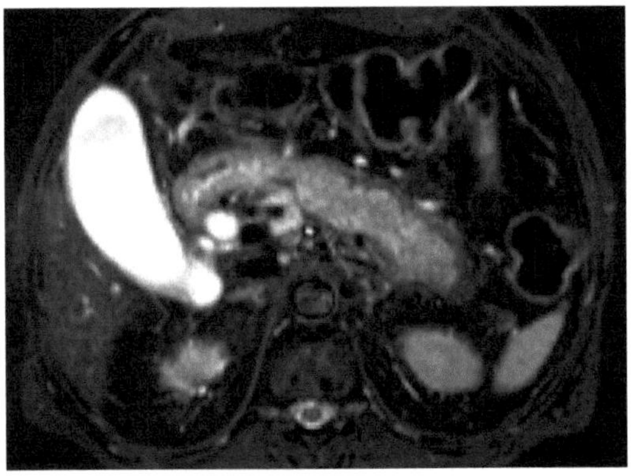

**Fig. 5.2** A 66-year-old male with autoimmune pancreatitis. T2-weighted MR image shows diffuse enlargement of the pancreas and capsule-like rim around the pancreas. Capsule-like rims are hypointense to the pancreatic parenchyma

area may cause biliary dilatation or may have abnormally decreased enhancement which are clues to the diagnosis.

The pancreas may appear normal in size or atrophic in 9–36 % of patients [3–5]. A normal-sized pancreas may result from a milder form of disease, but in such cases the enhancement pattern is usually altered [5]. Pancreatic atrophy is believed to represent a late burnt-out phase of the disease [2]. This appearance can also be seen after steroid therapy.

A capsule-like rim can been seen around the enlarged pancreas in 14–48 % of patients with AIP (Figs. 5.1a, and 5.2) [1, 2, 4, 5]. The capsule-like rim is low attenuation on contrast-enhanced CT and hypointense on both T1- and T2-weighted images and shows delayed enhancement on contrast-enhanced MR. The rim may diffusely surround the entire pancreas or only focal regions [5]. The rim is thought to represent peripancreatic extension of the characteristic inflammatory cell infiltration [1]. Mild peripancreatic stranding may also be present which is usually confined to the peripancreatic region with infrequent involvement of the mesentery and anterior pararenal fascia [2].

## Enhancement Characteristics

The enhancement pattern is a useful adjunct to the morphological changes of the pancreas, which is assessed by contrast-enhanced CT or

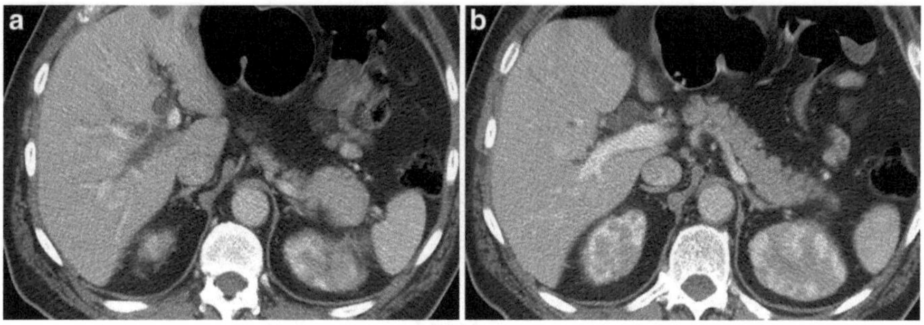


**Fig. 5.3** (**a**, **b**) A 68-year-old male with autoimmune pancreatitis. (**a**, **b**) Contrast-enhanced CT shows focal enlargement of the pancreatic tail. Remaining pancreas is normal. Multiple small low-density lesions are due to renal involvement of AIP

contrast-enhanced MRI using multiphasic technique. Irie et al. first described delayed enhancement in patients with diffuse changes of AIP; CT attenuation of the pancreas was higher at 6 min delayed scan compared to the 60 s delayed scan [1]. Qualitatively, CT attenuation of the pancreas in AIP is similar or higher than that of the liver and lower than that of spleen during the pancreatic phase and is similar or higher than that of the liver and higher than that of spleen in hepatic phase of biphasic CT [10, 13]. Quantitatively, mean CT attenuation value of the pancreatic parenchyma in AIP was significantly lower than that in normal controls during the pancreatic phase (AIP: 85 HU, normal pancreas: 104 HU; $p<0.05$), but not significantly different in the hepatic phase (AIP: 96 HU, normal pancreas: 89 HU; $p=0.6$) [7]. Similar enhancement pattern was observed on MR [8].

This enhancement pattern was also seen in patients with focal AIP: decreased enhancement during the pancreatic phase with delayed enhancement during the hepatic phase (Figs. 5.4a, b). On the other hand, pancreatic carcinoma shows decreased enhancement in the pancreatic phase with a minimal change in the enhancement in the hepatic phase (Figs. 5.5a, b). Wakabayashi et al. evaluated the CT enhancement pattern in 9 patients with focal AIP [9]. Of the 9 patients, 6 lesions were hypo-attenuating in the early phase but all were homogeneously iso-attenuating in the delayed phase. On the other hand, only 2 of 80 patients with pancreatic carcinoma had homogeneous enhancement in the delayed phase. Quantitatively, the mean CT attenuation value of focal AIP was not significantly different in the pancreatic phase (AIP: 71 HU, carcinoma: 59 HU; $p=0.06$), but significantly higher than that in carcinoma in the hepatic phase (AIP: 90 HU, carcinoma: 64 HU; $p<0.001$) [7]. Delayed enhancement of the mass or focally enlarged segment, defined as a 15-HU or greater increase from the pancreatic phase to the hepatic phase, was found in 7 of the 13 patients with focal AIP (54 %) and in 5 of 33 patients (15 %) with carcinoma ($p=0.02$).

## Diffusion-Weighted MR

Diffusion-weighted MR is a technique to evaluate the rate of microscopic water diffusion within tissues by using special magnetic gradients. Quantitative measurements of the diffusivity of water are described by the apparent diffusion coefficient. Kamisawa et al. showed that apparent diffusion coefficient values were significantly lower in AIP ($1.01 \pm 0.11 \times 10(-3)$ mm(2)/s) than in pancreatic cancer ($1.25 \pm 0.11 \times 10(-3)$ mm(2)/s) and normal pancreas ($1.49 \pm 0.16 \times 10(-3)$ mm(2)/s) ($P<0.001$) (Fig. 5.4c) [14]. Taniguchi et al. showed that apparent diffusion coefficient values were significantly lower in AIP ($0.97 \pm 0.18 \times 10(-3)$ mm(2)/s) compared to other types of chronic pancreatitis ($1.45 \pm 0.10 \times 10(-3)$ mm(2)/s) [15]. In addition, diffusion-weighted MR was helpful in reclassifying what appeared to be focal mass-forming AIP to diffuse AIP by

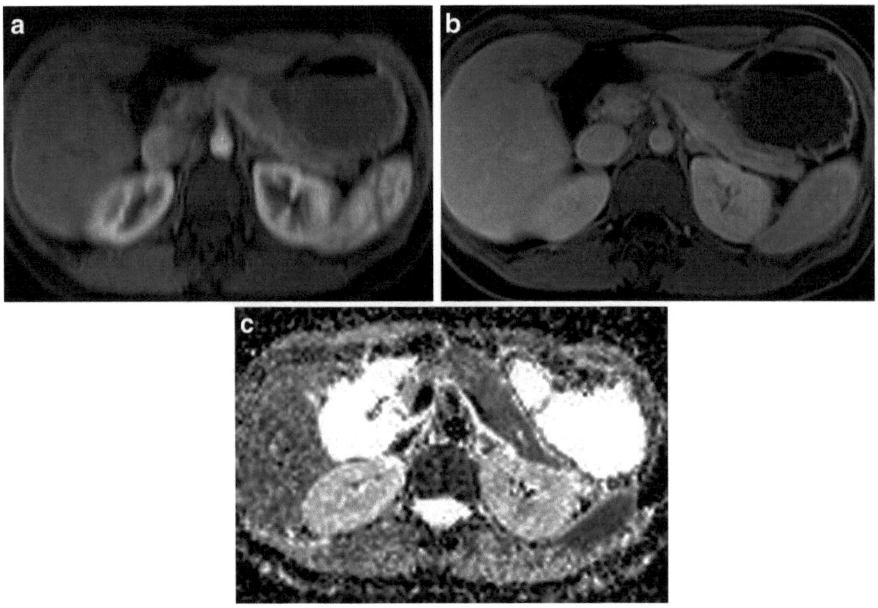

**Fig. 5.4** (**a**–**c**) A 30-year-old female with autoimmune pancreatitis, type II. (**a**, **b**) Contrast-enhanced MR images show segmental abnormality in the tail of the pancreas. The abnormal segment shows decreased enhancement during the early phase of contrast enhancement with delayed enhancement. (**c**) Diffusion-weighted images (ADC map) show restricted diffusion in abnormal segment

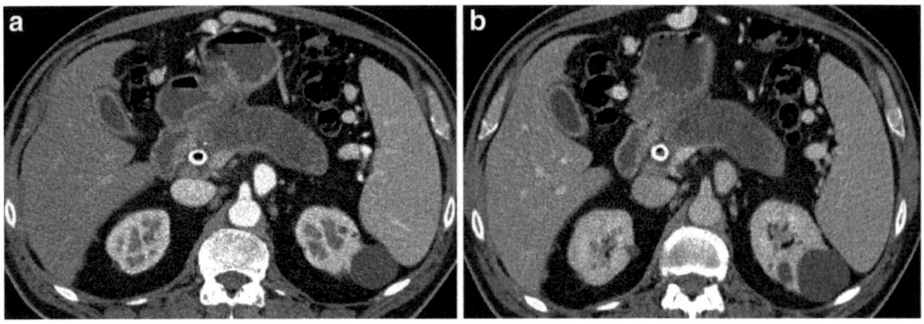

**Fig. 5.5** (**a**, **b**) An 83-year-old female with diffuse infiltrative pancreatic carcinoma. (**a**, **b**) Pancreas is diffusely enlarged and shows decreased enhancement. Unlike AIP, the abnormal pancreas does not show increased delayed enhancement. Note the rim of high density at the periphery of the pancreas

showing diffusely decreased apparent diffusion coefficient values in the non-enlarged pancreatic segment.

## Pancreatic Duct Changes

Diffuse or segmental narrowing of the main pancreatic duct is the characteristic ERCP finding [2, 16]. The pancreatic duct narrowing is often poorly seen on CT as the normal pancreatic duct is very small. MRCP is a preferred noninvasive method to assess the pancreatic ductal changes. Segmental narrowing of the main pancreatic duct may be seen as a poorly visualized segment on CT or MRCP compared to a normal-caliber pancreatic duct in uninvolved segments of pancreas [17, 18]. Mild pancreatic ductal dilation is commonly present upstream to the narrowed segment, and thus mild caliber changes of the main pancreatic duct are often detectable on CT or MR. The degree of main pancreatic duct dilation is usually milder than that seen in cases of pancreatic carcinoma. A relatively specific main pancreatic ductal change of AIP is multifocal narrowing, and this may be depicted on CT or MRCP [18, 19]. The duct-penetrating sign [20] may also be useful in differentiating AIP from pancreatic cancer. Secretin-stimulated MRCP may be helpful in the assessment of pancreatic duct-penetrating sign [19]. Enhancement of the pancreatic duct wall may be present in patients with AIP on portal phase or delayed phase CT [5].

## Other Pancreatic and Peripancreatic Findings

Pancreatic pseudocyst and/or calcification is typically associated with alcohol-induced chronic pancreatitis [9]. However, calcifications are seen in 14–32 % and cysts are seen in 10–12 % of patients with AIP [4, 5], especially in the late or post-acute phase; therefore, presence of calcifications or cysts should not exclude the possibility of AIP [21, 22]. Pancreatic pseudocysts associated with AIP typically shrink after steroid therapy [22]. Vessels are commonly involved by the extension of peripancreatic soft tissue in patients with AIP (44–68 %). Vascular involvement may be either arterial such as superior mesenteric artery (10 %) or venous such as splenic vein or portal vein (58 %) [4, 5] . Involved veins are often narrowed but occlusion may occur [5].

## Other Organ (Extrapancreatic) Involvement in the Abdomen

The most common site of extrapancreatic involvement is the biliary tree presenting with asymptomatic liver test abnormalities or jaundice [4]. On imaging, biliary involvement commonly appears as multifocal biliary strictures similar to primary sclerosing cholangitis. Rarely, it may form a mass which mimics cholangiocarcinoma. The kidneys are also commonly involved [23]. Radiographically, renal lesions are commonly bilateral and multiple, predominantly involving the renal cortex (Fig. 5.3b). Renal parenchymal lesions can be classified as small peripheral cortical nodules, round or wedge-shaped lesions, and diffuse patchy involvement. Renal lesions may present as a large solitary mass which mimic primary renal neoplasm. Retroperitoneal fibrosis is seen in 10 % of cases. Biliary or renal involvement and retroperitoneal fibrosis are exclusively seen in type 1 AIP. On the other hand, type 2 AIP is commonly associated with inflammatory bowel disease such as Crohn's disease or ulcerative colitis [24].

## Other Imaging Modalities

On PET, the pancreas shows increased 18F-fluorodeoxyglucose (FDG) uptake in almost all cases [25–29]. Although FDG uptake is commonly seen in pancreatic cancer (73–82 %), the pattern of uptake is usually different [26, 29]. FDG uptake in AIP is usually diffuse, segmental, or multifocal, while uptake in pancreatic carcinoma is usually focal. FDG uptake in extrapancreatic tissues such as the lacrimal gland, salivary gland, biliary tree, periaortic region, kidneys, prostate, and lymph nodes is common and specific for AIP [26, 27, 29]. On transabdominal US, the pancreas is diffusely or focally enlarged and hypoechoic. On contrast-enhanced US, the involved pancreatic segment commonly shows moderated to marked enhancement [30, 31].

## Differentiating AIP from Pancreatic Malignancy and Other Types of Pancreatitis

Differentiating AIP from pancreatic carcinoma on CT or MR can be difficult. AIP is one of the most common benign disease processes for which pancreatic resection is performed for suspected pancreatic carcinoma. AIP represents 31 % of tumefactive chronic pancreatitis patients who undergo pancreatic resection [32], and 2–6 % of patients who undergo pancreatic resection for suspected pancreatic cancer [32, 33]. Focal enlargement of the pancreas or low-attenuation mass formation is not uncommon in patients with AIP [2, 4, 9]. Moreover, pancreatic carcinoma may present as an iso-attenuating mass in approximately 10 % [34]. Findings that are useful in differentiating AIP from pancreatic carcinoma and its frequency are shown in Table 5.1 and Table 5.2 [35, 36]. Highly specific findings of AIP include diffuse pancreatic enlargement, capsule-like rim around the pancreas, other organ involvement (bile duct, kidney, retroperitoneum), and delayed enhancement of the pancreatic lesion. A low-density mass, distal pancreatic duct cutoff, or atrophy can be occasionally seen in AIP; given the much higher prevalence of pancreatic carcinoma, presence of such findings are highly suggestive of pancreatic carcinoma.

Although diffuse enlargement of the pancreas is highly suggestive of AIP, it is not without differential diagnosis. Diffuse infiltrating pancreatic malignancies such as lymphoma and pancreatic carcinoma should also be considered. While the pancreas of AIP typically shows delayed enhancement, lymphoma often shows washout of contrast on delayed scan [37]. A high-attenuation rim, which represents compressed normal parenchyma by carcinoma, is a helpful sign of diffuse infiltrating pancreatic carcinoma [38] (Figs. 5.5a, b). When the pancreas is focally enlarged but without findings suggestive of carcinoma (low-density mass, distal pancreatic duct cutoff, or atrophy), the finding is indeterminate and further investigation is necessary to make correct diagnosis (Fig. 5.3a) [35].

The morphology of the normal pancreas can vary even in subjects without pancreatic disease, thus assessing morphological changes in AIP such as diffuse enlargement is not always easy. In such cases, ancillary findings such as enhancement pattern (peak enhancement during pancreatic phase), lobulated contour, fatty marble, and absence of pancreatic duct irregularity are helpful to differentiate normal pancreas from AIP. Acute pancreatitis may present with diffuse enlargement of the gland with or without decreased enhancement. However, the clinical presentation is usually different. When pancreatic atrophy, calcifications, and/or pseudocyst formation is present, other forms of chronic pancreatitis must be considered in the differential diagnosis. These findings could be seen in the burnt-out phase of autoimmune pancreatitis.

**Table 5.1** Frequency of CT findings in AIP and pancreatic carcinoma

| CT findings | | |
|---|---|---|
| Diffuse pancreatic enlargement without (a), (b), or (c) | 52 % | 0 % |
| Capsule-like rim around the pancreas | 38 % | 0 % |
| Other organ involvement | 58 % | 2 % |
| Focal enlargement without (a), (b), or (c) or normal-sized pancreas | 31 % | 5 % |
| Low-density mass (a) | 15 % | 89 % |
| Pancreatic duct cutoff (b) | 8 % | 67 % |
| Distal pancreatic atrophy (c) | 17 % | 53 % |
| Liver lesions suggestive of metastases | 17 % | 18 % |

Modified from Chari et al.

**Table 5.2** Frequency of CT findings in focal AIP and pancreatic carcinoma

| CT findings | | |
|---|---|---|
| Delayed enhancement | 100 % | 6 % |
| Capsule-like rim around the pancreas | 35 % | 1 % |
| Wall thickening of the bile duct | 47 % | 6 % |
| Wall thickening of the gallbladder | 29 % | 4 % |
| Retroperitoneal fibrosis | 12 % | 0 % |
| Atrophy of the pancreatic body or tail | 0 % | 61 % |

Modified from Kamisawa et al.

## Differences in Type 1 and Type 2 AIP

Little has been reported regarding the differences between type 1 and type 2 AIP on cross-sectional imaging (Fig. 5.4a–c). In a recent study, Deshpande et al. reviewed resected cases of type 1 ($n = 11$) and type 2 ($n = 18$) AIP [39]. Pancreatic tail cutoff sign was exclusively seen in type 2 disease (4/10). Other imaging features such as diffuse swelling of the pancreas, pancreatic stranding, capsule-like rim, and common bile duct strictures were seen in both types of AIP and were not helpful in distinguishing from one another. An international multicenter survey showed that diffuse swelling of the pancreas was more common in type 1 compared to type 2 AIP (40 % vs. 25 %) [24]. The pattern of extra-pancreatic organ involvement is distinct between the two types and helpful when present [24]. Biliary or renal involvement and retroperitoneal fibrosis are seen in type 1 AIP, whereas inflammatory bowel disease is commonly associated with type 2 AIP.

## Posttreatment Changes and Relapse

Steroid therapy often results in disease remission with resolution of clinical symptoms. Enlarged pancreatic parenchyma commonly normalizes or becomes atrophic (Figs. 5.1c, d) [8, 10]. Improvement of pancreatic duct stricture may be evident on CT or MR. Abnormal signal changes on T1, T2, or diffusion-weighted MR images improve completely or partially. Delayed enhancement changes on contrast-enhanced CT or MR usually normalize after steroid treatment. A pancreas with diffuse enlargement or capsule-like rim may respond to steroid more favorably [6].

## Key Points

- Diffuse parenchymal enlargement of the pancreas is a characteristic feature of AIP seen in 24–73 % of patients. However, it may present as focal or segmental enlargement of pancreas or low-density mass.
- Capsule-like rim is a specific finding of AIP and seen in 14–48 % of patients with AIP.
- The pancreatic parenchyma commonly shows decreased enhancement during the early phase contrast administration and shows increased enhancement during the delayed phase.
- Presence of other organ (extrapancreatic) involvement is helpful in making the correct diagnosis of AIP.
- FDG-PET and MRI with diffusion-weighted imaging may be helpful when CT findings are inconclusive.

## References


1. Irie H, Honda H, Baba S, et al. Autoimmune pancreatitis: CT and MR characteristics. AJR Am J Roentgenol. 1998;170(5):1323–7.
2. Sahani DV, Kalva SP, Farrell J, et al. Autoimmune pancreatitis: imaging features. Radiology. 2004; 233(2):345–52.
3. Church NI, Pereira SP, Deheragoda MG, et al. Autoimmune pancreatitis: clinical and radiological features and objective response to steroid therapy in a UK series. Am J Gastroenterol. 2007;102(11):2417–25.
4. Takahashi N, Fletcher JG, Fidler JL, Hough DM, Kawashima A, Chari ST. Dual-phase CT of autoimmune pancreatitis: a multireader study. AJR Am J Roentgenol. 2008;190(2):280–6.
5. Suzuki K, Itoh S, Nagasaka T, Ogawa H, Ota T, Naganawa S. CT findings in autoimmune pancreatitis: assessment using multiphase contrast-enhanced multisection CT. Clin Radiol. 2010;65(9):735–43.
6. Sahani DV, Sainani NI, Deshpande V, Shaikh MS, Frinkelberg DL, Fernandez-del CC. Autoimmune pancreatitis: disease evolution, staging, response assessment, and CT features that predict response to corticosteroid therapy. Radiology. 2009;250(1): 118–29.
7. Takahashi N, Fletcher JG, Hough DM, et al. Autoimmune pancreatitis: differentiation from pancreatic carcinoma and normal pancreas on the basis of enhancement characteristics at dual-phase CT. AJR Am J Roentgenol. 2009;193(2):479–84.
8. Manfredi R, Frulloni L, Mantovani W, Bonatti M, Graziani R, Pozzi MR. Autoimmune pancreatitis: pancreatic and extrapancreatic MR imaging-MR cholangiopancreatography findings at diagnosis, after steroid therapy, and at recurrence. Radiology. 2011;260(2):428–36.
9. Wakabayashi T, Kawaura Y, Satomura Y, et al. Clinical and imaging features of autoimmune pancreatitis with focal pancreatic swelling or mass formation: comparison with so-called tumor-forming pancreatitis and pancreatic carcinoma. Am J Gastroenterol. 2003;98(12):2679–87.
10. Manfredi R, Graziani R, Cicero C, et al. Autoimmune pancreatitis: CT patterns and their changes after steroid treatment. Radiology. 2008;247(2):435–43.
11. Van Hoe L, Gryspeerdt S, Ectors N, et al. Nonalcoholic duct-destructive chronic pancreatitis: imaging findings. AJR Am J Roentgenol. 1998;170(3):643–7.
12. Kajiwara M, Kojima M, Konishi M, et al. Autoimmune pancreatitis with multifocal lesions. J Hepatobiliary Pancreat Surg. 2008;15(4):449–52.
13. Yang DH, Kim KW, Kim TK, et al. Autoimmune pancreatitis: radiologic findings in 20 patients. Abdom Imaging. 2006;31(1):94–102.
14. Kamisawa T, Takuma K, Anjiki H, et al. Differentiation of autoimmune pancreatitis from pancreatic cancer by diffusion-weighted MRI. Am J Gastroenterol. 2010;105(8):1870–5.

15. Taniguchi T, Kobayashi H, Nishikawa K, et al. Diffusion-weighted magnetic resonance imaging in autoimmune pancreatitis. Jpn J Radiol. 2009;27(3):138–42.
16. Horiuchi A, Kawa S, Hamano H, Hayama M, Ota H, Kiyosawa K. ERCP features in 27 patients with autoimmune pancreatitis. Gastrointest Endosc. 2002;55(4):494–9.
17. Kamisawa T, Tu Y, Egawa N, et al. Can MRCP replace ERCP for the diagnosis of autoimmune pancreatitis? Abdom Imaging. 2009;34(3):381–4.
18. Park SH, Kim MH, Kim SY, et al. Magnetic resonance cholangiopancreatography for the diagnostic evaluation of autoimmune pancreatitis. Pancreas. 2010;39(8):1191–8.
19. Carbognin G, Girardi V, Biasiutti C, et al. Autoimmune pancreatitis: imaging findings on contrast-enhanced MR, MRCP and dynamic secretin-enhanced MRCP. Radiol Med. 2009;114(8):1214–31.
20. Ichikawa T, Sou H, Araki T, et al. Duct-penetrating sign at MRCP: usefulness for differentiating inflammatory pancreatic mass from pancreatic carcinomas. Radiology. 2001;221(1):107–16.
21. Nishimura T, Masaoka T, Suzuki H, Aiura K, Nagata H, Ishii H. Autoimmune pancreatitis with pseudocysts. J Gastroenterol. 2004;39(10):1005–10.
22. Muraki T, Hamano H, Ochi Y, et al. Corticosteroid-responsive pancreatic cyst found in autoimmune pancreatitis. J Gastroenterol. 2005;40(7):761–6.
23. Takahashi N, Kawashima A, Fletcher JG, Chari ST. Renal involvement in patients with autoimmune pancreatitis: CT and MR imaging findings. Radiology. 2007;242(3):791–801.
24. Kamisawa T, Chari ST, Giday SA, et al. Clinical profile of autoimmune pancreatitis and its histological subtypes: an international multicenter survey. Pancreas. 2011;40(6):809–14.
25. Nakamoto Y, Saga T, Ishimori T, et al. FDG-PET of autoimmune-related pancreatitis: preliminary results. Eur J Nucl Med. 2000;27(12):1835–8.
26. Ozaki Y, Oguchi K, Hamano H, et al. Differentiation of autoimmune pancreatitis from suspected pancreatic cancer by fluorine-18 fluorodeoxyglucose positron emission tomography. J Gastroenterol. 2008;43(2):144–51.
27. Matsubayashi H, Furukawa H, Maeda A, et al. Usefulness of positron emission tomography in the evaluation of distribution and activity of systemic lesions associated with autoimmune pancreatitis. Pancreatology. 2009;9(5):694–9.
28. Nakajo M, Jinnouchi S, Fukukura Y, Tanabe H, Tateno R, Nakajo M. The efficacy of whole-body FDG-PET or PET/CT for autoimmune pancreatitis and associated extrapancreatic autoimmune lesions. Eur J Nucl Med Mol Imaging. 2007;34(12):2088–95.
29. Lee TY, Kim MH, Park do H, et al. Utility of 18F-FDG PET/CT for differentiation of autoimmune pancreatitis with atypical pancreatic imaging findings from pancreatic cancer. AJR Am J Roentgenol. 2009;193(2):343–8.
30. Numata K, Ozawa Y, Kobayashi N, et al. Contrast-enhanced sonography of autoimmune pancreatitis: comparison with pathologic findings. J Ultrasound Med. 2004;23(2):199–206.
31. D'Onofrio M, Zamboni G, Tognolini A, et al. Mass-forming pancreatitis: value of contrast-enhanced ultrasonography. World J Gastroenterol. 2006;12(26):4181–4.
32. Yadav D, Notahara K, Smyrk TC, et al. Idiopathic tumefactive chronic pancreatitis: clinical profile, histology, and natural history after resection. Clin Gastroenterol Hepatol. 2003;1(2):129–35.
33. Hardacre JM, Iacobuzio-Donahue CA, Sohn TA, et al. Results of pancreaticoduodenectomy for lymphoplasmacytic sclerosing pancreatitis. Ann Surg. 2003;237(6):853–8.
34. Prokesch RW, Chow LC, Beaulieu CF, Bammer R, Jeffrey Jr RB. Isoattenuating pancreatic adenocarcinoma at multi-detector row CT: secondary signs. Radiology. 2002;224(3):764–8.
35. Chari ST, Takahashi N, Levy MJ, et al. A diagnostic strategy to distinguish autoimmune pancreatitis from pancreatic cancer. Clin Gastroenterol Hepatol. 2009;7(10):1097–103.
36. Kamisawa T, Imai M, Yui Chen P, et al. Strategy for differentiating autoimmune pancreatitis from pancreatic cancer. Pancreas. 2008;37(3):e62–7.
37. Ishigami K, Tajima T, Nishie A, et al. MRI findings of pancreatic lymphoma and autoimmune pancreatitis: a comparative study. Eur J Radiol. 2010;74(3):e22–8.
38. Choi YJ, Byun JH, Kim JY, et al. Diffuse pancreatic ductal adenocarcinoma: characteristic imaging features. Eur J Radiol. 2008;67(2):321–8.
39. Deshpande V, Gupta R, Sainani N, et al. Subclassification of autoimmune pancreatitis: a histologic classification with clinical significance. Am J Surg Pathol. 2011;35(1):26–35.

# EUS Features

# 6

Michael J. Levy and William R. Brugge

## Introduction

AIP has historically been considered a rare disorder, but it is increasingly recognized due to an evolving understanding of the diverse nature of this protean disorder. It is now realized that the pancreatic manifestations are but one of often many manifestations of a systemic fibroinflammatory process. A low threshold is needed for diagnosis and AIP should be considered in patients presenting with unexplained pancreatic disease, especially those with a current or prior history of obstructive jaundice. The diagnosis should also be entertained in patients with a pancreatic mass or enlargement, pancreatic atrophy, or exocrine insufficiency. AIP is seldom the cause of pancreatitis. While many patients with AIP present with vague abdominal pain, routinely searching for AIP in patients predominantly complaining of abdominal pain is of low yield.

The Japan Pancreas Society established the first set of AIP diagnostic criteria that required (1) diffuse pancreatic enlargement and (2) diffuse, irregular main pancreatic duct narrowing. Diagnosis also requires any of the following: (1) increased immunoglobulin G (IgG) level, (2) presence of autoantibodies (antinuclear antibody or rheumatoid factor), and/or (3) fibrosis and lymphoplasmacytic infiltration within tissue specimens. Creation of the Japanese criteria was an important step in the diagnosis and management of patients with AIP. Worldwide experience led to differing and somewhat conflicting sets of diagnostic criteria [12–16]. While variation exists among the classification schemes, they each consider an array of clinical, laboratory, and imaging findings to accurately establish the diagnosis [4, 15, 17, 18]. Chari and colleagues [18] incorporated many cardinal features of AIP to establish the Mayo Clinic HISORt criteria that rely on histology, imaging, serology, other organ involvement, and response to steroid therapy [14, 19–24]. Incorporation of these criteria into a diagnostic algorithm has been shown to enhance diagnostic sensitivity without sacrificing specificity.

Even when the diagnosis is considered, diagnostic uncertainty often remains [25–27]. Incomplete or inadequate evaluation risks unnecessary surgery for a benign disorder that tends to have a fluctuating course often with complete resolution of all manifestations with or without immunosuppressive therapy [4, 28]. Due to limitations of prior diagnostic algorithms, the Mayo Clinic HISORt criteria were established, which enhance the sensitivity of AIP diagnosis without sacrificing specificity [29]. Despite proper use of existing diagnostic algorithms, there is still often substantial delay in the diagnosis and use of

M.J. Levy, M.D. (✉)
Division of Gastroenterology and Hepatology, Mayo Clinic, 200 First Street SW, Rochester, MN 55905, USA
e-mail: levy.michael@mayo.eu

W.R. Brugge
Harvard Medical School, Massachusetts General Hospital, Boston, MA, USA

M.J. Levy and S.T. Chari (eds.), *Autoimmune (IgG4-related) Pancreatitis and Cholangitis*,
DOI 10.1007/978-1-4419-6430-4_6, © Springer Science+Business Media New York 2013

unnecessary interventions. In addition, a subset of patients with suspected AIP remain undiagnosed, leading to diagnostic steroid trials that often add to the diagnostic confusion and risk patient safety. There is clear need to further refine the diagnostic approach to these patients [30].

## Historical Role of EUS

Pancreatic imaging is a key component of all AIP diagnostic criteria. However, existing diagnostic criteria consider only the findings of computed tomography (CT), magnetic resonance imaging (MRI), and endoscopic retrograde cholangiopancreatography (ERCP) [31–33]. Notably absent from all the algorithms is the use of EUS. EUS, with its ability to provide high-definition imaging of the pancreas and ability to acquire tissue, could potentially play a major role in definitive diagnosis of AIP and exclusion of cancer. While the ability of EUS to diagnose pancreatic cancer is well studied, there is absence of quality data supporting the role of EUS for definitive diagnosis of AIP. It is unclear if EUS imaging alone provides sufficient accuracy to establish or even reliably suggest the diagnosis of AIP. While EUS may serve as a means of tissue acquisition, the general inability of fine-needle aspiration (FNA) to establish the diagnosis and the difficulty of obtaining Tru-Cut biopsy (TCB) specimens in most centers limit even this use of EUS.

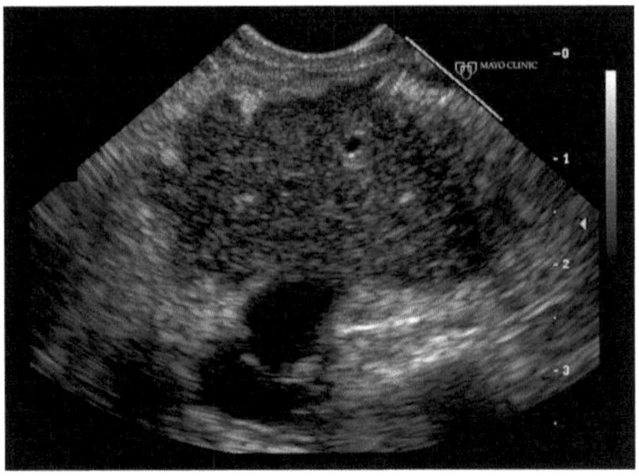

**Fig. 6.1** Classic EUS appearance of AIP including hypoechoic diffuse (sausage-shape) pancreatic enlargement with hypoechoic, coarse, patchy, heterogeneous parenchyma

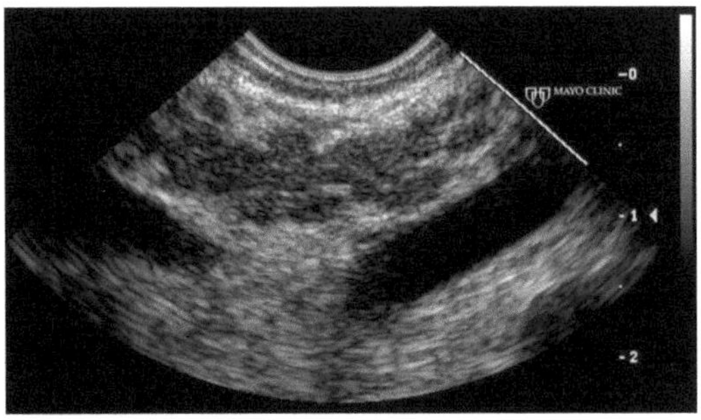

**Fig. 6.2** EUS reveals a hypoechoic, course, pancreas in which the features are patchy and heterogeneous, in the absence of a diffusely enlarged ("sausage-shape") gland

## Endoscopic Ultrasound Imaging Features

There are emerging data that suggest the potential utility of EUS imaging for the diagnosis of AIP [34–39]. However, these reports are mostly descriptive and lack the necessary methodology to determine the predictive value of EUS imaging alone. In the absence of such data, we provide opinion based on review of the limited published reports and our clinical experience.

Unfortunately, there are no pathognomonic EUS findings of AIP. We regard the most characteristic and "classic" EUS AIP findings to be diffuse (sausage-shaped) pancreatic enlargement with hypoechoic, coarse, patchy, and heterogeneous appearing parenchyma (Fig. 6.1). In our experience when patients have all these features, there is a high probability of AIP. However, patients often fail to demonstrate one or more of these features (Figs. 6.2 and 6.3), which may limit the accuracy of EUS. More problematic are patients who present with EUS evidence of a mass lesion that can mimic pancreatic carcinoma (Fig. 6.4). At times this process may appear to result in vascular invasion and perception of unresectable neoplasia (Fig. 6.5). Also, the EUS features of AIP often overlap with other pancreatic disorders such as usual or "nonspecific" chronic pancreatitis (Fig. 6.6). And finally, EUS may demonstrate a normal appearing pancreas falsely suggesting the absence of any pathology.

There are no studies that have directly compared EUS to CT or MRI, and it remains unclear

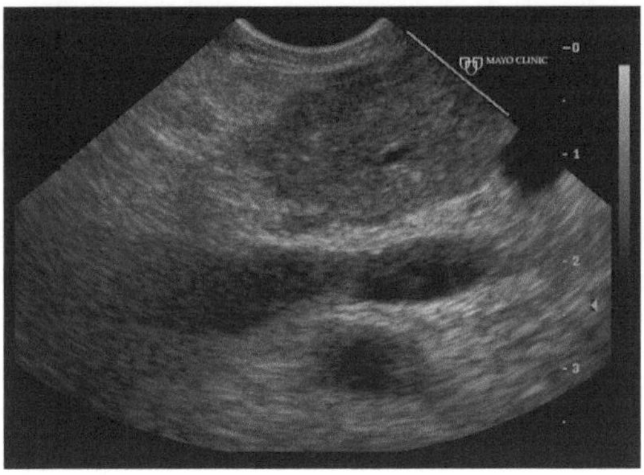

**Fig. 6.3** EUS appearance of a hypoechoic diffusely enlarged ("sausage-shape") gland, without the course and heterogeneous features

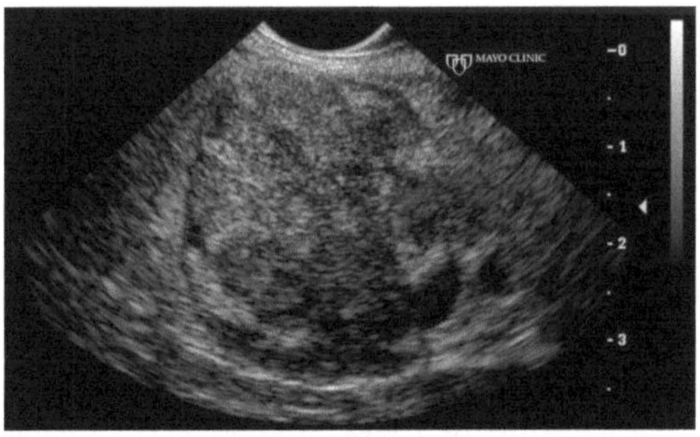

**Fig. 6.4** EUS finding of a mass-like lesion in a patient with AIP

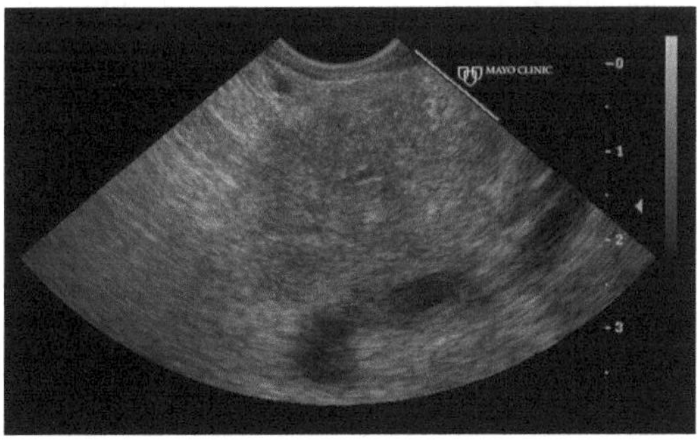

**Fig. 6.5** EUS finding of a mass-like lesion in a patient with AIP that may be confused with an "unresectable" pancreatic ductal carcinoma

as to the additive value of EUS imaging when CT or MRI raise no concern for AIP or findings are nondiagnostic. However, pertinent information may be obtained among a cohort of 48 patients

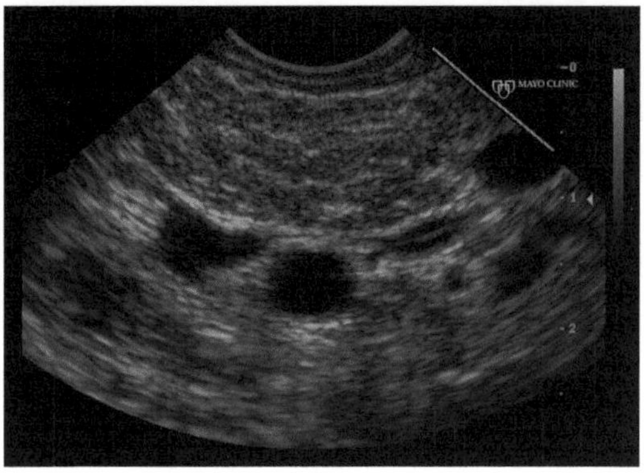

**Fig. 6.6** EUS features of nonspecific chronic pancreatitis in a patient with AIP

with AIP diagnosed by HISORt criteria who underwent pancreatic EUS imaging and TCB from our center [37, 40]. The diagnosis of AIP was strongly suspected prior to EUS in 14 patients as a result of their clinical, laboratory, imaging, and laboratory findings. For 22 patients, the diagnosis was considered pre-EUS as part of a broader differential, and in 12 patients the EUS appearance alone led to the initial suspicion of AIP. These data suggest that EUS imaging alone may increase the diagnostic accuracy for AIP in patients with negative or nondiagnostic CT or MRI.

While some features appear "characteristic" of AIP, none have proven useful when used in isolation to diagnose AIP. In addition the presence of these perceived "characteristic" features in other pancreatic disorders limits their diagnostic specificity. The lack of pathognomonic features and diverse spectrum of EUS findings limits the utility of EUS imaging alone. This has driven the pursuit of safe methods for obtaining tissue to enhance diagnostic accuracy.

## Endoscopic Ultrasound-Guided Tissue Acquisition

### Fine-Needle Aspiration

Despite few reports diagnosing AIP using FNA specimens alone, there are no broadly accepted criteria for the cytologic diagnosis, and there is great reluctance by most pathologists to rely on FNA specimens [41–43]. FNA commonly yields a diminutive tissue sample and results in a loss of tissue architecture, thereby interfering with the histologic evaluation. Although some report the ability to obtain core specimens with standard FNA needles, such efforts have not been adequately studied or validated.

Due to the inability to obtain adequate core specimens with standard FNA needles, some advocate the use of less rigorous or incomplete pathology definitions for the cytologic diagnosis of AIP. These less stringent criteria may rely on the presence of a lymphoplasmacytic infiltrate alone without the need to find such infiltrate positioned in a periductal location [41–43]. Similarly, the need for preservation of ductules, venules, or arterioles within the collected specimens appears to vary among individual endosonographers and their pathologists [41–43]. While "softening" the pathology criteria may enhance the diagnostic sensitivity of FNA for AIP, doing so is sure to compromise diagnostic specificity. This is particularly problematic for pancreatic carcinoma, which is often associated with a lymphoplasmacytic infiltration. Placing too much value on the significance of a negative FNA with the perception that an underlying malignancy has been excluded can be dangerous given the 10–40 % false negative rate of FNA for cancer even among expert centers [44–47].

## Tru-Cut Biopsy

To overcome limitations associated with FNA needles, large caliber cutting biopsy needles have been developed that acquire samples with preserved tissue architecture, thereby permitting histological examination [48–55]. The EUS Tru-Cut biopsy device (Quick-Core, Wilson-Cook, Winston-Salem, North Carolina) incorporates a disposable 19-gauge needle with a tissue tray and sliding sheath that is designed for the capture of a tissue core. This device has been shown to be particularly useful for the diagnosis of stromal tumors, lymphoma, and well-differentiated, desmoplastic, and/or vascular tumors that are often difficult to diagnose by cytology alone [56–60]. Although characteristic histologic findings of AIP exist, until recently it has been impractical to use histology to definitively establish the diagnosis preoperatively. We initially reported the utility in using EUS TCB to acquire core specimens adequate to demonstrate the full spectrum of histologic features in the diagnosis of AIP [37].

The classic constellation of histologic finding in AIP is termed lymphoplasmacytic sclerosing pancreatitis (LPSP) that consists of (1) a lymphoplasmacytic infiltrate that surrounds (a) medium and large size interlobular pancreatic ducts and (b) pancreatic venules (obliterative phlebitis) while sparing arterioles and (2) swirling fibrosis centered around pancreatic ducts (storiform fibrosis) [61, 62]. The specimens obtained with TCB are of sufficient size and quality to reveal each of these features and may be used to distinguish AIP from usual chronic pancreatitis and pancreatic carcinoma [25, 63, 64]. The evaluation is enhanced through IgG4 immunostaining of tissue samples to identify IgG4-positive plasma cells. The finding of either moderate (11–30 cells/HPF) or dense infiltration (>30 cells/HPF) is considered diagnostic [38, 65]. These findings distinguish AIP from alcohol-induced pancreatitis and the peri-tumoral inflammation associated with ductal carcinoma [38]. While traditionally a histopathologic diagnosis required review of resected pancreatic specimens, the recent introduction of EUS-guided Tru-Cut biopsy can greatly simplify the diagnosis [37].

We recently updated our experience at the Mayo Clinic in patients with a final HISORt diagnosis of AIP in order to determine the safety and diagnostic sensitivity of EUS TCB. We identified 48 patients [38 male, 10 female; mean age 59.7 years (range 18–87)] in whom a mean of 2.9 EUS TCBs (range 1–7) were performed. Histologic examination of the EUS TCB specimens provided a diagnosis in 35 (73 %) patients. The diagnostic sensitivity varied among the 5 endosonographers from 33 % to 90 %. Nondiagnostic cases were found to have chronic pancreatitis ($n=8$), nonspecific histology ($n=2$), or a failed tissue acquisition ($n=3$). EUS FNA–TCB (mean 3.4 passes, range 1–7 passes) was performed in 37 of the 48 patients, failing to establish or suggest the diagnosis in any patient. Complications included mild transient abdominal pain ($n=3$) and self-limited intra-procedural bleeding ($n=1$). It is unclear if TCB and/or FNA attributed to these complications. No patient required hospitalization or therapeutic intervention. Of note, the serum IgG4 was >2x the upper limit of normal in only 23 % of patients. None of the patients with EUS TCB diagnosis of AIP required surgical intervention for diagnosis. Over a mean follow-up of 2.6 years, no false negative diagnoses of pancreatic cancer were identified. Prior to EUS, the diagnosis of AIP was strongly suspected in 14 patients as a result of their clinical, laboratory, imaging, and laboratory findings. For 22 patients the diagnosis was considered pre-EUS as part of a broader differential. Our data suggest the potential utility of EUS imaging to the initial suspicion of AIP in 12 patients, thereby initiating pancreatic TCB and subsequent clinical evaluation for AIP.

EUS TCB appears safe and provides sufficient material to definitively diagnose AIP with high sensitivity. EUS TCB obviates the need for surgical intervention in this medically treatable disease. Our findings are consistent with the expert panel deliberations held at the 2009 Honolulu Meeting, sponsored by the American Pancreatic Association and Japan Pancreas Society [43]. The panel noted that although pancreatic FNA has little or no role in diagnosing AIP, TCB specimens may be sufficient for diagnosis.

## AIP Subtypes (Types 1 and 2)

This chapter has thus far provided a general discussion regarding the role of EUS in AIP, almost all of which applies to the most widely recognized and most common form of AIP: lymphoplasmacytic sclerosing pancreatitis (LPSP), the histologic pattern seen in type 1 AIP [20, 66–68]. The Japanese, Korean, and HISORt criteria were designed to diagnose type 1, but not type 2, AIP [69]. There are few data pertaining to the less common variant of AIP, type 2 that is referred to as idiopathic duct centric chronic pancreatitis (IDCP) [20, 70–72].

Differences in the age at presentation, gender, results of $IgG_4$ staining, and presence of associated disorders may provide clues to the presence of type 1 or 2 AIP. However, the disease subtypes are most reliably distinguished by histologic features [20, 63]. Given the paucity of diagnostic clues and the need for histologic review of large core biopsies, until recently the definitive diagnosis of type 2 AIP was only possible from surgical pancreatic biopsy or resected specimens. While our initial experience using EUS TCB offered the promise of enhanced diagnosis for type 1 AIP, [37] until recently there were no data pertaining to the use of EUS TCB in the setting of type 2 disease.

We recently reported our experience with EUS TCB [40] in this patient cohort using blinded pathology review of TCB specimens in 5 patients [4 male; mean age 39.6 years (range 25–71)] with a final diagnosis of type 2 AIP based on complete clinical, laboratory, imaging, and follow-up data [4, 15, 17]. Patients presented with obstructive jaundice ($n=2$), abdominal pain ($n=2$), and recurrent acute pancreatitis ($n=1$). The serum $IgG_4$ level was marginally elevated in only 1 of 4 patients in whom it was measured. Pre-EUS CT ($n=4$) and MRI ($n=1$) revealed diffuse pancreatic enlargement ($n=3$), a focal pancreatic head mass ($n=1$), and a normal pancreas ($n=1$). One patient had ulcerative colitis. Based on all pre-EUS data, the diagnosis of AIP (of either subtype) was not specifically suspected in any of the 5 patients, but was considered as part of a broad differential in 3 patients. In the remaining 2 patients, the EUS imaging alone raised suspicion for the presence of AIP and led to subsequent TCB.

EUS revealed a diffusely hypoechoic pancreas ($n=5$), and a focal pancreatic head mass was present in one patient. A mean of 3.6 TCB (range 2–7) passes were used to secure a histology diagnosis in 4 patients. In one patient, the clinical and imaging response to steroids helped enable diagnosis. No patient required surgical intervention for diagnosis or management. Four patients underwent a mean of 2.25 FNA passes (range 2–3) that demonstrated pancreatic acinar cells, without evidence of neoplasia or AIP of either subtype. No complications developed.

## Summary

Although personal opinion and limited data suggest that EUS imaging alone may improve AIP diagnosis, there are few data to substantiate this view. The lack of pathognomonic imaging features, considerable variation in pancreatic imaging, and a diverse spectrum of clinical disease highlight the need for safe and reliable measures for acquiring pancreatic biopsies to enhance the diagnostic accuracy of AIP.

While FNA cytologic specimens can be examined for lymphocytes and plasma cells, their presence in other disorders limits specificity, risking mismanagement of an unrecognized pancreatic carcinoma. Tissue samples collected via FNA lack preservation of tissue architecture which most pathologists consider necessary for a diagnosis of AIP. As such, until data show otherwise, reliance on FNA to establish the diagnosis of AIP is discouraged. Instead TCB should be used with histologic evaluation and IgG4 immunostaining [29, 63]. We perform EUS TCB for patients with a compatible clinical presentation in whom there is diagnostic uncertainty and when the finds are likely to alter management. Doing so may prevent misdiagnosis of pancreatic carcinoma risking lost opportunity for potentially curative resection while avoiding unnecessary surgical interventions for those with AIP. Unfortunately, it may not be possible to obtain pancreatic core biopsies due to technical, anatomical, or personnel limitations. In such patients, it is even more critical to consider all diagnostic criteria in a manner that often allows diagnosis even in the absence of histologic evaluation. Further study is needed to determine the sensitivity and specificity of EUS imaging alone as well as for FNA and TCB. New imaging technologies including elastography and contrast-enhanced ultrasound, as well as new biopsy needles under development, may offer additional promise.

## References

1. Sarles H, Sarles JC, Muratore R, Guien C. Chronic inflammatory sclerosis of the pancreas–an autonomous pancreatic disease? Am J Dig Dis. 1961;6: 688–98.
2. Yoshida K, Toki F, Takeuchi T, Watanabe S, Shiratori K, Hayashi N. Chronic pancreatitis caused by an autoimmune abnormality. Proposal of the concept of autoimmune pancreatitis. Dig Dis Sci. 1995;40:1561–8.
3. Ito T, Nakano I, Koyanagi S, Miyahara T, Migita Y, Ogoshi K, Sakai H, Matsunaga S, Yasuda O, Sumii T, Nawata H. Autoimmune pancreatitis as a new clinical entity. Three cases of autoimmune pancreatitis with effective steroid therapy. Dig Dis Sci. 1997;42:1458–68.
4. Okazaki K, Chiba T. Autoimmune related pancreatitis. Gut. 2002;51:1–4.
5. Zhang L, Smyrk TC. Autoimmune pancreatitis and IgG4-related systemic diseases. Int J Clin Exp Pathol. 2010;3:491–504.
6. Maire F, Le Baleur Y, Rebours V, Vullierme MP, Couvelard A, Voitot H, Sauvanet A, Hentic O, Levy P, Ruszniewski P, Hammel P. Outcome of patients with type 1 or 2 autoimmune pancreatitis. Am J Gastroenterol. 2010;106:151–6.
7. Takuma K, Kamisawa T, Tabata T, Inaba Y, Egawa N, Igarashi Y. Short-term and long-term outcomes of autoimmune pancreatitis. Eur J Gastroenterol Hepatol. 2011;23:146–52.
8. Takuma K, Kamisawa T, Igarashi Y. Autoimmune pancreatitis and IgG4-related sclerosing cholangitis. Curr Opin Rheumatol. 2011;23:80–7.
9. Sah RP, Chari ST. Clinical hypothyroidism in autoimmune pancreatitis. Pancreas. 2010;39:1114–6.
10. Goldsmith PJ, Cockbain AJ, Smith AM. Spontaneous resolution of pulmonary nodules in autoimmune pancreatitis. Jop: J Pancreas [Electronic Resource]. 2010; 11:630–2.
11. Triantopoulou C, Malachias G, Maniatis P, Anastopoulos J, Siafas I, Papailiou J. Renal lesions associated with autoimmune pancreatitis: CT findings. Acta Radiol. 2010;51:702–7.
12. Ryu JK, Chung JB, Park SW, Lee JK, Lee KT, Lee WJ, Moon JH, Cho KB, Kang DW, Hwang J-H, Yoo K-S, Yoo BM, Lee DH, Kim HK, Moon YS, Lee J, Lee HS, Choi HS, Lee SK, Kim Y-T, Kim CD, Kim SJ, Hahm JS, Yoon YB. Review of 67 patients with autoimmune pancreatitis in Korea: a multicenter nationwide study. Pancreas. 2008;37:377–85.
13. Okazaki K, Kawa S, Kamisawa T, Naruse S, Tanaka S, Nishimori I, Ohara H, Ito T, Kiriyama S, Inui K, Shimosegawa T, Koizumi M, Suda K, Shiratori K, Yamaguchi K, Yamaguchi T, Sugiyama M, Otsuki M, Research Committee of Intractable Diseases of the P. Clinical diagnostic criteria of autoimmune pancreatitis: revised proposal. J Gastroenterol. 2006;41:626–31.
14. Chari ST, Smyrk TC, Levy MJ, Topazian MD, Takahashi N, Zhang L, Clain JE, Pearson RK, Petersen BT, Vege SS, Farnell MB. Diagnosis of autoimmune pancreatitis: the Mayo Clinic experience. Clin Gastroenterol Hepatol. 2006;4:1010–6. quiz 934.

15. Pearson RK, Longnecker DS, Chari ST, Smyrk TC, Okazaki K, Frulloni L, Cavallini G. Controversies in clinical pancreatology: autoimmune pancreatitis: does it exist? Pancreas. 2003;27:1–13.
16. Society JP. Diagnostic criteria for autoimmune pancreatitis by the Japan Pancreas Society. J Jpn Pancreas Soc. 2002;17:585–7.
17. Kloppel G, Luttges J, Lohr M, Zamboni G, Longnecker D. Autoimmune pancreatitis: pathological, clinical, and immunological features. Pancreas. 2003;27:14–9.
18. Chari ST, Smyrk TC, Levy MJ, Topazian MD, Takahashi N, Clain JE, Pearson RK, Petersen BT, Swaroop VS, Farnell MB. Autoimmune pancreatitis: diagnosis using histology, imaging, serology, other organ involvement and response to steroids. 2006: Pending publication.
19. Ghazale A, Chari ST, Smyrk TC, Levy MJ, Topazian MD, Takahashi N, Clain JE, Pearson RK, Pelaez-Luna M, Petersen BT, Vege SS, Farnell MB. Value of serum IgG4 in the diagnosis of autoimmune pancreatitis and in distinguishing it from pancreatic cancer. Am J Gastroenterol. 2007;102:1646–53.
20. Notohara K, Burgart LJ, Yadav D, Chari S, Smyrk TC. Idiopathic chronic pancreatitis with periductal lymphoplasmacytic infiltration: clinicopathologic features of 35 cases.[see comment]. Am J Surg Pathol. 2003;27:1119–27.
21. Takahashi N, Kawashima A, Fletcher JG, Chari ST. Renal involvement in patients with autoimmune pancreatitis: CT and MR imaging findings. Radiology. 2007;242:791–801.
22. Zhang L, Notohara K, Levy MJ, Chari ST, Smyrk TC. IgG4-positive plasma cell infiltration in the diagnosis of autoimmune pancreatitis. Mod Pathol. 2007;20:23–8.
23. Ghazale A, Chari ST. Optimising corticosteroid treatment for autoimmune pancreatitis. Gut. 2007;56:1650–2.
24. Chari ST, Takahashi N, Levy MJ, Smyrk TC, Clain JE, Pearson RK, Petersen BT, Topazian MA, Vege SS. A diagnostic strategy to distinguish autoimmune pancreatitis from pancreatic cancer. Clin Gastroenterol Hepatol. 2009;7:1097–103.
25. Yadav D, Notahara K, Smyrk TC, Clain JE, Pearson RK, Farnell MB, Chari ST. Idiopathic tumefactive chronic pancreatitis: clinical profile, histology, and natural history after resection. Clin Gastroenterol Hepatol. 2003;1:129–35.
26. Kamisawa T, Egawa N, Nakajima H, Tsuruta K, Okamoto A, Kamata N. Clinical difficulties in the differentiation of autoimmune pancreatitis and pancreatic carcinoma. Am J Gastroenterol. 2003;98:2694–9.
27. Taniguchi T, Tanio H, Seko S, Nishida O, Inoue F, Okamoto M, Ishigami S, Kobayashi H. Autoimmune pancreatitis detected as a mass in the head of the pancreas without hypergammaglobulinemia, which relapsed after surgery: case report and review of the literature. Dig Dis Sci. 2003;48:1465–71.
28. Kojima E, Kimura K, Noda Y, Kobayashi G, Itoh K, Fujita N. Autoimmune pancreatitis and multiple bile duct strictures treated effectively with steroid. J Gastroenterol. 2003;38:603–7.
29. Chari ST, Smyrk TC, Takahashi N, Clain JE, Farnell MB, Levy MJ, Pearson RK, Petersen BT, Topazian M, Vege SS. Autoimmune pancreatitis: diagnosis using histology, imaging, serology, other organ involvement and response to steroids. Pancreas. 2005;31:435–6.
30. Sadler R, Chapman RW, Simpson D, Soonawalla ZF, Waldegrave EL, Burden JM, Misbah SA, Ferry BL. The diagnostic significance of serum IgG4 levels in patients with autoimmune pancreatitis: a UK study. Eur J Gastroenterol Hepatol. 2010;23:139–45.
31. Park SH, Kim M-H, Kim SY, Kim HJ, Moon S-H, Lee SS, Byun JH, Lee SK, Seo DW, Lee M-G. Magnetic resonance cholangiopancreatography for the diagnostic evaluation of autoimmune pancreatitis. Pancreas. 2010;39:1191–8.
32. Ishigami K, Tajima T, Nishie A, Ushijima Y, Fujita N, Asayama Y, Kakihara D, Irie H, Ito T, Igarashi H, Nakamura M, Honda H. MRI findings of pancreatic lymphoma and autoimmune pancreatitis: a comparative study. Eur J Radiol. 2010;74:e22–8.
33. Nishino T, Oyama H, Toki F, Shiratori K. Differentiation between autoimmune pancreatitis and pancreatic carcinoma based on endoscopic retrograde cholangiopancreatography findings. J Gastroenterol. 2010;45:988–96.
34. Levy MJ, Wiersema MJ, Chari ST. Chronic pancreatitis: focal pancreatitis or cancer? Is there a role for FNA/biopsy? Autoimmune pancreatitis. Endoscopy. 2006;38 Suppl 1:S30–5.
35. Finkelberg DL, Sahani D, Deshpande V, Brugge WR. Autoimmune pancreatitis. N Eng J Med. 2006;355:2670–6.
36. Farrell JJ, Garber J, Sahani D, Brugge WR. EUS findings in patients with autoimmune pancreatitis. Gastrointest Endosc. 2004;60:927–36.
37. Levy MJ, Reddy RP, Wiersema MJ, Smyrk TC, Clain JE, Harewood GC, Pearson RK, Rajan E, Topazian MD, Yusuf TE, Chari ST, Petersen BT. EUS-guided trucut biopsy in establishing autoimmune pancreatitis as the cause of obstructive jaundice. Gastrointest Endosc. 2005;61:467–72.
38. Zhang L, Chari ST, Levy MJ, SMyrk TC. Pancreatic IgG4 stain for diagnosing autoimmune pancreatitis (AIP) and for distinguishing AIP subtypes. Gastroenterology. 2005;128:A474.
39. Hocke M, Ignee A, Dietrich CF. Contrast-enhanced endoscopic ultrasound in the diagnosis of autoimmune pancreatitis. Endoscopy. 2011;43:163–5.
40. Levy MJ, Smyrk TC, Takahashi N, Zhang L, Chari ST. Idiopathic duct-centric pancreatitis: disease description and endoscopic ultrasonography-guided trucut biopsy diagnosis. Pancreatology. 2011;11:76–80.
41. Mizuno N, Bhatia V, Hosoda W, Sawaki A, Hoki N, Hara K, Takagi T, Ko SBH, Yatabe Y, Goto H, Yamao K. Histological diagnosis of autoimmune pancreatitis

using EUS-guided trucut biopsy: a comparison study with EUS-FNA. J Gastroenterol. 2009;44:742–50.
42. Deshpande V, Mino-Kenudson M, Brugge WR, Pitman MB, Fernandez-del Castillo C, Warshaw AL, Lauwers GY. Endoscopic ultrasound guided fine needle aspiration biopsy of autoimmune pancreatitis: diagnostic criteria and pitfalls. Am J Surg Pathol. 2005;29:1464–71.
43. Chari ST, Kloeppel G, Zhang L, Notohara K, Lerch MM, Shimosegawa T, Autoimmune Pancreatitis International Cooperative Study G. Histopathologic and clinical subtypes of autoimmune pancreatitis: the Honolulu consensus document. Pancreas. 2010;39: 549–54.
44. Voss M, Hammel P, Molas G, Palazzo L, Dancour A, O'Toole D, Terris B, Degott C, Bernades P, Ruszniewski P. Value of endoscopic ultrasound guided fine needle aspiration biopsy in the diagnosis of solid pancreatic masses. Gut. 2000;46:244–9.
45. Eloubeidi MA, Tamhane A. EUS-guided FNA of solid pancreatic masses: a learning curve with 300 consecutive procedures. Gastrointest Endosc. 2005; 61:700–8.
46. Mitsuhashi T, Ghafari S, Chang CY, Gu M. Endoscopic ultrasound-guided fine needle aspiration of the pancreas: cytomorphological evaluation with emphasis on adequacy assessment, diagnostic criteria and contamination from the gastrointestinal tract. Cytopathology. 2006;17:34–41.
47. Turner BG, Cizginer S, Agarwal D, Yang J, Pitman MB, Brugge WR. Diagnosis of pancreatic neoplasia with EUS and FNA: a report of accuracy. Gastrointest Endosc. 2009;71:91–8.
48. Piccinino F, Sagnelli E, Pasquale G, Giusti G. Complications following percutaneous liver biopsy. A multicentre retrospective study on 68,276 biopsies. J Hepatol. 1986;2:165–73.
49. Kovalik EC, Schwab SJ, Gunnells JC, Bowie D, Smith SR. No change in complication rate using spring-loaded gun compared to traditional percutaneous renal allograft biopsy techniques. Clin Nephrol. 1996;45:383–5.
50. Brandt KR, Charboneau JW, Stephens DH, Welch TJ, Goellner JR. CT- and US-guided biopsy of the pancreas. Radiology. 1993;187:99–104.
51. Welch TJ, Sheedy 2nd PF, Johnson CD, Johnson CM, Stephens DH. CT-guided biopsy: prospective analysis of 1,000 procedures. Radiology. 1989;171:493–6.
52. Harrison BD, Thorpe RS, Kitchener PG, McCann BG, Pilling JR. Percutaneous Trucut lung biopsy in the diagnosis of localised pulmonary lesions. Thorax. 1984;39:493–9.
53. Ingram DM, Sheiner HJ, Shilkin KB. Operative biopsy of the pancreas using the Trucut needle. Aust N Z J Surg. 1978;48:203–6.
54. Lavelle MA, O'Toole A. Trucut biopsy of the prostate. Br J Urol. 1994;73:600.
55. Ball AB, Fisher C, Pittam M, Watkins RM, Westbury G. Diagnosis of soft tissue tumours by Tru-Cut biopsy. Br J Surg. 1990;77:756–8.
56. Wiersema MJ, Levy MJ, Harewood GC, Vazquez-Sequeiros E, Jondal ML, Wiersema LM. Initial experience with EUS-guided trucut needle biopsies of perigastric organs. Gastrointest Endosc. 2002;56: 275–8.
57. Levy MJ, Jondal ML, Clain J, Wiersema MJ. Preliminary experience with an EUS-guided trucut biopsy needle compared with EUS-guided FNA. Gastrointest Endosc. 2003;57:101–6.
58. Levy MJ, Wiersema MJ. EUS-guided trucut biopsy. Gastrointest Endosc. 2005;62:417–26.
59. Levy MJ, Smyrk TC, Reddy RP, Clain JE, Harewood GC, Kendrick ML, Pearson RK, Petersen BT, Rajan E, Topazian MD, Wang KK, Wiersema MJ, Yusuf TE, Chari ST. Endoscopic ultrasound-guided trucut biopsy of the cyst wall for diagnosing cystic pancreatic tumors. Clin Gastroenterol Hepatol. 2005;3: 974–9.
60. Gines A, Wiersema MJ, Clain JE, Pochron NL, Rajan E, Levy MJ. Prospective study of a Trucut needle for performing EUS-guided biopsy with EUS-guided FNA rescue. Gastrointest Endosc;62.
61. Abraham SC, Wilentz RE, Yeo CJ, Sohn TA, Cameron JL, Boitnott JK, Hruban RH. Pancreaticoduodenectomy (Whipple resection) in patients without malignancy: are they all chronic pancreatitis? Am J Surg Pathol. 2003;27:110–20.
62. Kloppel G, Luttges J, Sipos B, Capelli P, Zamboni G. Autoimmune pancreatitis: pathological findings. Jop: J Pancreas [Electronic Resource]. 2005;6:97–101.
63. Zamboni G, Luttges J, Capelli P, Frulloni L, Cavallini G, Pederzoli P, Leins A, Longnecker D, Kloppel G. Histopathological features of diagnostic and clinical relevance in autoimmune pancreatitis: a study on 53 resection specimens and 9 biopsy specimens. Virchows Arch. 2004;445:552–63.
64. Suda K, Takase M, Fukumura Y, Ogura K, Ueda A, Matsuda T, Suzuki F. Histopathologic characteristics of autoimmune pancreatitis based on comparison with chronic pancreatitis. Pancreas. 2005;30:355–8.
65. Kamisawa T. IgG4-positive plasma cells specifically infiltrate various organs in autoimmune pancreatitis. Pancreas. 2004;29:167–8.
66. Kawaguchi K, Koike M, Tsuruta K, Okamoto A, Tabata I, Fujita N. Lymphoplasmacytic sclerosing pancreatitis with cholangitis: a variant of primary sclerosing cholangitis extensively involving pancreas. Hum Pathol. 1991;22:387–95.
67. Kloppel G. Chronic pancreatitis, pseudotumors and other tumor-like lesions. Mod Pathol. 2007;20 Suppl 1:S113–31.
68. Kamisawa T, Takuma K, Tabata T, Inaba Y, Egawa N, Tsuruta K, Hishima T, Sasaki T, Itoi T. Serum IgG4-negative autoimmune pancreatitis. J Gastroenterol. 2010;46:108–16.
69. Naitoh I, Nakazawa T, Ohara H, Ando T, Hayashi K, Okumura F, Miyabe K, Yoshida M, Sano H, Takada H, Kanematsu T, Joh T. Comparative evaluation of the Japanese diagnostic criteria for autoimmune pancreatitis. Pancreas. 2010;39:1173–9.

70. Kloppel G, Detlefsen S, Chari ST, Longnecker DS, Zamboni G. Autoimmune pancreatitis: the clinicopathological characteristics of the subtype with granulocytic epithelial lesions. J Gastroenterol. 2010;45: 787–93.
71. Deshpande V, Gupta R, Sainani N, Sahani DV, Virk R, Ferrone C, Khosroshahi A, Stone JH, Lauwers GY. Subclassification of autoimmune pancreatitis: a histologic classification with clinical significance. Am J Surg Pathol. 2010;35:26–35.
72. Kamisawa T, Notohara K, Shimosegawa T. Two clinicopathologic subtypes of autoimmune pancreatitis: LPSP and IDCP. Gastroenterology. 2010;139: 22–5.

# ERCP Features

# 7

Terumi Kamisawa

## Introduction

In 1992, Toki et al. from Tokyo Women's Medical University group reported four cases of peculiar pancreatitis showing diffuse irregular narrowing of the entire main pancreatic duct (MPD) on endoscopic retrograde pancreatography (ERP) [1]. Three years later, Yoshida et al., from the same group, proposed a new entity of autoimmune pancreatitis (AIP) based on their experience [2]. Thus, AIP was originally defined in Japan based on the unique MPD features. Therefore, in the Japanese diagnostic criteria for AIP pancreatography, showing diffuse or segmental irregular narrowing of the MPD is mandatory [3].

## Endoscopic Pancreatographic Findings Suggesting AIP

In AIP patients, unlike other causes of pancreatic duct obstruction or stenosis, MPD narrowing involves a greater extent of the duct, manifest by extensive narrowing and irregularity without upstream dilation. In typical AIP cases, more than one-third of the entire length of the MPD is narrowed. Diffuse irregular narrowing of the MPD is rather specific to AIP (Fig. 7.1) [3–5]. In our study [6] comparing endoscopic pancreatography (ERP) findings of AIP and pancreatic cancer, the length of the narrowed portion of the MPD was 6.7 ± 3.2 (mean ± SD) cm in AIP patients, which was significantly longer than in pancreatic cancer patients (2.6 ± 0.8 cm; $p < 0.01$). The length of the narrowed portion of the MPD on ERP was longer than 3 cm in 76 % of AIP patients, which was significantly higher than in pancreatic cancer patients (20 %; $p < 0.01$). In AIP patients, the degree of MPD narrowing may vary in the same patient, and skipped narrowed lesions of the MPD were detected in 35 % of AIP versus 0 % of patients with pancreatic cancer, ($p < 0.01$) (Fig. 7.2). In AIP patients with segmental narrowing of the MPD, secondary upstream dilatation of the MPD is less often noted than in pancreatic cancer. The maximal diameter of the upstream MPD was 2.9 ± 0.7 mm in segmental AIP patients, which was significantly smaller than in pancreatic head cancer patients (7.1 ± 1.9 mm; $p < 0.01$). The maximal diameter of the upstream MPD was < 5 mm in 94 % of segmental AIP patients, compared to 18 % of pancreatic cancer patients (18 %; $p < 0.01$). In addition, side branches were more often visualized emanating from the narrowed portions of the MPD in AIP patients (65 %) than in pancreatic cancer patients (25 %; $p < 0.05$) (Fig. 7.2). Obstruction of the MPD was detected more often in pancreatic cancer patients (60 %) than in AIP patients (6 %; $p < 0.01$).

Histopathological features for most patients diagnosed with AIP in Japan include dense

T. Kamisawa, MD, Ph.D. (✉)
Department of Internal Medicine,
Tokyo Metropolitan Komagome Hospital, 3-18-22
Honkomagome, Bunkyo-ku/Tokyo 113-8677, Japan
e-mail: kamisawa@cick.jp

M.J. Levy and S.T. Chari (eds.), *Autoimmune (IgG4-related) Pancreatitis and Cholangitis*,
DOI 10.1007/978-1-4419-6430-4_7, © Springer Science+Business Media New York 2013

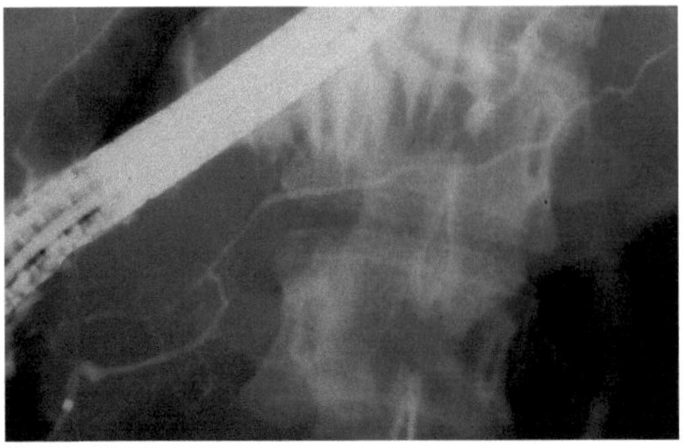

**Fig. 7.1** ERP feature of AIP showing diffuse narrowing of the main pancreatic duct (With permission from Terumi Kamisawa, et al. Clinical difficulties in the differentiation of autoimmune pancreatitis from pancreatic carcinoma. Am J Gastroenterology. 2003; 98 (12); 2694–2699)

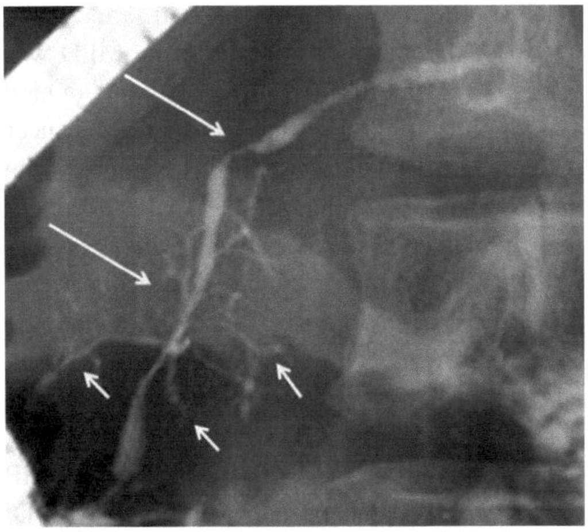

**Fig. 7.2** ERP feature of AIP showing skipped narrowed lesions of the main pancreatic duct (*long arrows*). Many side branches were derived from the narrowed lesions (*short arrows*)

pancreatic lymphoplasmacytic infiltration and fibrosis, which is termed lymphoplasmacytic sclerosing pancreatitis. Typically an abundant lymphoplasmacytic infiltrate and fibrosis surrounds interlobular pancreatic ducts as well as the MPD. Although the periductal inflammation is usually extensive and distributed throughout the entire pancreas, the degree and extent of periductal inflammation differ from duct to duct according to the location of the involved pancreas. The infiltrate is primarily subepithelial with the epithelium only rarely infiltrated by inflammatory cells. This process encompasses the pancreatic ducts and narrows their lumen [7–9]. On the other hand, pancreatic cancer typically infiltrates and destroys the epithelium of the bile ducts and main pancreatic duct and side branches, resulting in ductal obstruction. These differences in periductal histopathological features likely account for the variance in pancreatographic findings between AIP and pancreatic cancer. Pancreatographic findings such as absence of MPD obstruction, skip lesions of the MPD, side branch derivation from the narrowed portion of the MPD, MPD involvement over >3 cm, and maximal upstream MPD diameter of <5 mm are each suggestive of AIP rather than pancreatic cancer [6].

Nishino et al. also reported three ERP findings including the presence/absence of side branches, the length of the narrowed MPD, and the maximal diameter of the upstream MPD could be used to distinguish AIP from pancreatic cancer in most cases [10]. In an international multicenter study, the presence of extensive MPD narrowing or multiple separate narrowed regions of the MPD was the most specific (≥97 %) but the least sensitive (≤ 38 %) of the four key pancreatographic features (long narrowing, lack of upstream dilatation, multiple narrowing, and side branch derivation) of AIP [11].

It is difficult to differentiate a short narrowing of the MPD in AIP from stenosis in pancreatic cancer (Fig. 7.3a). There are some pancreatic cancer cases showing pancreatographic findings similar to those of AIP [10].

## Endoscopic Cholangiographic Findings Suggesting AIP

On endoscopic retrograde cholangiography, stenosis of the distal extrahepatic bile duct is detected frequently in both AIP and pancreatic cancer patients. In our recent study [12], stenosis of the distal bile duct was smooth in 87 % of AIP patients but irregular in 65 % of pancreatic cancer patients ($p<0.01$) (Fig. 7.4). Left-side deviation of the lower bile duct was detected in both groups. Stenosis of the intrahepatic or hilar bile duct was detected in only AIP patients (16 %, $p<0.01$) (Fig. 7.5).

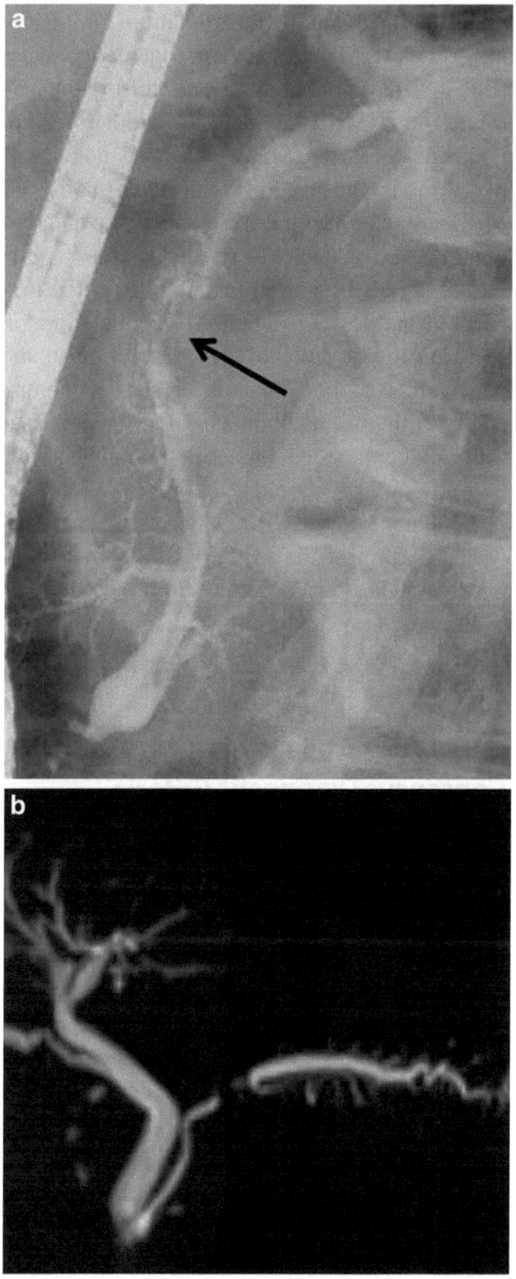


**Fig. 7.3** (**a**) ERP feature of AIP showing a short narrowing of the main pancreatic duct (*arrow*). (**b**) The narrowed portion is not visualized on MRCP. Upstream dilatation of the MPD is less than that of pancreatic cancer

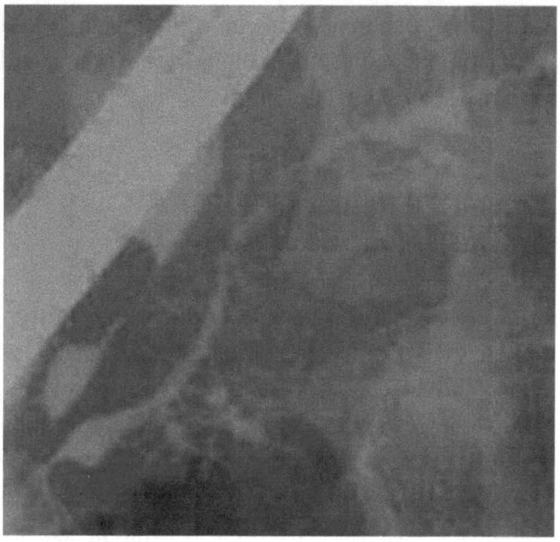

**Fig. 7.4** ERCP feature of AIP showing stenosis of the lower bile duct

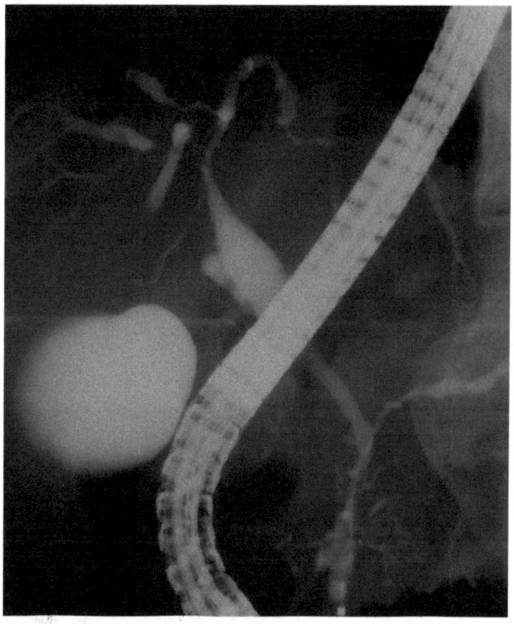

**Fig. 7.5** ERCP feature of AIP showing stenosis of the hilar and intrahepatic bile duct (With permission from Terumi Kamisawa, Naoto Egawa, Kouji Tsuruta, Atsutake Okamoto, Nobuaki Funata. Primary sclerosing cholangitis may be overestimated in Japan. Journal of Gastroenterology. 2005; Volume 40, Issue 3: 318–319)

When the inflammatory process affects the pancreatic head, it usually also involves the distal bile duct, leading to stenosis and wall thickening secondary to fibrosis and lymphoplasmacytic infiltration.The epithelium of the bile duct is well preserved. Stenosis of the intrahepatic or hilar bile duct is considered evidence of other organ involvement and supports the diagnosis of AIP rather than pancreatic cancer, although it should be distinguished from cholangiocarcinoma and primary sclerosing cholangitis.

## Can MRCP Replace ERCP for the Diagnosis of AIP?

Although pancreatographic findings may differentiate AIP from pancreatic cancer, ERCP can cause adverse events such as pancreatitis. Magnetic resonance cholangiopancreatography (MRCP) is replacing diagnostic ERCP in many pancreatobiliary diseases. In the new Korean diagnostic criteria, AIP can be diagnosed by MRCP without the need for ERCP [13].

The major drawback in use of MRCP for diagnosing AIP is the inability to reliably detect MPD narrowing due to the inferior resolution of MRCP compared with ERCP. In our study [12], diffuse narrowing of the MPD on ERCP appeared as skipped nonvisualized lesions in 50 % (Fig. 7.6), faint visualization in 19 %, and nonvisualization in 31 % on MRCP. Segmental narrowing of the MPD seen on ERCP was not visualized in 86 % on MRCP, and distinguishing between AIP and pancreatic cancer was difficult with MRCP (Fig. 7.3b). However, less pronounced upstream MPD dilatation on MRCP may suggest AIP rather than pancreatic cancer (Fig. 7.3b). Side branch derivation from the narrowed portion of the MPD is another feature poorly assessed by MRCP. Skipped nonvisualized lesions and a faintly visualized, narrowed MPD associated with diffuse pancreatic enlargement may be valuable CT or MRCP clues to AIP. Park et al. also reported that skipped MPD narrowing and less upstream MPD dilatation on MRCP suggest AIP [14]. As resolution of the pancreatic and bile ducts after steroid therapy can be fully evaluated on MRCP, MRCP is useful to judge the effect of steroid therapy and follow-up after steroid therapy. With the development of MRCP models, visualized narrowed portion of the MPD has been increased. Secretin-MRCP is reported to improve MPD examination and may allow accurate diagnosis of AIP [15].

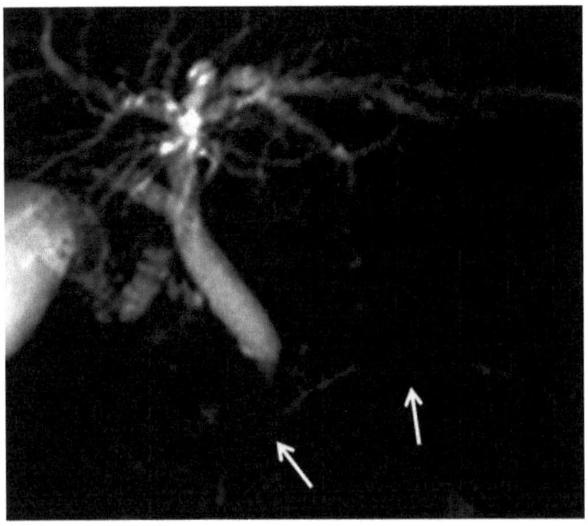

**Fig. 7.6** MRCP feature of diffuse-type AIP showing skipped nonvisualized lesions of the main pancreatic duct (*arrows*)

## Role of ERCP in International Consensus Diagnostic Criteria for AIP

Local expertise and practice patterns in the use of various tests vary considerably worldwide. The major initial presenting manifestation of AIP is obstructive jaundice due to associated sclerosing cholangitis or mass effect [16]. Endoscopic biliary drainage is often performed to manage obstructive jaundice along with brush cytology and intraductal biopsy to help exclude a neoplastic process [17]. ERP is routinely used for investigating obstructive jaundice in Japan and Korea, but injecting the pancreatic duct is generally avoided in patients with obstructive jaundice to minimize the risk of post-ERP pancreatitis in Western countries [11]. As previously noted, ERP may help establish the diagnosis of AIP and is a key imaging modality in Japan and Korea. However, the use of other criteria is critical to diagnose AIP in centers that do not rely on ERP in this setting as a result of concern regarding safety and/or lack of experience.

## Endoscopic Observation and Biopsy from the Major Duodenal Papilla

The major duodenal papilla is sometimes swollen in AIP patients (Fig. 7.7) [18, 19] and may histologically demonstrate dense IgG4-positive plasma cells and lymphocyte infiltration with fibrosis. In our study [18] of IgG4 immunostaining of biopsy specimens from the major duodenal papilla, severe infiltration of IgG4-positive plasma cells (≥10/HPF (high power field)) was observed in the papilla of all eight AIP patients with pancreatic head involvement. Moderate infiltration of IgG4-positive plasma cells (9–4/HPF) was detected in one patient with pancreatic head cancer, but there were rare (≤3/HPF) IgG4-positive plasma cells infiltrating the papilla in two AIP patients who only had pancreatic body and/or tail involvement, in nine patients with pancreatic cancer, and in ten patients with papillitis. IgG4 immunostaining of biopsy specimens obtained from the major duodenal papilla is useful for supporting a diagnosis of AIP with pancreatic head involvement.

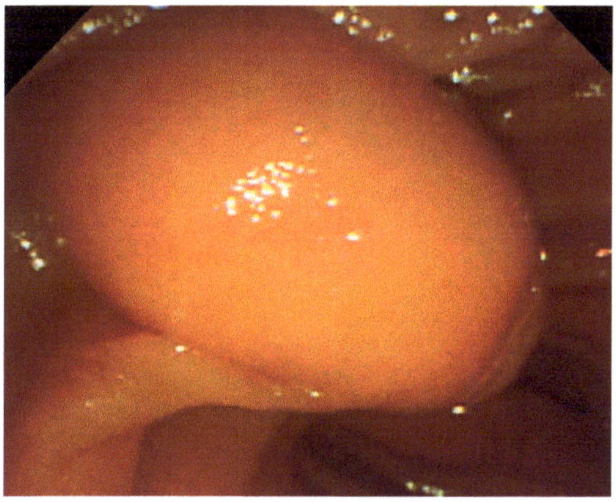

**Fig. 7.7** Endoscopic feature of AIP showing a markedly swollen major duodenal papilla (With permission from Terumi Kamisawa, et al. Disappearance of an ampullary pseudotumor after steroid therapy for autoimmune pancreatitis. Gastrointestinal Endoscopy. 2010; 71 (4): 847–848)

## Conclusions

Several ERP findings may be used when evaluating AIP and provide reasonable accuracy among physicians familiar with these features. MRCP does not replace ERCP in initial diagnosis, but may have a role in the follow-up of patients with AIP.

## References


1. Toki F, Kozu T, Oi I, et al. An unusual type of chronic pancreatitis showing diffuse irregular narrowing of the entire main pancreatic duct on ERCP – a report of four cases. Endoscopy. 1992;24:640.
2. Yoshida K, Toki F, Takeuchi T, et al. Chronic pancreatitis caused by an autoimmune abnormality. Proposal of the concept of autoimmune pancreatitis. Dig Dis Sci. 1995;40:1561–8.
3. Okazaki K, Kawa S, Kamisawa T, et al. Clinical diagnostic criteria of autoimmune pancreatitis: revised proposal. J Gastroenterol. 2006;41:626–31.
4. Okazaki K, Kawa S, Kamisawa T, et al. Japanese consensus guidelines for autoimmune pancreatitis: I. Concept and diagnosis of autoimmune pancreatitis. J Gastroenterol. 2010;45:249–65.
5. Kamisawa T, Anjiki H, Takuma K, et al. Endoscopic approach for diagnosing autoimmune pancreatitis. World J Gastrointest Endosc. 2010;2:20–4.
6. Kamisawa T, Imai M, Chen PY, et al. Strategy for differentiating autoimmune pancreatitis from pancreatic cancer. Pancreas. 2008;37:e62–7.
7. Kamisawa T, Funata N, Hayashi Y, et al. Close relationship between autoimmune pancreatitis and multifocal fibrosclerosis. Gut. 2003;52:683–7.
8. Kloppel G, Sipos B, Zamboni G, Kojima M, Morohoshi T. Autoimmune pancreatitis: histo- and immunopathological features. J Gastroenterol. 2007; 42(Suppl):28–31.
9. Chandan VS, Iacobuzio-Donalue C, Abraham SC. Patchy distribution of pathologic abnormalities in autoimmune pancreatitis. Implications for preoperative diagnosis. Am J Surg Pathol. 2008;32:1762–9.
10. Nishino T, Oyama H, Toki F, et al. Differentiation between autoimmune pancreatitis and pancreatic carcinoma based on endoscopic retrograde cholangiopancreatography findings. J Gastroenterol. 2010;45: 988–96.
11. Sugumar A, Levy MJ, Kamisawa T, et al. Endoscopic retrograde pancreatography criteria to diagnose autoimmune pancreatitis: an international multicentre study. Gut. 2011;60:666–70.
12. Takuma K, Kamisawa T, Tabata T, et al. Utility of pancreatography for diagnosing autoimmune pancreatitis. World J Gastroenterol. 2011;17:2332–7.

13. Otsuki M, Chung JB, Okazaki K, et al. Asian diagnostic criteria for autoimmune pancreatitis: consensus of the Japan-Korea Symposium on Autoimmune Pancreatitis. J Gastroenterol. 2008;43:403–8.
14. Park SH, Kim MH, Kim SY, et al. Magnetic resonance cholangiopancreatography for the diagnostic evaluation of autoimmune pancreatitis. Pancreas. 2010;39:1191–8.
15. Carbognin G, Girardi V, Biasiutti C, et al. Autoimmune pancreatitis: imaging findings on contrast-enhanced MR, MRCP and dynamic secretin-enhanced MRCP. Radiol Med. 2009;114:1214–31.
16. Kamisawa T, Takuma K, Egawa N, et al. Autoimmune pancreatitis and IgG4-related sclerosing disease. Nat Rev Gastroenterol Hepatol. 2010;7:401–9.
17. Kamisawa T, Okazaki K, Kawa S, et al. Japanese consensus guidelines for management of autoimmune pancreatitis: III. Treatment and prognosis of AIP. J Gastroenterol. 2010;45:471–7.
18. Kamisawa T, Tu Y, Egawa N, et al. A new diagnostic endoscopic tool for autoimmune pancreatitis. Gastrointest Endosc. 2008;68:358–61.
19. Kim MH, Moon SH, Kamisawa T. Major duodenal papilla in autoimmune pancreatitis. Dig Surg. 2010;27:110–4.

# 8 Clinical Features

Timothy B. Gardner and Chris E. Forsmark

## Introduction

As the pancreatic manifestation of an apparent systemic disorder which may affect multiple organs, autoimmune pancreatitis (AIP) is generally considered a form of chronic pancreatitis that has distinct pathological, histological, and clinical characteristics [1, 2]. The clinical manifestations of AIP are quite variable, although there appear to be a few common presentations. Identifying and categorizing the broad range of clinical and subclinical manifestations of AIP is quite challenging, as little is known of the natural history, presymptomatic stage, and spectrum of disease. The descriptions of the clinical manifestations of AIP come from small retrospective cohorts, case series, and case reports. This highly selected population inevitably represents patients with more severe or advanced or unusual clinical presentations. In the absence of a characteristic and easily available diagnostic test, it will remain difficult or impossible to categorize the full spectrum of clinical illness associated with AIP. Finally, it is beginning to appear that the two different subtypes of AIP, lymphoplasmacytic sclerosing pancreatitis (LPSP—type 1) and idiopathic duct-centric chronic pancreatitis or AIP with granulocytic epithelial lesionsGELs—type 2), have distinct clinical spectrums of disease. Therefore, when highlighting the clinical features of AIP, it is likely to be important that type 1 and 2 disease be considered as similar, but distinct, entities. This chapter will focus on each type of AIP, recognizing that clinical overlap between the two does exist.

## Prevalence

Data on the prevalence of AIP are very limited, with virtually all data reported from Japan. It is important to consider that although AIP appears to be a worldwide phenomenon, different regions appear to have differences in the relative prevalence of type 1 and type 2 AIP. For example, in Japan, type 1 appears to be the predominant form of AIP while in Western countries such as the United States and Europe, a mix of types 1 and 2 is encountered [3–5]. AIP has been described in both first-world and developing countries, as well as immigrants from Eastern countries to the West [6].

Despite a dramatic increase in research interest and publications on AIP in recent years, the true prevalence of AIP is unknown. This is primarily due to the absence of a reliable and available diagnostic test. This is similar to the situation with

T.B. Gardner, M.D. (✉)
Gastroenterology and Hepatology, Dartmouth Medical School, One Medical Center Drive, Lebanon, NH 03756, USA
e-mail: timothy.b.gardner@hitchcock.org

C.E. Forsmark, M.D.
Division of Gastroenterology, Hepatology, and Nutrition, University of Florida, Gainesville, FL, USA

M.J. Levy and S.T. Chari (eds.), *Autoimmune (IgG4-related) Pancreatitis and Cholangitis*,
DOI 10.1007/978-1-4419-6430-4_8, © Springer Science+Business Media New York 2013 

celiac disease prior to the availability of sensitive and specific serology. After an accurate diagnostic test was introduced, the full spectrum of celiac disease was able to be elucidated and the non-gastrointestinal and subclinical manifestations became apparent and estimates of overall prevalence increased dramatically. It seems likely that the prevalence of AIP is also underestimated. The prevalence of AIP is also difficult to determine due to the relative rarity of the disease, the confusion over classification in regard to clinical subtypes, under-recognition of disease, and underreporting. One of the first studies of prevalence surveyed Japanese hospitals to determine how many patients admitted with pancreatitis had AIP based on the diagnostic criteria for AIP proposed by the Japanese Pancreas Society [7]. The authors estimated AIP prevalence in Japan to be 0.82 per 100,000. Other authors from Japan and Korea report prevalence rates of 5–6 % of all patients with a diagnosis of chronic pancreatitis [4, 8].

There are extremely limited data in regard to AIP prevalence in Western countries. In addition, the fact that Western countries are believed to have a greater percentage of type 2 patients makes estimations of prevalence prone to underestimation. It has been noted in retrospective case series of patients in the United States who have undergone operative resection for presumed pancreatic malignancy that a small fraction of these patients have AIP. In one series, 43 of 1,808 (2.4 %) patients who underwent pancreatic resections for presumed malignancy were found to have type 1 on histological evaluation of resected specimens [9]. In 245 pathology specimens of patients who underwent pancreatic resection for benign pancreatic disease at the Mayo Clinic, 11 % were subsequently found to have AIP [10]. These very limited data provide no reliable estimate of prevalence and there are no data at all on incidence.

## Demographics

Type 1 AIP tends to be a disease of elderly males, as most patients (up to 85 %) with it are older than 50 years [11, 12]. However, AIP has been reported in patients as young as the preteen years, although it is unclear if the entity at this age represents type 1 or 2 [13, 14]. Although the age of onset is typically in the sixth decade, type 1 AIP has been histologically confirmed in patients as young as 30. The male to female predominance is approximately 2:1 [7]. Type 1 has also been described as an incidental finding at autopsy [15].

In young patients (less than 40 years old), type 2 AIP appears to be more prevalent than type 1 and the male to female predominance remains approximately 2:1 [5, 16]. These data are supported by the fact that the clinical characteristics of AIP in the young tend to be more consistent with type 2 than type 1. For example, one study from Japan stratifying AIP patients by age demonstrated that young patients show different clinical features from middle-aged or elderly patients with AIP; young patients are more likely to have abdominal pain and serum amylase elevations [17]. However, until further prevalence studies in Western countries of type 2 AIP are performed, more definitive conclusions about demographics of this subtype cannot be made.

## Serology

A hallmark of type 1 AIP is an increasing amount of circulating immunoglobulins, specifically immunoglobulin subclass 4 [18–21].Type 2 AIP does not as yet have a serologic biomarker. Hamano et al. published the initial landmark study in which they demonstrated than an elevated serum IgG4 level was both highly sensitive (95 %) and specific (97 %) for AIP [18]. Subsequently, further evaluation of IgG4 levels in AIP has not demonstrated such robust test characteristics. In a study of 510 patients from the Mayo clinic, 45 patients had AIP, 135 had pancreatic adenocarcinoma, 268 had other pancreatic diseases, and 62 had no pancreatic disease, the sensitivity, specificity, and positive predictive values for elevated serum IgG4 (>140 mg/dL) for diagnosis of AIP were 76 %, 93 %, and 36 %, respectively [19]. See Table 8.1. Serum IgG4 levels, even in the presence of classic

**Table 8.1** IgG4 level in patients with different diseases of the pancreas[a]

| | AIP | Normal Pancreas | Pancreatic Cancer | Benign pancreatic Tumor | Chronic Pancreatitis |
|---|---|---|---|---|---|
| Number[b] | 45 | 62 | 135 | 64 | 79 |
| Mean IgG4 ± SM | 550 ± 99 | 49 ± 6 | 68 ± 9 | 47 ± 5 | 46 ± 5 |
| Range | 16–2,890 | 3–263 | 3–1,140 | 3–195 | 3–231 |
| Proportion elevated >140 mg/dL | 76 % | 4.8 % | 9.6 % | 4.7 % | 6.3 % |

Reprinted with permission [1]
[a]Adopted from [19]
[b]Based on 510 patients referred to the Mayo Clinic for evaluation of pancreatic disease from 1/05 to 6/06

histological findings of type 1, can be normal [2]. However, serum IgG4 elevations are usually not seen in patients with pancreatic malignancy [22]. In addition, although patients with type 2 may have elevated serum IgG4 levels, it is likely a less common finding than in type 1 [16, 23].

A meta-analysis of 159 patients with AIP and 1099 controls were described in seven selected papers reporting the usefulness of serum IgG4 in diagnosing AIP. In total, 304 controls had pancreatic cancer, 96 had autoimmune diseases, and the remaining 699 had other conditions. Serum IgG4 showed fair accuracy in distinguishing between AIP and the overall controls, pancreatic cancer, and other autoimmune diseases (area under the curve [+/− SE]: 0.920 +/−0.073, 0.914 +/−0.191, and 0.949 +/−0.024, respectively) [20].

Levels of total IgG and gamma globulins may also be increased in AIP, although it is unusual to have elevated serum levels of IgG or gamma globulins without elevation of serum IgG4 levels [24]. Lower serum IgM and IgA have also been reported in patients with AIP [25]. Additionally, levels of IgG4 can fluctuate during the course of disease, depending on remission status [26]. Given the lack of sensitivity and specificity in regard to total immunoglobulin and IgG4 level, these tests should not be used as the sole diagnostic test for AIP.

Elevated titers of many other autoantibodies have been described in AIP, including rheumatoid factor (RF) and antinuclear antibody (ANA) [1]. Autoantibodies against carbonic anhydrase II and IV as well as lactoferrin are detected in some patients with AIP [27, 28]. Involvement of antinuclear and antismooth muscle antibodies, as well as autoantibodies to the pancreatic secretory trypsin inhibitor, has been described. A novel peptide (AIP 1–7), which demonstrates homology with an amino acid sequence of plasminogen-binding protein (PBP) of Helicobacter pylori and with ubiquitin-protein ligase E3 component n-recognin 2 (UBR2), was positive in 33 of 35 patients with autoimmune pancreatitis (94 %) and in 5 of 110 patients with pancreatic cancer (5 %) [29]. An increased frequency of peripheral eosinophilia has been described in AIP, although this finding is clearly not specific to this disease [30]. It is not clear that these antibodies, including IgG4, have an important pathophysiologic role or are simply markers of disease. One recent study described complement deposition along with IgG4 along the basement membrane of pancreatic ductal cells and acini, suggesting the IgG4 may play a direct role in immune-complex mediated injury [31]. The antigenic target of the IgG4 remains unknown.

## Clinical Features

AIP has diverse clinical symptoms, due in part to the difference between type 1 and type 2 (Table 8.2). The "classic" type 1 clinical presentation is painless jaundice in an elderly male—this occurs in up to 80 % of patients with a new presentation of type 1 [1, 32]. The jaundice is secondary to inflammation of the pancreas entrapping the intrapancreatic portion of the common bile duct. See Fig. 8.1. The degree of

**Table 8.2** Clinical spectrum of type 1 and type 2 AIP

| Feature | Type 1[a] | Type 2[b] |
|---|---|---|
| Most common presenting complaint | Obstructive jaundice (80–90 %) | Obstructive jaundice (50–60 %) |
| Presenting with acute pancreatitis | (10–15 %) | (30–40 %) |
| Mean age at presentation | 60–70 | 40–50 |
| Male to female predominance | 2:1 | 2:1 |
| Elevated serum IgG4 | Often elevated | Occasionally elevated |
| Associated with inflammatory bowel disease | No | Yes |
| Relapse | 40–50 % | Rare |

[a]Type 1 = "lymphoplasmacytic sclerosing pancreatitis"
[b]Type 2 = "idiopathic duct-centric chronic pancreatitis"

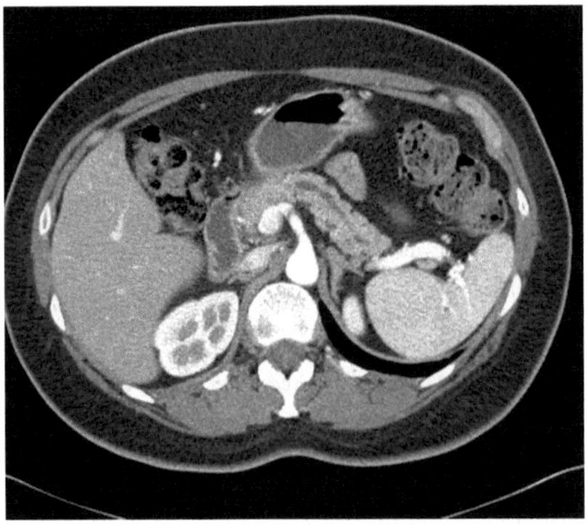

**Fig. 8.2** Pancreas-phase CT scan from a 42-year-old patient with recurrent acute pancreatitis and type 2 AIP. Note that the pancreatic duct is dilated proximal to a focal stricture in the neck

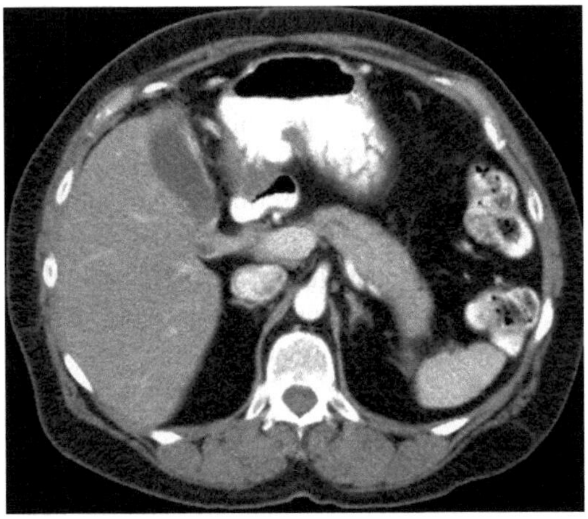

**Fig. 8.1** Pancreas-phase CT of a 57-year-old female with type 1 who presented with painless jaundice. The pancreas is diffusely enlarged with a classic "sausage-shaped" appearance. Also note that pancreatic duct is diminutive

pancreatic inflammation can be diffuse or localized, and thus some patients will present with a focal pancreatic mass [33]. The primary clinical challenge in this setting is distinguishing AIP from pancreatic malignancy. The biliary manifestation of $IgG_4$-related disease ($IgG_4$-RD) will be addressed in subsequent chapters, but there is often clinical overlap between this entity and AIP [34]. Patients presenting with obstructive jaundice may have just a stricture of the intrapancreatic bile duct but may also have coexistent strictures of more proximal biliary ducts due to $IgG_4$-related sclerosing cholangitis ($IgG_4$-SC). See Figs. 8.2 and 8.3. This may have clinical importance as clinical relapse after successful therapy may be much more common in those with more extensive biliary strictures.

Patients with type 1 can sometimes present with weight loss and new onset glucose intolerance, making the distinction even more difficult between AIP and pancreatic malignancy [5, 9]. Like other forms of benign pancreatic disease, pancreatic adenocarcinoma has been reported in the context of underlying type 1, although this relationship has not been firmly or completely established [35, 36].

A subset of patients may present with abdominal pain, back pain, or recurrent vomiting [2, 32]. Initially, it was felt that although AIP patients can present with acute pancreatitis, this was a relatively rare phenomenon [37]. However, more recently, a large case-control study from the Mayo Clinic determined that 35 % of newly diagnosed AIP patients had features of either acute or chronic pancreatitis at the time of presentation and that all patients treated with corticosteroids responded to treatment [38]. In another study

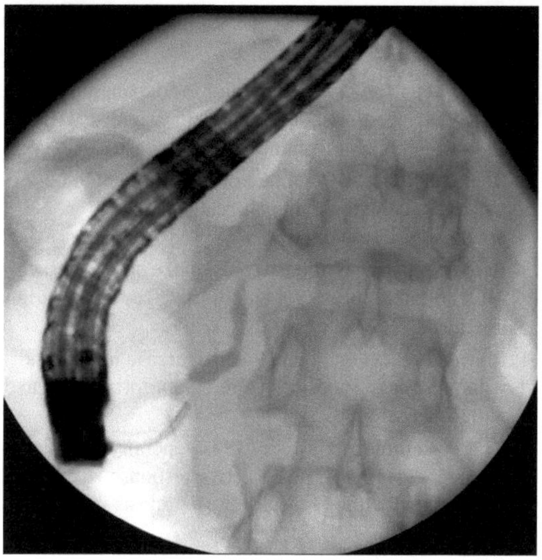

**Fig. 8.3** Pancreatogram from the same 42-year-old patient with type 2 AIP obtained at ERCP demonstrating a stricture in the pancreatic neck with proximal ductal dilation

from a single center in France, acute pancreatitis was more prevalent in patients with type 2, although when compared to patients with type 1, this result was not statistically significant [5]. Endocrine or exocrine failure directly attributable to AIP, however, appears to be relatively rare, especially in type 2 [5, 39]. Patients with type 1 can also present with large pancreatic pseudocysts [40]. Thus, the pancreatic manifestations of type 1 can mimic pancreatic malignancy, painless chronic pancreatitis, or acute pancreatitis but are less likely to mimic unexplained pancreatic insufficiency

The recognition of type 2 as a distinct clinical entity has led to more focus on distinguishing the cardinal clinical features of this AIP subset. Patients with type 2 tend to be younger and have less association with extrapancreatic disease, with the exception of inflammatory bowel disease [16]. Colitis has been reported in up to 30 % of patients with type 2, and the finding of IgG4-positive cells on colon biopsy suggests that IBD may represent an extrapancreatic manifestation of AIP [12, 41]. Patients with type 2 tend to present more often with acute pancreatitis than do type 1 patients but also do present with obstructive jaundice at high frequencies [16, 42]. Further study is needed to better define the clinical profile of type 2 disease.

In addition to the pancreatic manifestations and presentations of AIP, a number of extrapancreatic organs may be involved in those with $IgG_4$-RD. These are discussed in more detail in subsequent chapters but a few observations are appropriate. These extrapancreatic manifestations often provide important clues in reaching a confident diagnosis of AIP. Some of these findings may be present and visible on standard radiographic imaging obtained in the evaluation of a patient with pancreatitis or pancreatic mass. Retroperitoneal fibrosis, focal areas of renal parenchymal changes suggestive of tubulointerstitial nephritis, and pseudotumors of various intra-abdominal organs are all consistent with underlying $IgG_4$-RD. In addition, the coexistence of enlarged salivary or lacrimal glands; pseudotumors in the lung, orbit, or thyroid; or other rare conditions noted in subsequent chapters also should increase clinical suspicion that AIP is present.

## Distinguishing AIP from Malignancy

The classic clinical presentation of AIP often closely mimics that of pancreatic adenocarcinoma—painless jaundice in an elderly male—sometimes associated with weight loss and new onset or worsening glucose intolerance. In addition, imaging can demonstrate focal pancreatic and biliary strictures, as well as a pancreatic parenchymal mass. It is important therefore for clinicians to distinguish between these two entities due to vastly different prognostic and therapeutic considerations [43]. The diagnostic criteria from multiple societies and institutions (Japan, Asian, Mayo HiSORT) are discussed elsewhere in the text. However, it is important to recognize that each of the classifications systems has its strengths and weaknesses and none has been prospectively validated specifically as a tool to distinguish between malignant and inflammatory disease [44].

Clinicians must first keep in mind that compared to pancreatic adenocarcinoma, AIP is a rare disease. It is also important to remember that all focal pancreatic masses should be sampled histologically prior to a consideration of AIP and a negative initial biopsy does not preclude the diagnosis of subsequent malignancy [45]. A diagnosis of AIP should never be made in the context of a pancreatic mass unless histological sampling has definitively ruled out malignancy.

However, clinical features, in addition to pancreatic imaging and serology, can help to distinguish AIP from malignancy. Symptoms such as fluctuating jaundice or pain are seen more frequently in AIP than in malignancy [46]. In addition, a 2-week trial of corticosteroids has been advocated as a means of differentiating the two clinical entities [47]. However, it is very important to set an objective measurement of response, such as resolution of imaging findings, and not rely on symptom improvement to distinguish benign from malignant etiologies.

Not only does misdiagnosis occur in patients treated inappropriately with corticosteroids for pancreatic adenocarcinoma, it also occurs in patients with functional pain syndromes treated with prolonged courses of corticosteroids without evidence of AIP. Often this occurs in the context of positive serologic tests without any other corroborating evidence. Furthermore, multiple patients have undergone operative interventions, such as pancreatic head resection or partial hepatectomy, without consideration of autoimmune disease.

It is therefore incumbent on the clinician to consider AIP in the differential diagnosis of patients with chronic pancreatitis or biliary strictures. However, exquisite care must be taken to assure that a proper diagnosis, especially in cases of malignancy, is made. Clinical pearls to help avoid misdiagnosis are shown in Table 8.3.

**Table 8.3** Clinical pearls to help avoid misdiagnosis in AIP

| |
|---|
| 1. Utilize the Mayo HISORt and/or the Japanese Pancreas Society Guidelines to help diagnose AIP and differentiate it from malignant disease |
| 2. Remember that AIP is a rare disease thought to be much less common than pancreatic adenocarcinoma or cholangiocarcinoma |
| 3. Before initiating corticosteroids, make sure a marker is identified to follow for an objective response during treatment |
| 4. Elevated serum IgG4 levels can decrease in patients with pancreatic cancer who are inappropriately treated with corticosteroids |
| 5. Corticosteroid response in AIP is generally seen within 2–4 weeks. If no objective response is documented within 4 weeks, the diagnosis is unlikely to be AIP |
| 6. Corticosteroids often cause subjective improvement in symptoms even in patients without AIP |
| 7. Serum IgG4 levels are elevated in 5 % of patients without pancreatic disease, 10 % of pancreatic cancer, and 6 % of chronic pancreatitis—an increased IgG4 level is not specific for AIP |
| 8. All focal pancreatic masses should be sampled prior to initiating corticosteroids |

From [45]. Review

## Natural History

The true natural history of AIP is unknown because of its relatively new description, overall small numbers of patients, and different subsets of disease. However, there are studies, mostly from Japan, that have attempted to address this issue. Uchida and colleagues followed 21 patients with AIP and observed them at a mean interval of 40.8 months (range, 18–130 months) [48]. Three of the patients underwent surgical therapy, 12 patients received methylprednisolone (PSL) treatment, and the 6 remaining patients received no treatment. At the conclusion of follow-up, 7 of the 21 patients showed pancreatic atrophy, of whom 2 were non-PSL-treated patients. Three patients developed chronic pancreatitis. One patient was diagnosed with pancreatic cancer after 50 months of PSL therapy. A study of 51 patients with type 1 found recurrence in 21 (41 %) patients and pancreatic stone formation in 9 (18 %) patients [49].

Studies to evaluate the natural history of disease without corticosteroid intervention are limited. However, 12 patients with type 1 in Japan were followed for more than 6 months after the diagnosis of AIP without being given steroids. Six patients were later treated with steroids due to exacerbation of AIP. Five of them developed obstructive jaundice due to bile duct stenosis.

Spontaneous improvement occurred in three patients. Four asymptomatic patients with segmental pancreatic enlargement demonstrated no changes without steroid therapy [50].

More effort has been made to try and differentiate the natural history of type 1 and type 2. The most obvious difference thus far reported has been that patients with type 1 disease have a relapse rate of approximately 50 %, where patients with type 2 disease rarely have relapsing disease [16, 33]. In a single institution in France, 16 out of 28 patients with type 1 disease developed diabetes, compared with one patient out of 16 patients who had type 2 disease [5]. In that same study, 10 out 28 patients with type 1 and 5 out of 16 patient developed exocrine pancreatic insufficiency. However, this study was retrospective analysis and not all patients were treated with corticosteroids.

## Prognosis of AIP

There is a little information about the long-term prognosis of patients treated for AIP [51]. The disease is almost always responsive to treatment with corticosteroids, and patients with inflammatory disease tend to respond more favorably than those with fibrotic disease [52]. However, spontaneous remission does occur and it is unknown whether treatment helps to change the natural history of disease [53, 54]. Often, patients treated for AIP develop pancreatic atrophy, although the development of pancreatic endocrine and exocrine insufficiency does not always follow [55]. In a survey of 167 patients admitted to hospitals in Japan in 2002, 67 % had AIP complicated by DM. Approximately half of those patients demonstrated improvement of diabetes following corticosteroid treatment and only 20 % of total patients developed worsening glucose intolerance due to the corticosteroids [56].

Hirano et al. published the most comprehensive evaluation of prognosis in AIP [57]. Of 42 patients with AIP, 19 were treated with corticosteroids and 23 were not. In patients not treated, after an average observation period of 25 months, 16 patients (70 %) developed unfavorable events including obstructive jaundice as a result of distal bile duct stenosis in four, growing pseudocyst in one, sclerogenic changes of extrapancreatic bile duct in nine, hydronephrosis as a result of retroperitoneal fibrosis in one, and interstitial nephritis in one. In the patients treated with corticosteroids, after an average observation period of 23 months, six patients (32 %) developed unfavorable events consisting of interstitial pneumonia in three and a recurrence of obstructive jaundice in three. They concluded that corticosteroids could reduce AIP-related unfavorable events and recommended their early introduction [57].

At this time, given the relatively recent description of the disease, there are no data in regard to the mortality rate associated with AIP. In addition, no information in regard to AIP's effect on life expectancy is available.

## Summary and Future Directions

The clinical spectrum varies widely in AIP depending on the type (type 1 or type 2) of disease. Most commonly patients with type 1 AIP are older males presenting with painless jaundice and an elevated IgG4 level. In type 2 AIP, the classic clinical presentation has not yet been defined, but these patients tend to be younger and comparatively more often present with acute pancreatitis and normal IgG4 levels. With further clinical experience, areas of clinical overlap and separation will be better defined.

Future clinical investigation should focus on the natural history of AIP, including asymptomatic patients. Whether or not patients with different clinical manifestations of IgG4-related disease have unique or different prognoses also needs to be evaluated. Efforts to find a more accurate serologic marker also need to be explored, so that autoimmune disease can be better differentiated from malignancy at presentation. Eventually, with more robust experience with the two AIP subtypes, refinement of the clinical spectrum will allow for more optimal treatment recommendations in this disease.

## Key Points

- The two clinical subtypes of AIP (type 1 and type 2) have both overlapping and separate clinical characteristics.
- Patients with type 1 most commonly present as older males with obstructive jaundice.
- Patients with type 2 are younger and more frequently present with painful acute or chronic pancreatitis.
- Although not completely accurate for diagnosis of AIP, IgG4 currently is the most widely used serum test for AIP.
- AIP and pancreatic malignancy frequently present with similar symptoms; it is essential to rule out malignancy before considering the diagnosis of AIP.
- The long-term natural history of AIP is unknown; however patients with type 2 are less likely to relapse after treatment.
- More clinical experience with these two entities is needed before the clinical spectrum of disease can be completely defined.

## References

1. Gardner TB, Chari ST. Autoimmune pancreatitis. Gastroenterol Clin North Am. 2008;37:439–60, vii.
2. Chari ST, Smyrk TC, Levy MJ, Topazian MD, Takahashi N, Zhang L, Clain JE, Pearson RK, Petersen BT, Vege SS, Farnell MB. Diagnosis of autoimmune pancreatitis: the Mayo Clinic experience. Clin Gastroenterol Hepatol. 2006;4:1010–16.
3. Kloppel G, Detlefsen S, Chari ST, Longnecker DS, Zamboni G. Autoimmune pancreatitis: the clinicopathological characteristics of the subtype with granulocytic epithelial lesions. J Gastroenterol. 2010;45:787–93.
4. Kim KP, Kim MH, Lee SS, Seo DW, Lee SK. Autoimmune pancreatitis: it may be a worldwide entity. Gastroenterology. 2004;126:1214.
5. Maire F, Le Baleur Y, Rebours V, Vullierme MP, Couvelard A, Voitot H, Sauvanet A, Hentic O, Levy P, Ruszniewski P, Hammel P. Outcome of patients with type 1 or 2 autoimmune pancreatitis. Am J Gastroenterol. 2011;106:151–6.
6. Varadarajulu S, Cotton PB. Autoimmune pancreatitis: is it relevant in the west? Gastroenterology. 2003;125:1557.
7. Nishimori I, Tamakoshi A, Otsuki M. Prevalence of autoimmune pancreatitis in Japan from a nationwide survey in 2002. J Gastroenterol. 2007;42 Suppl 18:6–8.
8. Okazaki K. Autoimmune pancreatitis is increasing in Japan. Gastroenterology. 2003;125:1557–8.
9. Weber SM, Cubukcu-Dimopulo O, Palesty JA, Suriawinata A, Klimstra D, Brennan MF, Conlon K. Lymphoplasmacytic sclerosing pancreatitis: inflammatory mimic of pancreatic carcinoma. J Gastrointest Surg. 2003;7:129–37; discussion 137–9.
10. Yadav D, Notahara K, Smyrk TC, Clain JE, Pearson RK, Farnell MB, Chari ST. Idiopathic tumefactive chronic pancreatitis: clinical profile, histology, and natural history after resection. Clin Gastroenterol Hepatol. 2003;1:129–35.
11. Raina A, Yadav D, Krasinskas AM, McGrath KM, Khalid A, Sanders M, Whitcomb DC, Slivka A. Evaluation and management of autoimmune pancreatitis: experience at a large US center. Am J Gastroenterol. 2009;104:2295–306.
12. Park DH, Kim MH, Chari ST. Recent advances in autoimmune pancreatitis. Gut. 2009;58:1680–9.
13. Gargouri L, Ponsot P, Viala J, Belarbi N, Martinez C, Bellaiche M, Mougenot JF, Hugot JP, Belghiti J, Cezard JP. Recurrent autoimmune pancreatitis in a 10-year-old boy. J Pediatr Gastroenterol Nutr. 2009;48:374–7.
14. Fukumori K, Shakado S, Miyahara T, Fukuizumi K, Takemoto R, Nishi H, Sakai H, Muranaka T, Sata M. Atypical manifestations of pancreatitis with autoimmune phenomenon in an adolescent female. Intern Med. 2005;44:886–91.
15. Kitano Y, Matsumoto K, Chisaka K, Imazawa M, Takahashi K, Nakade Y, Okada M, Aso K, Yokoyama K, Yamamoto M, Yoshie M, Ogawa K, Haneda M. An autopsy case of autoimmune pancreatitis. JOP. 2007;8:621–7.
16. Sah RP, Chari ST, Pannala R, Sugumar A, Clain JE, Levy MJ, Pearson RK, Smyrk TC, Petersen BT, Topazian MD, Takahashi N, Farnell MB, Vege SS. Differences in clinical profile and relapse rate of type 1 versus type 2 autoimmune pancreatitis. Gastroenterology. 2010;139:140–8.
17. Kamisawa T, Wakabayashi T, Sawabu N. Autoimmune pancreatitis in young patients. J Clin Gastroenterol. 2006;40:847–50.
18. Hamano H, Kawa S, Horiuchi A, Unno H, Furuya N, Akamatsu T, Fukushima M, Nikaido T, Nakayama K, Usuda N, Kiyosawa K. High serum IgG4 concentrations in patients with sclerosing pancreatitis. N Engl J Med. 2001;344:732–8.
19. Ghazale A, Chari ST, Smyrk TC, Levy MJ, Topazian MD, Takahashi N, Clain JE, Pearson RK, Pelaez-Luna M, Petersen BT, Vege SS, Farnell MB. Value of serum IgG4 in the diagnosis of autoimmune pancreatitis and in distinguishing it from pancreatic cancer. Am J Gastroenterol. 2007;102:1646–53.
20. Morselli-Labate AM, Pezzilli R. Usefulness of serum IgG4 in the diagnosis and follow up of autoimmune pancreatitis: a systematic literature review and meta-analysis. J Gastroenterol Hepatol. 2009;24:15–36.
21. Kang P, Lee KT, Sinn DH, Kim BJ, Lee JS, Lee JK, Rhee JC. Clinical usefulness of serum immunoglobulin

G and G4 level in the diagnosis of autoimmune pancreatitis. Korean J Gastroenterol. 2008;52:304–9.
22. Raina A, Krasinskas AM, Greer JB, Lamb J, Fink E, Moser AJ, Zeh 3rd HJ, Slivka A, Whitcomb DC. Serum immunoglobulin G fraction 4 levels in pancreatic cancer: elevations not associated with autoimmune pancreatitis. Arch Pathol Lab Med. 2008;132:48–53.
23. Pace A, Topalidis T, Blaker M, Guthoff A, de Weerth A, Lohse AW. Autoimmune pancreatitis with normal IgG4-Levels: 4 case reports and review of the literature. Z Gastroenterol. 2007;45:1245–51.
24. Song TJ, Kim MH, Moon SH, Eum JB, Park do H, Lee SS, Seo DW, Lee SK. The combined measurement of total serum IgG and IgG4 may increase diagnostic sensitivity for autoimmune pancreatitis without sacrificing specificity, compared with IgG4 alone. Am J Gastroenterol. 2010;105:1655–60.
25. Taguchi M, Kihara Y, Nagashio Y, Yamamoto M, Otsuki M, Harada M. Decreased production of immunoglobulin M and A in autoimmune pancreatitis. J Gastroenterol. 2009;44:1133–9.
26. Egawa N, Irie T, Tu Y, Kamisawa T. A case of autoimmune pancreatitis with initially negative autoantibodies turning positive during the clinical course. Dig Dis Sci. 2003;48:1705–8.
27. Nishi H, Tojo A, Onozato ML, Jimbo R, Nangaku M, Uozaki H, Hirano K, Isayama H, Omata M, Kaname S, Fujita T. Anti-carbonic anhydrase II antibody in autoimmune pancreatitis and tubulointerstitial nephritis. Nephrol Dial Transplant. 2007;22:1273–5.
28. Nishimori I, Miyaji E, Morimoto K, Nagao K, Kamada M, Onishi S. Serum antibodies to carbonic anhydrase IV in patients with autoimmune pancreatitis. Gut. 2005;54:274–81.
29. Frulloni L, Lunardi C, Simone R, Dolcino M, Scattolini C, Falconi M, Benini L, Vantini I, Corrocher R, Puccetti A. Identification of a novel antibody associated with autoimmune pancreatitis. N Engl J Med. 2009;361:2135–42.
30. Wang Q, Lu CM, Guo T, Qian JM. Eosinophilia associated with chronic pancreatitis. Pancreas. 2009;38:149–53.
31. Detlefsen S, Bräsen JH, Zamboni G, Capelli P, Klöppel G. Deposition of complement C3c, immunoglobulin (Ig)G4 and IgG at the basement membrane of pancreatic ducts and acini in autoimmune pancreatitis. Histopathology. 2010;57(6):825–35.
32. Church NI, Pereira SP, Deheragoda MG, Sandanayake N, Amin Z, Lees WR, Gillams A, Rodriguez-Justo M, Novelli M, Seward EW, Hatfield AR, Webster GJ. Autoimmune pancreatitis: clinical and radiological features and objective response to steroid therapy in a UK series. Am J Gastroenterol. 2007;102:2417–25.
33. Frulloni L, Scattolini C, Falconi M, Zamboni G, Capelli P, Manfredi R, Graziani R, D'Onofrio M, Katsotourchi AM, Amodio A, Benini L, Vantini I. Autoimmune pancreatitis: differences between the focal and diffuse forms in 87 patients. Am J Gastroenterol. 2009;104:2288–94.
34. Ghazale A, Chari ST, Zhang L, Smyrk TC, Takahashi N, Levy MJ, Topazian MD, Clain JE, Pearson RK, Petersen BT, Vege SS, Lindor K, Farnell MB. Immunoglobulin G4-associated cholangitis: clinical profile and response to therapy. Gastroenterology. 2008;134:706–15.
35. Motosugi U, Ichikawa T, Yamaguchi H, Nakazawa T, Katoh R, Itakura J, Fujii H, Sato T, Araki T, Shimizu M. Small invasive ductal adenocarcinoma of the pancreas associated with lymphoplasmacytic sclerosing pancreatitis. Pathol Int. 2009;59:744–7.
36. Witkiewicz AK, Kennedy EP, Kennyon L, Yeo CJ, Hruban RH. Synchronous autoimmune pancreatitis and infiltrating pancreatic ductal adenocarcinoma: case report and review of the literature. Hum Pathol. 2008;39:1548–51.
37. Takayama M, Hamano H, Ochi Y, Saegusa H, Komatsu K, Muraki T, Arakura N, Imai Y, Hasebe O, Kawa S. Recurrent attacks of autoimmune pancreatitis result in pancreatic stone formation. Am J Gastroenterol. 2004;99:932–7.
38. Sah RP, Pannala R, Chari ST, Sugumar A, Clain JE, Levy MJ, Pearson RK, Smyrk TC, Petersen BT, Topazian MD, Takahashi N, Vege SS. Prevalence, diagnosis, and profile of autoimmune pancreatitis presenting with features of acute or chronic pancreatitis. Clin Gastroenterol Hepatol. 2010;8:91–6.
39. Ito T, Kawabe K, Arita Y, Hisano T, Igarashi H, Funakoshi A, Sumii T, Yamanaka T, Takayanagi R. Evaluation of pancreatic endocrine and exocrine function in patients with autoimmune pancreatitis. Pancreas. 2007;34:254–9.
40. Welsch T, Kleeff J, Esposito I, Buchler MW, Friess H. Autoimmune pancreatitis associated with a large pancreatic pseudocyst. World J Gastroenterol. 2006;12:5904–6.
41. Ravi K, Chari ST, Vege SS, Sandborn WJ, Smyrk TC, Loftus Jr EV. Inflammatory bowel disease in the setting of autoimmune pancreatitis. Inflamm Bowel Dis. 2009;15:1326–30.
42. Pezzilli R. Acute recurrent pancreatitis: an autoimmune disease? World J Gastroenterol. 2008;14:999–1006.
43. Law R, Bronner M, Vogt D, Stevens T. Autoimmune pancreatitis: a mimic of pancreatic cancer. Cleve Clin J Med. 2009;76:607–15.
44. Sugumar A, Chari ST. Distinguishing pancreatic cancer from autoimmune pancreatitis: a comparison of two strategies. Clin Gastroenterol Hepatol. 2009;7:S59–62.
45. Gardner TB, Levy MJ, Takahashi N, Smyrk TC, Chari ST. Misdiagnosis of autoimmune pancreatitis: a caution to clinicians. Am J Gastroenterol. 2009;104:1620–3.
46. Kamisawa T, Imai M, Yui Chen P, Tu Y, Egawa N, Tsuruta K, Okamoto A, Suzuki M, Kamata N.

Strategy for differentiating autoimmune pancreatitis from pancreatic cancer. Pancreas. 2008;37:e62–7.
47. Moon SH, Kim MH, Park DH, Hwang CY, Park SJ, Lee SS, Seo DW, Lee SK. Is a 2-week steroid trial after initial negative investigation for malignancy useful in differentiating autoimmune pancreatitis from pancreatic cancer? A prospective outcome study. Gut. 2008;57:1704–12.
48. Uchida K, Yazumi S, Nishio A, Kusuda T, Koyabu M, Fukata M, Miyoshi H, Sakaguchi Y, Fukui T, Matsushita M, Takaoka M, Okazaki K. Long-term outcome of autoimmune pancreatitis. J Gastroenterol. 2009;44:726–32.
49. Kawa S, Hamano H, Ozaki Y, Ito T, Kodama R, Chou Y, Takayama M, Arakura N. Long-term follow-up of autoimmune pancreatitis: characteristics of chronic disease and recurrence. Clin Gastroenterol Hepatol. 2009;7:S18–22.
50. Kamisawa T, Anjiki H, Takuma K, Egawa N, Kubota N. The natural course of autoimmune pancreatitis. Hepatogastroenterology. 2009;56:866–70.
51. Okazaki K. Is outcome of autoimmune pancreatitis similar to conventional types of chronic pancreatitis? Intern Med. 2006;45:571–2.
52. Pannala R, Chari ST. Corticosteroid treatment for autoimmune pancreatitis. Gut. 2009;58:1438–9.
53. Ozden I, Dizdaroglu F, Poyanli A, Emre A. Spontaneous regression of a pancreatic head mass and biliary obstruction due to autoimmune pancreatitis. Pancreatology. 2005;5:300–3.
54. Goldsmith PJ, Cockbain AJ, Smith AM. Spontaneous resolution of pulmonary nodules in autoimmune pancreatitis. JOP. 2010;11:630–2.
55. Kamisawa T, Egawa N, Inokuma S, Tsuruta K, Okamoto A, Kamata N, Nakamura T, Matsukawa M. Pancreatic endocrine and exocrine function and salivary gland function in autoimmune pancreatitis before and after steroid therapy. Pancreas. 2003;27:235–8.
56. Nishimori I, Tamakoshi A, Kawa S, Tanaka S, Takeuchi K, Kamisawa T, Saisho H, Hirano K, Okamura K, Yanagawa N, Otsuki M. Influence of steroid therapy on the course of diabetes mellitus in patients with autoimmune pancreatitis: findings from a nationwide survey in Japan. Pancreas. 2006;32:244–8.
57. Hirano K, Tada M, Isayama H, Yagioka H, Sasaki T, Kogure H, Nakai Y, Sasahira N, Tsujino T, Yoshida H, Kawabe T, Omata M. Long-term prognosis of autoimmune pancreatitis with and without corticosteroid treatment. Gut. 2007;56:1719–24.

# 9 Approach to Diagnosis

Raghuwansh P. Sah and Suresh T. Chari

## Introduction

Autoimmune pancreatitis (AIP) closely mimics the presentation of pancreatic cancer (PC). However, unlike pancreatic cancer, AIP responds to steroid treatment [1, 2]. A correct and timely diagnosis of AIP can avert unnecessary surgery as well as ease patient anxiety related to the suspicion of PC. Similarly misdiagnosing PC as AIP can lead to significant delay in diagnosis of PC and inappropriate treatment with steroids. Thus, distinguishing AIP from pancreatic cancer is of great clinical significance.

Both AIP and PC most commonly present with obstructive jaundice [3]. AIP is generally painless or associated with mild abdominal pain. Persistent narcotic-requiring pain is highly suggestive of PC. Infrequently, severe pain and pancreatitis may be present at presentation of AIP although this is often followed by jaundice which becomes the overshadowing symptom thereafter [4]. PC can also present with painless jaundice. Constitutional features like weight loss, anorexia, or fatigue occur in both AIP and PC. Thus, in most patients clinical features alone are not sufficient to differentiate AIP from PC.

AIP is a rare disease [5, 6] although its recognition is increasing worldwide. Pancreatic cancer is relatively more common [7]. Only about 3–5 % of patients undergoing resection for suspected pancreatic cancer were found to have AIP [8]. Therefore, a high index of suspicion is required to diagnose AIP although overdiagnosis is a real possibility. Differentiating AIP from PC is a challenging task even at the expert centers. In this chapter, we describe a validated approach to diagnosis of AIP based on the international consensus diagnostic criteria (ICDC) [9]. Misdiagnosing AIP or PC could be largely avoided with careful application of this approach.

## The International Consensus Diagnostic Criteria (ICDC)

The international consensus diagnostic criteria (ICDC) [9] were developed as a unified framework for diagnosis of AIP taking into account multiple previously published diagnostic criteria [10–15]. Each feature is classified as strong (*level 1*) or supportive (*level 2*) diagnostic evidence. The diagnosis of AIP is made by specific combinations of these features described below.

### Pancreatic Histology

Diagnostic histology for type 1 AIP requires at least three of the following:

R.P. Sah, MBBS (✉)
Internal Medicine, Mayo Clinic Rochester,
200 1st ST., SW, Rochester, MN 55905, USA
e-mail: sah.raghuwansh@mayo.edu

S.T. Chari, MD
Division of Gastroenterology and Hepatology,
Internal Medicine, Mayo Clinic College of Medicine,
200 First Street SW, Rochester, MN 55905, USA

M.J. Levy and S.T. Chari (eds.), *Autoimmune (IgG4-related) Pancreatitis and Cholangitis*,
DOI 10.1007/978-1-4419-6430-4_9, © Springer Science+Business Media New York 2013

1. Periductal lymphoplasmacytic infiltrate without granulocyte infiltration
2. Obliterative phlebitis
3. Storiform fibrosis
4. Abundant (>10 cells/HPF) IgG4-positive cells

Type 2 AIP may demonstrate lymphoplasmacytic infiltrate with storiform fibrosis on histology, but it is considered diagnostic in the presence of both of the following:

1. Granulocytic infiltration of duct wall (GEL) with or without granulocytic acinar inflammation
2. Absent or scant (0–10 cells/HPF) IgG4-positive cells

## Parenchymal Imaging

The following features, which are similar in both AIP subtypes, may be seen on pancreatic parenchymal imaging with a CT/MRI scan:

1. Diffuse enlargement of the pancreas (also called "sausage-shaped" pancreas) with delayed enhancement (considered *typical imaging*). A capsule-like rim surrounding the diffusely enlarged gland can sometimes be seen.
2. Focal/segmental enlargement with delayed enhancement (considered *supportive imaging*).
3. *Atypical* features (low-density mass, upstream duct dilatation, pancreatic duct cutoff, and distal atrophy) which are strongly suggestive of pancreatic cancer. Normal-looking pancreas (*indeterminate imaging*) can be seen occasionally.

## Ductal Imaging

ERP features of long (> 1/3 length of the main pancreatic duct) or multiple strictures without marked upstream dilatation (duct size < 5 mm) are strongly suggestive of type 1 AIP, while segmental/focal narrowing without marked upstream dilatation are supportive.

## Serology (S)

Serum IgG4 elevations are associated with type 1, but not type 2, AIP which may be as follows:

1. Strong *(level 1)* evidence if IgG4 ≥2 X ULN.
2. Supportive (*level 2*) evidence if IgG4 <2 X ULN. This may also be seen in up to 10 % of PC.

## Other Organ Involvement (OOI)

Evidence of extrapancreatic involvement (OOI) in type 1 AIP could be as follows:

1. Strong (*level 1*) evidence: radiological evidence of proximal bile duct involvement or retroperitoneal fibrosis or demonstration of ≥3/4 histological features described above in an extrapancreatic organ
2. Supportive (*level 2)* evidence: radiological evidence of kidney involvement or clinical evidence of salivary/lacrimal gland enlargement or demonstration of 2/4 histological features described above in an extrapancreatic organ

## Steroid Responsiveness

Dramatic radiological improvement at 2 weeks of steroid treatment constitutes a positive response [9, 16].

# Diagnostic Approach

Pancreatic imaging with CT/MRI is recommended as the first basis of decision making (Fig. 9.1). In patients with *supportive/indeterminate imaging* for AIP, the next steps in the diagnostic strategy should be considered only after a negative work-up for PC. In patients with any features of PC (such as *atypical imaging* features described above), negative work-up for PC must include a negative FNA before proceeding further.

The next step is to look for collateral evidence: (1) clinical assessment for salivary/lacrimal glands and radiological review for proximal biliary strictures, retroperitoneal fibrosis, and renal involvement (**OOI**) and (2) obtain IgG4 serology (**S**). Collateral evidence may be strong, moderate, and mild or absent as described in Fig. 9.1.

Based on these noninvasive data, diagnosis of type 1 AIP can be made in many patients (clinical

**Diagnosis of AIP**

| Collateral Evidence<br>• IgG4 serology<br>• Other organ involvement | Imaging Findings: *Typical* | Imaging Findings: *Indeterminate Atypical** | Diagnosis |
|---|---|---|---|
| ***Strong***<br>Both Level 1 | ✔ | ✔ | Type 1 AIP |
| ***Moderate***<br>One Level 1 | ✔ | ✔ if<br>Response to steroids | Type 1 AIP |
| ***Weak***<br>No level 1;<br>≥1 Level 2 | ✔ | ✔ if<br>LPSP on pancreas biopsy<br>Or<br>ERP + Response to steroids | Type 1 AIP |
| ***None*** | ✔ if pancreas biopsy shows LPSP | | Type 1 AIP |
| ***None*** | ✔ if Pancreas biopsy shows IDCP | | Type 2 AIP |

✔ = Diagnostic criteria fulfilled

* In presence of atypical imaging features, negative work-up for pancreatic cancer including FNA required

**Fig. 9.1** The diagnosis of AIP based on International Consensus Diagnostic Criteria. Details of each diagnostic feature are described in the text. LPSP: Lymphoplasmacytic sclerosing pancreatitis, ICDP: Idiopathic duct centric pancreatitis

diagnosis). In others, further assessment of pancreatic histology using EUS biopsy, response to steroid treatment, or pancreatic ductal imaging with ERP may be required for diagnosis. Currently, type 2 AIP, which lacks OOI or serology, can only be diagnosed on the basis of histology.

## Clinical Diagnosis

AIP is diagnosed based on clinical features alone in these two groups which include about 50 % of type 1 AIP patients:

(A) *Typical imaging* with any collateral evidence
(B) *Supportive/atypical imaging* with strong collateral evidence

## Biopsy

In the absence of any collateral features (about 20 % of type 1 AIP patients), diagnosis of AIP can be made based on histology. Pancreatic tissue can be obtained by endoscopic ultrasound (EUS)-guided core biopsies for which referral to centers with experience in this procedure may be necessary. Fine-needle aspiration cytology (FNAC), routinely done for evaluation of pancreatic cancer, is not sufficient for histological confirmation of AIP [10, 17, 18].

## Steroid Trial

In patients with supportive/atypical imaging, diagnosis of AIP can be established through a diagnostic steroid trial in the presence of the following:

(A) Moderate collateral evidence
(B) Mild collateral evidence with consistent ERP features

It cannot be overemphasized that diagnostic steroid trial is to be used sparingly by an experienced pancreatologist only in patients with appropriate collateral evidence to confirm a suspicion of AIP. It should not be a means to diagnose AIP with the intention "if it responds to steroids, it must be AIP."

## Controversies and Pitfalls

### Utility of ERP

Diagnostic ERP has been extensively used in Japan and Korea for the diagnosis of AIP [11, 12] although this is infrequently done in the setting of obstructive jaundice in the West. ERP features can be useful in AIP but require significant training and expertise [19]. Its diagnostic utility and the inter-user agreement for AIP were poor among Western readers [19]. We found that AIP can be diagnosed in 90 % patients without ERP. Only in the subgroup of patients with moderate collateral evidence, ERP was required for diagnosis. For Western centers, we recommend the use of EUS biopsy as an alternate approach in this small subgroup.

## Ampullary Biopsies and OOI

Ampullary biopsies with IgG4 stain have been proposed as a diagnostic test for AIP although its diagnostic utility remains controversial [20–22]. In ICDC, ampullary biopsy may provide collateral evidence of other organ involvement if ≥2/4 histological features described earlier are present. We found that clinical and radiological review for OOI was sufficient in most cases and the routine use of ampullary biopsy is currently not recommended.

## False Diagnoses

One piece of mild collateral evidence may be seen in up to 12 % PC patients (mostly elevation in serum IgG4, rarely OOI in the form of renal or liver involvement with metastasis) [15]. Since PC is much more common, this subgroup of PC may be encountered commonly in practice. One may be easily misled to attempt steroid trial in such patients. Steroids can transiently lead to symptomatic improvement even in cases of PC. Thus, steroid trial should be used judiciously as discussed above. Further, reduction of IgG4 levels or subjective improvement (such as feeling better, resolution of constitutional symptoms) should not be regarded as responsiveness to steroid treatment which should be followed radiologically.

## Seronegative Type 1 AIP Versus Type 2 AIP

About 20 % of type 1 AIP patients lack any collateral evidence in the form of OOI or IgG4 seropositivity. Thus, lack of collateral features does not necessarily imply a diagnosis of type 2 AIP. These two groups have different prognosis and risk of relapse [23], and histology is necessary for a definitive diagnosis in these cases. These patients get classified as AIP-NOS or probable AIP in the absence of a diagnostic histology either due to indiscriminate steroid trial or a nondiagnostic histology.

## Conclusion

AIP is a recently recognized, rare pancreatic disease that mimics pancreatic cancer but has a benign prognosis. International consensus diagnostic criteria can be used to diagnose AIP and distinguish it from pancreatic cancer.

## References

1. Sah RP, Chari ST, Pannala R, et al. Differences in clinical profile and relapse rate of type 1 versus type 2 autoimmune pancreatitis. Gastroenterology. 2010;139(1):140–8. quiz e12-3.
2. Hart PA, Kamisawa T, Brugge WR, et al. Long-term outcomes of autoimmune pancreatitis: a multicentre, international analysis. Gut. 2012. doi:10.1136/gutjnl-2012-303617.
3. Kamisawa T, Chari ST, Giday SA, et al. Clinical profile of autoimmune pancreatitis and its histological subtypes: an international multicenter survey. Pancreas. 2011;40(6):809–14.
4. Sah RP, Pannala R, Chari ST, et al. Prevalence, diagnosis, and profile of autoimmune pancreatitis presenting with features of acute or chronic pancreatitis. Clin Gastroenterol Hepatol. 2010;8(1):91–6.
5. Nishimori I, Tamakoshi A, Otsuki M. Prevalence of autoimmune pancreatitis in Japan from a nationwide survey in 2002. J Gastroenterol. 2007;42 Suppl 18:6–8.
6. Kanno A, Nishimori I, Masamune A, et al. Nationwide epidemiological survey of autoimmune pancreatitis in Japan. Pancreas. 2012;41(6):835–9.

7. Siegel R, Naishadham D, Jemal A. Cancer statistics, 2012. CA Cancer J Clin. 2012;62(1):10–29.
8. Wolfson D, Barkin JS, Chari ST, et al. Management of pancreatic masses. Pancreas. 2005;31(3):203–17.
9. Shimosegawa T, Chari ST, Frulloni L, et al. International consensus diagnostic criteria for autoimmune pancreatitis: guidelines of the International Association of Pancreatology. Pancreas. 2011;40(3):352–8.
10. Chari ST, Smyrk TC, Levy MJ, et al. Diagnosis of autoimmune pancreatitis: the Mayo Clinic experience. Clin Gastroenterol Hepatol. 2006;4(8):1010–6. quiz 934.
11. Okazaki K, Kawa S, Kamisawa T, et al. Japanese consensus guidelines for management of autoimmune pancreatitis: I. Concept and diagnosis of autoimmune pancreatitis. J Gastroenterol. 2010;45(3):249–65.
12. Otsuki M, Chung JB, Okazaki K, et al. Asian diagnostic criteria for autoimmune pancreatitis: consensus of the Japan-Korea symposium on autoimmune pancreatitis. J Gastroenterol. 2008;43(6):403–8.
13. Frulloni L, Scattolini C, Falconi M, et al. Autoimmune pancreatitis: differences between the focal and diffuse forms in 87 patients. Am J Gastroenterol. 2009;104(9):2288–94.
14. Schneider A, Lohr JM, Singer MV. The M-ANNHEIM classification of chronic pancreatitis: introduction of a unifying classification system based on a review of previous classifications of the disease. J Gastroenterol. 2007;42(2):101–19.
15. Chari ST, Takahashi N, Levy MJ, et al. A diagnostic strategy to distinguish autoimmune pancreatitis from pancreatic cancer. Clin Gastroenterol Hepatol. 2009;7(10):1097–103.
16. Moon SH, Kim MH, Park DH, et al. Is a 2-week steroid trial after initial negative investigation for malignancy useful in differentiating autoimmune pancreatitis from pancreatic cancer? A prospective outcome study. Gut. 2008;57(12):1704–12.
17. Mizuno N, Bhatia V, Hosoda W, et al. Histological diagnosis of autoimmune pancreatitis using EUS-guided trucut biopsy: a comparison study with EUS-FNA. J Gastroenterol. 2009;44(7):742–50.
18. Iwashita T, Yasuda I, Doi S, et al. Use of samples from endoscopic ultrasound-guided 19-gauge fine-needle aspiration in diagnosis of autoimmune pancreatitis. Clin Gastroenterol Hepatol. 2012;10(3):316–22.
19. Sugumar A, Levy MJ, Kamisawa T, et al. Endoscopic retrograde pancreatography criteria to diagnose autoimmune pancreatitis: an international multicentre study. Gut. 2011;60(5):666–70.
20. Moon SH, Kim MH, do Park H, et al. IgG4 immunostaining of duodenal papillary biopsy specimens may be useful for supporting a diagnosis of autoimmune pancreatitis. Gastrointest Endosc. 2010;71(6):960–6.
21. Kamisawa T, Tu Y, Egawa N, et al. A new diagnostic endoscopic tool for autoimmune pancreatitis. Gastrointest Endosc. 2008;68(2):358–61.
22. Rebours V, Le Baleur Y, Cazals-Hatem D, et al. IgG4 immunostaining of gastric, duodenal or colonic biopsies is not helpful for the diagnosis of autoimmune pancreatitis. Clin Gastroenterol Hepatol. 2012; 10(1):91–4.
23. Balasubramanian G, Sugumar A, Smyrk TC, et al. Demystifying seronegative autoimmune pancreatitis. Pancreatology. 2012;12(4):289–94.

# 10 Surgical Implications

Clancy J. Clark, Carlos Fernandez-del Castillo,
and Michael B. Farnell

## Introduction

Autoimmune pancreatitis (AIP) frequently mimics pancreatic cancer and is challenging to diagnose without pathologic confirmation. For the surgeon, AIP is a rare diagnosis typically found after pancreatic resection for suspected pancreatic cancer. Given the dismal outcomes with pancreatic cancer and the dramatic effects of corticosteroids in the treatment of AIP, the desire to recognize a patient with AIP prior to surgery is high. In this chapter, we discuss the surgeon's role as a pragmatist in the diagnosis and management of autoimmune pancreatitis.

In 1961, Sarles et al. described "primary inflammatory sclerosis of the pancreas" [1]. It was not until the 1990s that autoimmune pancreatitis was recognized as a defined entity distinct from other forms of pancreatitis. The term "autoimmune pancreatitis" encompasses a multitude of histologic findings described as primary chronic pancreatitis, chronic sclerosing pancreatitis, nonalcoholic duct-destructive chronic pancreatitis, lymphoplasmacytic sclerosing pancreatitis, and duct-narrowing chronic pancreatitis [2]. Yoshida et al., in a 1995 case report, proposed steroid therapy as a treatment option for this rare pancreatic disorder [3].

Prior to the 1990s, surgeons performed pancreatic resection for suspected pancreatic adenocarcinoma and occasionally discovered "benign" pancreatitis on final pathology. Similarly, patients thought to have chronic pancreatitis complicated by biliary obstruction or refractory abdominal pain underwent pancreatic resection with final pathology confirming "chronic pancreatitis." Over the last decade, we have learned from retrospective single-institution studies that many of these patients had autoimmune pancreatitis [4, 5]. Since AIP is a rare and newly recognized entity, much of our understanding of the surgical implications of this disease is limited. Moreover, the literature is biased by dramatic resolution of the inflammatory process with steroid therapy in a limited number of highly selected patients.

## Presentation

Autoimmune pancreatitis frequently mimics pancreatic cancer with a typical presentation of weight loss and painless jaundice in an older male [2]. When imaging studies demonstrate a mass in the head of the pancreas, pancreatic cancer is the most likely diagnosis. With an overall 5-year survival under 5 % and surgical resection the only potentially curative therapy, surgeons have a responsibility to anticipate pancreatic

C.J. Clark, MD (✉)
Wake Forest Baptist Health, Medical Center Blvd., Winston-Salem, NC 27157, USA
e-mail: cjclark@wakehealth.edu

C.F.-d. Castillo, MD
Department of Surgery, Massachusetts General Hospital, Boston, MA, USA

M.B. Farnell, MD
Mayo Clinic, 200 1st ST SW, Rochester, MN 55905, USA

M.J. Levy and S.T. Chari (eds.), *Autoimmune (IgG4-related) Pancreatitis and Cholangitis*,
DOI 10.1007/978-1-4419-6430-4_10, © Springer Science+Business Media New York 2013

**Table 10.1** Clinical characteristics of autoimmune pancreatitis

| Parameter | Findings |
|---|---|
| Presentation | Jaundice<br>Weight loss<br>Abdominal pain<br>Malabsorption and steatorrhea |
| Past medical history | Diabetes<br>Inflammatory bowel disease<br>Sjogren's syndrome<br>Primary sclerosing cholangitis<br>Retroperitoneal fibrosis<br>Riedel's thyroiditis<br>Mediastinal adenopathy<br>Interstitial nephritis<br>No history of alcohol abuse |

resection in all patients with a resectable lesion in the pancreas. Improving our understanding of how AIP presents can help surgeons develop a preoperative evaluation strategy and facilitate counseling of patients on the likelihood of pancreatic cancer versus AIP. A summary of clinical characteristics of AIP is outlined in Table 10.1.

Although AIP is an inflammatory process of the pancreas, it does not typically present as acute or chronic pancreatitis. Sah et al. reported that 24 % of AIP patients presented with acute pancreatitis and 11 % presented as chronic pancreatitis [6].

In patients evaluated for acute or chronic pancreatitis at Mayo Clinic over an 18-month period, only 3.5 % (7 of 178) had autoimmune pancreatitis [6]. Both exocrine and endocrine dysfunctions of the pancreas, such as steatorrhea and diabetes, have been described in patients with AIP. Diffuse AIP may present with chronic pancreatitis-like symptoms, while focal AIP can present with a pseudotumor and biliary obstruction [2].

Up to 75 % of patients with known autoimmune pancreatitis will present with obstructive jaundice [6]. Abraham et al. reviewed the pancreaticoduodenectomy experience at Johns Hopkins and identified 9 % of patients (40 of 442) had benign disease despite preoperative suspicion for malignancy [5]. Of these patients, 68 % had a concerning mass, 40 % had common bile duct strictures, and 13 % had false-positive cytology. Half of these patients presented with jaundice. Autoimmune pancreatitis was identified in 23 % of patients (11 of 47) found to have benign disease on final pathology.

Weber et al. at Memorial Sloan-Kettering Cancer Center (MSKCC) examined their experience with AIP from 1985 to 2001 [7]. During this study period, 12 % of patients (159 of 1,287) that underwent pancreatic resection were found to have benign disease. AIP represented 23 % ($n=31$) of patients with benign disease. Only 6 of the 31 patients with AIP had a preoperative history suggestive of an autoimmune process.

Patients with a final diagnosis of either autoimmune pancreatitis or pancreatic cancer have similar clinical characteristics at presentation including age, weight loss, abdominal pain, incidence of diabetes, rate of alcohol abuse, and history of pancreatitis [4, 8]. In the Johns Hopkins series, none of the patients with autoimmune pancreatitis had a history of alcohol abuse or choledocholithiasis [4]. The only noticeable difference between AIP and pancreatic cancer patients was computed tomography (CT) imaging where discrete lesions were more common in the cancer group while autoimmune pancreatitis had more diffuse enlargement of the pancreas [4].

Recent reports have suggested two subtypes of AIP described by Park et al. as type 1 and type 2 [9, 10]. Type 1 AIP is likely a systemic IgG4-associated disease that may involve extrapancreatic organs as well. Serum IgG4 levels are typically elevated and immunohistochemical staining of pancreatic tissue for IgG4 is robust. Type 1 AIP can involve the bile duct, retroperitoneum, kidney, lymph nodes, and salivary glands [9]. When the biliary tree is involved with AIP, it frequently mimics primary sclerosing cholangitis or cholangiocarcinoma. IgG4-associated inflammatory disease can also spare the pancreas as described in case reports of IgG4 cholangitis [11–13].

Less is known about type 2 AIP. It occurs typically in younger patients (fourth decade) with equal distribution between the sexes. Type 2 AIP has been associated with inflammatory bowel disease. Unlike type 1, type 2 AIP is typically IgG4 seronegative. Currently, type 2 AIP has no surrogate biomarker and requires histologic evaluation for diagnosis [9, 10].

## Diagnosis

Three diagnostic criteria schemes exist for autoimmune pancreatitis: the Asian, Mayo HISORt, and Italian criteria. The Asian diagnostic criteria were developed at a consensus conference held in Seoul, Korea, in 2007 involving Japanese and Korean gastroenterologists. The Asian criteria require either radiographic evidence that supports AIP with hypergammaglobulinemia or abundant IgG4-positive cells on staining of pancreatic tissue [14]. The HISORt criteria outlined by Mayo Clinic combine histology, imaging, serology, and other organ involvement with clinical response to steroid treatment [8]. The Italian criteria require three of four diagnostic features in medically managed patients: (1) histology or cytology that should exclude pancreatic cancer and may reveal the presence of granulocyte epithelial lesion, (2) suggestive radiological findings, (3) association with other autoimmune diseases or extrapancreatic involvement, or (4) response to steroid therapy [15]. Currently, no simple diagnostic test exists for AIP. Preoperative indicators of autoimmune pancreatitis are outlined in Table 10.2.

**Table 10.2** Diagnostic features of autoimmune pancreatitis

| Parameter | Findings |
|---|---|
| Laboratory tests | Elevated IgG or IgG4 |
| CT/MRI | Diffusely enlarged pancreas |
| | Smooth contour of pancreas |
| | Capsule-like rim enhancement of pancreas |
| ERCP/MRCP | Small main pancreatic duct |
| | Stricture or narrowing of pancreatic duct |
| Histology | IgG4-positive staining cells (> 10/high power field) |
| | Storiform fibrosis |
| | Periductal lymphoplasmacytic infiltrate |
| | Obliterative phlebitis |

*CT* computed tomography, *MRI* magnetic resonance imaging, *ERCP* endoscopic retrograde cholangiopancreatography, *MRCP* magnetic resonance cholangiopancreatography

Laboratory studies are generally nonspecific for autoimmune pancreatitis. Sah et al. reported that liver function tests were abnormal at presentation in 86 % of patients (50 of 58) [6]. In a case series by Hardacre et al., CA 19-9 was elevated in both AIP ($n=17$, mean 145 U/mL) and pancreatic cancer ($n=25$, mean 369 U/mL), but CA19-9 levels were not statistically different [4]. However, Chari et al. from Mayo Clinic reported that CA 19-9 levels over 150 U/mL were less common in AIP patients (3 of 39, 8 %) compared to pancreatic cancer patients (56 of 91, 62 %) [8].

The laboratory hallmark of AIP is an elevated serum IgG4. In 2001, Hamano et al. described elevated serum IgG4 in AIP patients, while patients with other pancreaticobiliary disorders have levels of IgG4 similar to normal subjects [16]. Twenty patients with AIP and 70 patients with pancreatic cancer were included in the study. Diagnosis of AIP was based on main pancreatic duct narrowing and gland swelling that responded to glucocorticoid therapy. AIP was not confirmed with histology. With a serum cutoff of 135 mg/dL, IgG4 was 95 % sensitive and 97 % specific for the differentiation of AIP from pancreatic cancer [16]. Subsequent studies have not been able to achieve such high sensitivity or specificity. In a 2009 meta-analysis of the current literature on IgG4 testing, Morselli-Labate et al. found that sensitivities range from 67 % to 100 % and specificities are typically over 90 % except for one study that reported a specificity of 64 % [17]. Although IgG4 is a useful test for diagnosing AIP, it should be remembered that 10 % of patients with pancreatic cancer will have an elevated IgG4 [8].

High-quality multidetector contrast-enhanced computed tomography (CT) can differentiate AIP from pancreatic cancer in selected patients. Diffuse pancreatic enlargement is suggestive of AIP (Fig. 10.1). Other subtle findings of AIP include smooth contour of the pancreas, early capsule-like rim enhancement, and delayed but uniform pancreatic enhancement with a persisting rim of hyper-attenuation [2]. Although initial reports and diagnostic schemes from Japan and Korea suggested that entire gland involvement was necessary for the diagnosis of AIP, focal and segmental involvement have been reported and

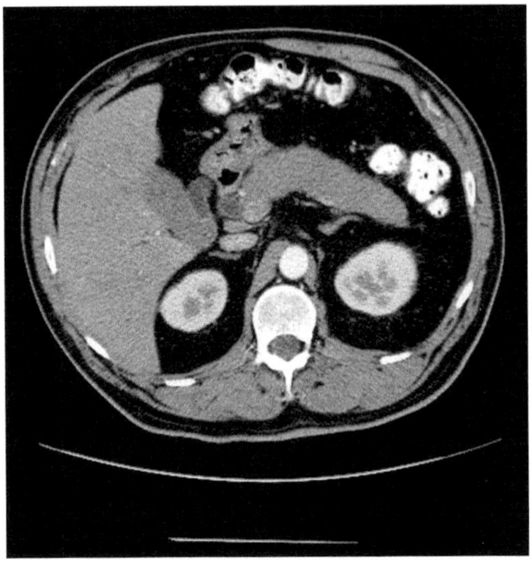

**Fig. 10.1** CT image of diffuse pancreatic enlargement in a patient with autoimmune pancreatitis

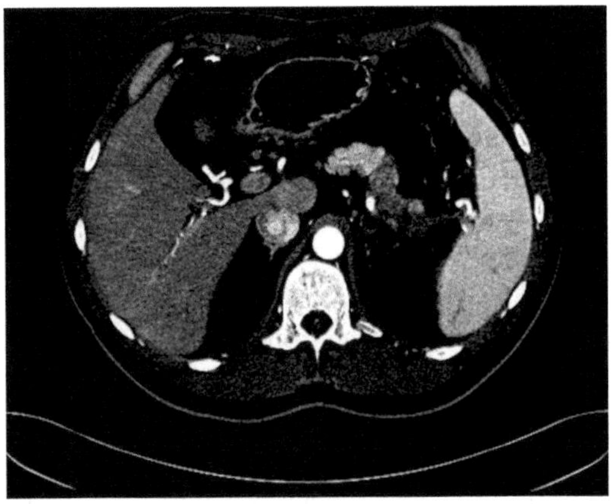

**Fig. 10.2** Autoimmune pancreatitis mimicking pancreatic cancer on CT. Hypodense mass in tail of pancreas

are readily visible on imaging. In many cases, focal AIP shares similar features on CT with pancreatic cancer making the diagnosis of AIP impossible by CT alone (Fig. 10.2). In the MSKCC series of 31 resected AIP patients, Weber et al. noted that the most common radiographic findings were a pancreatic mass (61 %) or biliary stricture (23 %) both of which are features worrisome for malignancy [7].

Unlike acute or chronic pancreatitis, CT imaging should not demonstrate fluid collections, fat stranding, necrosis, pseudocysts, calcifications, or a dilated pancreatic duct. Likewise, CT findings concerning for pancreatic cancer should not be present, such as suspicious liver lesions, pancreatic duct cutoff, or distal pancreatic atrophy [8].

Imaging based on magnetic resonance cholangiopancreatography (MRCP) or endoscopic retrograde cholangiopancreatography (ERCP) is limited in their ability to differentiate carcinoma from benign strictures. Distal bile duct strictures of AIP may present with characteristics typical of adenocarcinoma, with an irregular or shelf-like contour or more segmental as seen in primary sclerosing cholangitis; by contrast, biliary strictures in chronic (non-autoimmune) pancreatitis usually have a smooth contour. As outlined in the Asian diagnostic criteria for AIP, pancreatic duct stenosis and narrowing are important radiographic findings. As described in the Johns Hopkins series, distal common bile duct involvement was common (7 of 11, 72.7 %) in AIP patients who had pancreaticoduodenectomy for suspected malignancy [5].

Although elevated serum levels of IgG4 and imaging characteristics may suggest autoimmune pancreatitis, histologic evaluation remains the gold standard for diagnosis. Pancreatic and bile duct brushings do not provide sufficient tissue architecture to diagnose AIP but may confirm a diagnosis of pancreatic or biliary malignancy. Brush cytology is very specific for pancreaticobiliary malignancies but can be very insensitive (26–89 %) [18]. Brush cytology and endoscopic evaluation of the pancreatic and biliary ducts should be limited to patients presenting with obstructive jaundice that require biliary drainage.

Given the proximity of the stomach and duodenum to the pancreas, endoscopic ultrasound (EUS) provides detailed images of the pancreas enabling assessment of the main pancreatic duct, side branches, solid and cystic lesions, and local adenopathy. EUS-guided fine-needle aspiration (FNA) can provide sufficient sampling to facilitate a diagnosis of pancreatic cancer. Recently studies have proposed the use of core needle biopsy of pancreatic parenchyma to facilitate the diagnosis of AIP [8]. EUS-guided core needle biopsy appears to be safe with a complication rate of 2.4 % (6 of 247) [19]. Currently, we have limited experience with EUS-guided core needle biopsy, and its role in preoperative evaluation of AIP versus pancreatic cancer is not known. In addition, EUS-guided core needle biopsy is limited to body and tail lesions.

In the preoperative assessment, the main goal of brushing cytology, FNA, or core needle biopsy should be to facilitate a diagnosis of pancreaticobiliary malignancy. The absence of malignant cells neither confirms a diagnosis of AIP nor excludes underlying malignancy. Abundance of IgG4-positive cells is required for the diagnosis of AIP using the Asian criteria. However, AIP may be IgG4 positive in only 50 % of patients [2]. In addition, sampling error maybe a significant issue given the potential patchy distribution of AIP [20]. Chandan et al. reexamined 39 pancreatic resection specimens for parenchymal sparing and distribution of AIP within the specimen. They identified 82 % of specimens had histologically unremarkable (spared) parenchyma abutting classic changes of AIP. Positive IgG4 staining was correlated with histologic evidence of AIP, while areas of parenchymal sparing lacked IgG4 staining ($p<0.0001$). This study suggests that FNA and core needle biopsy could easily miss AIP during a preoperative evaluation.

The final step in fulfilling the criteria for a diagnosis of AIP is a trial period of steroid therapy. Moon et al. investigated a 2-week trial of steroid therapy in 22 consecutive patients that had a suspected diagnosis of AIP and a negative workup for malignancy. In this study, all patients who did not demonstrate response to steroids (7 of 22) during a 2-week trial were diagnosed with pancreatic adenocarcinoma [21]. Importantly, Moon et al. reported that during the study period, 1091 patients were diagnosed with pancreatic cancer and 348 patients underwent major pancreatic resections. This would indicate after careful selection only 2 % of patients were considered candidates for a trial of steroids.

At this time, we strongly discourage attempting a steroid trial to confirm a diagnosis of AIP unless a multidisciplinary team has exhausted all efforts to diagnosis pancreatic cancer. Tissue sampling should have been obtained on two separate occasions. A steroid trial should be limited to 2 weeks and strict objective criteria for continued therapy must be outlined with the managing team and the patient prior to starting steroid therapy. Importantly, response to steroid therapy alone does not confirm a diagnosis of AIP, since inflammatory changes adjacent to adenocarcinoma may respond to steroid therapy leading to an error in diagnosis. Response to steroid therapy should complement other collateral evidence of AIP.

## Indications for Surgical Intervention

No specific guidelines exist for the surgical management of AIP. Conventional wisdom would suggest that painless jaundice and a resectable mass in the head of the pancreas (with double duct sign) require no further evaluation and resection is warranted. In light of the growing understanding of AIP, Chari et al. have proposed an algorithm to guide surgeons and gastroenterologists in the evaluation of AIP patients [8]. Significant emphasis in the evaluation of suspected AIP is interpretation of imaging studies. Application of such an algorithm depends on a multidisciplinary team interested in pancreatology and pancreatic imaging.

In patients with uncertain diagnosis or any suspicion for malignancy, operative intervention is indicated. After a 2-week trial of steroids, failure to demonstrate objective improvement (e.g., resolution of main duct narrowing and decrease in size of pancreatic mass) also mandates surgical intervention. Surgical resection is then diagnostic and potentially therapeutic. Since AIP may represent a systemic process, diagnosis of AIP at the time of resection should guide subsequent follow-up. Likewise, recognition of AIP as a separate entity from chronic pancreatitis provides opportunity for nonoperative treatment strategies if recurrence is noted in the remnant pancreas.

Steroid therapy is generally successful with 87–98 % in remission by 3 months. Relapsing

AIP occurs in 6–54 % of patients [2, 22]. Patients who develop complications associated with long-term corticosteroid therapy may be candidates for operative therapy. With a confirmed diagnosis of AIP, surgical intervention does not require resection. Biliary bypass, such as hepaticoduodenostomy or hepaticojejunostomy, should be considered in AIP patients with persistent jaundice or those who have become dependent on biliary stents. Long-term outcomes in patients treated with medical therapy are currently not known. Also, indications for surgical intervention in recurrent or relapsing AIP are not yet defined.

## Operative Considerations

Unless the surgeon has histologic confirmation of AIP, a pancreatic resection should be approached using oncologic principles. All specimens should be resected with adequate margins and with an appropriate lymphadenectomy. The specimen should be oriented and inked for evaluation by pathology. Intraoperative biopsies are not necessary because important diagnostic information (e.g., IgG4 staining) is not immediately available.

Our current understanding of pancreatic resection for AIP is based on a retrospective review of operative notes. The difficulty of pancreatectomy is likely dependent on the location and extent of pancreatic involvement. The majority of resected patients in published series were managed with pancreaticoduodenectomy. In the MSKCC series, Weber et al. reported that 79 % (23 or 29) had pancreaticoduodenectomy, 14 % (4 of 29) had distal pancreatectomy, and 7 % (2 of 29) had total pancreatectomy [7]. At the time of operation, two additional patients were not resected due to encasement of the superior mesenteric artery and portal vein.

In a retrospective review of operative notes for autoimmune pancreatitis at Johns Hopkins, pancreaticoduodenectomy was considered difficult in 71 % of patients compared with 44 % of patients with pancreatic cancer [4]. Patients with AIP had more intraoperative blood loss (1,290 mL [range 250–5,200] vs. 832 mL [range 250–3,000]; $p < 0.05$) compared with pancreatic cancer patients but similar postoperative morbidity and mortality. In a small series of eight patients, Schnelldorfer et al. found no significant difference in operative times, blood loss, or perioperative morbidity in patients with AIP compared to control patients who underwent resection for chronic pancreatitis [23].

## Surgical Experience at Mayo and Massachusetts General Hospital

In a retrospective review of the surgical experience at Mayo Clinic Rochester and Massachusetts General Hospital from 1986 to 2011, 69 patients underwent pancreatic resection for autoimmune pancreatitis. Sixty-eight percent ($n=47$) of patients were male with a median age of 60 (IQR 46–68). Preoperative diagnosis included concern for malignancy 78.3 % ($n=54$), pancreatitis 13.0 % ($n=9$), preoperative biopsy or fine-needle aspiration positive for malignancy 5.8 % ($n=4$), or unknown 2.9 % ($n=2$). One patient (1.5 %) underwent distal pancreatectomy for autoimmune pancreatitis refractory to medical therapy. Autoimmune pancreatitis was considered in the preoperative differential in four patients (5.8 %). The majority of patients underwent standard pancreaticoduodenectomy ($n=36$, 52.2 %) or pylorus-preserving pancreaticoduodenectomy ($n=18$, 26.1 %). Distal pancreatectomy was performed in 13 patients (18.8 %) and total pancreatectomy in two patients (2.9 %). Operative details are outlined in Table 10.3. Thirty patients (43.5 %) had a postoperative complication in the first 30 days and one postoperative death. Five patients (7.3 %) developed a postoperative pancreatic fistula (ISGPF grade A, $n=3$, 4.4 %; grade B, $n=1$, 1.5 %; grade C, $n=1$, 1.5 %).

For patients who underwent pancreatic resection for autoimmune pancreatitis, median follow-up was 58.4 months ($n=58$, IQR 24.8–115.3 months). Eighteen (26.1 %) patients have developed postoperative diabetes mellitus and 24 (34.8 %) patients have exocrine insufficiency with steatorrhea requiring pancreatic enzyme replacement. Postoperatively, 15 (21.7 %) patients have been

**Table 10.3** Operative details for pancreatic resection at Mayo Clinic Rochester and Massachusetts General Hospital ($n=69$)

| Variable | n (%) |
|---|---|
| Operation | |
| Standard pancreaticoduodenectomy | 36 (52.2) |
| Pylorus-preserving pancreaticoduodenectomy | 18 (26.1) |
| Distal pancreatectomy with splenectomy | 8 (11.6) |
| Distal pancreatectomy without splenectomy | 5 (7.2) |
| Total pancreatectomy | 2 (2.9) |
| Operative time, min, median (IQR) | 337 (236–408) |
| Estimated blood loss, mL, median (IQR) | 600 (300–1,170) |
| Blood transfuse within 24 h of operation | 16 (23.2) |
| Difficult operation per operative note | 34 (49.3) |
| Intraoperative complication | 16 (23.2) |
| Portal vein/SMV repair or reconstruction | 16 (23.5) |

*IQR* interquartile range

treated with glucocorticoids. Late reoperation (> 30 days) was required in 6 (8.7 %) patients and endoscopic intervention required in seven patients (pancreatic stent, $n=3$, 4.4 %; biliary stent, $n=4$, 5.8 %). Overall 5- and 10-year survival were 89.1 % and 80.5 %, respectively.

## Recurrent Disease and Quality of Life After Resection

Perioperative morbidity is comparable between pancreatic cancer and AIP patients who undergo pancreatic resection. Less is known about long-term outcomes. Should the surgeon and patient celebrate or are we trading a lethal disease with a chronic disease? At MSKCC, eight of 29 (28 %) patients who underwent resection for AIP developed recurrent symptoms requiring intervention [7]. Patients who presented without a discrete pancreatic mass and those treated with distal pancreatectomy were more likely to have recurrent symptoms (Fig. 10.3). Nearly all patients (7 of 8) with recurrent symptoms were managed with endoscopic or percutaneous biliary drainage. Only one patient was treated with steroid therapy to control recurrent disease. No patients required surgical intervention.

Schnelldorfer et al. reported that two of the eight patients with AIP treated with pancreatic resection developed recurrent jaundice [23]. One presented with biliary sepsis early in the postoperative period and the second patient developed recurrence at 6 months. No patients received postoperative steroid therapy. However, two patients with persistent abdominal pain received trial corticosteroids with no benefit. No patients required reoperation in this series.

In the Johns Hopkins series of 37 patients, no patients developed recurrent jaundice and only one patient developed recurrent episodes of abdominal pain and pancreatitis [4]. Median follow-up was 33 months. Eleven percent of patients (4 of 37) required subsequent operations for bowel obstruction or ventral hernia.

Quality of life after pancreatic resection for AIP has not been well investigated. Hardacre et al. conducted follow-up telephone interviews with 24 AIP patients treated with pancreaticoduodenectomy. In this series, 68 % of patients reported an improvement in quality of life, 18 % no change, and 14 % had a decrease in quality of life [4]. In a small series of eight patients with mean 5-year follow-up, Schnelldorfer et al. reported that 57 % of patients (4 of 7) had good quality of life based on SF-36 questionnaires [23].

## Conclusion

The surgeon's role in diagnosing and managing AIP is to provide a conservative and realistic perspective. The majority of patients suspected of AIP will have pancreatic cancer. A multidisciplinary team can facilitate the diagnosis of AIP in the preoperative period and should focus on high-quality imaging, serum IgG4, and histologic confirmation. A short 2-week course of corticosteroids should be tested only on carefully selected patients. Pathologic evaluation of a pancreatic resection specimen remains the gold standard for diagnosing AIP. The role of pancreatic resection for known AIP is not well defined. In the limited

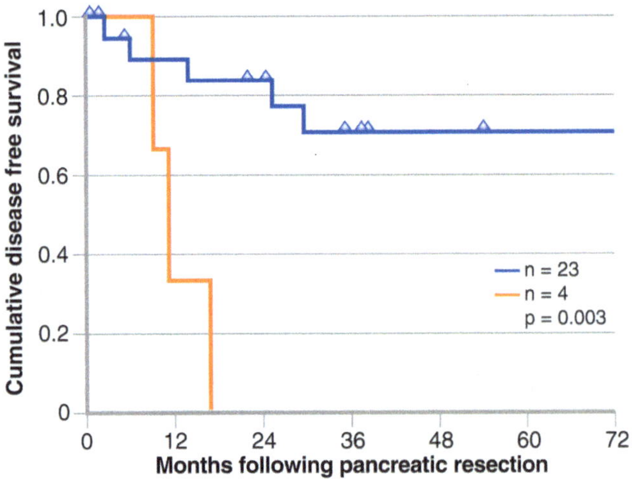


**Fig. 10.3** Time to recurrent symptoms of autoimmune pancreatitis according to type of resection. Distal pancreatectomy (*dash line*) versus pancreaticoduodenectomy (*solid line*) ([7]. Permission to reproduce being requested from JOGS/Springer)

number of studies, the diagnosis of AIP does not increase the morbidity or mortality of pancreatic resection. Surgeons should anticipate significant inflammation with loss of planes and adherence to adjacent structures (e.g., portal vein) during the resection of pancreatic specimens. Although relapsing AIP is not infrequent, only a minority (0–28 %) of patients will develop recurrent symptoms after resection. Since AIP is a clinically distinct entity from chronic pancreatitis, we must carefully monitor these patients after resection. Steroid therapy has not been investigated in resected patients but may play some role in controlling the disease and suppressing symptoms. Lastly, with limited long-term follow-up, the role of the surgeon has not been defined for patients that fail steroid therapy, develop multiple recurrences, or have continued bile or pancreatic duct obstructive symptoms despite steroid therapy. Care for patients with AIP requires careful individualized care by a team of surgeons, radiologists, and gastroenterologists interested in this disease.

## References

1. Sarles H, Sarles JC, Muratore R, Guien C. Chronic inflammatory sclerosis of the pancreas–an autonomous pancreatic disease? Am J Dig Dis. 1961;6:688–98.
2. Buscarini E, Frulloni L, De Lisi S, et al. Autoimmune pancreatitis: a challenging diagnostic puzzle for clinicians. Dig Liver Dis. 2010;42(2):92–8.
3. Yoshida K, Toki F, Takeuchi T, et al. Chronic pancreatitis caused by an autoimmune abnormality. Dig Dis Sci. 1995;40(7):1561–8.
4. Hardacre JM, Iacobuzio-Donahue CA, Sohn TA, et al. Results of pancreaticoduodenectomy for lymphoplasmacytic sclerosing pancreatitis. Ann Surg. 2003;237(6):853–8. discussion 858-9.
5. Abraham SC, Wilentz RE, Yeo CJ, et al. Pancreaticoduodenectomy (Whipple resections) in patients without malignancy: are they all "chronic pancreatitis"? Am J Surg Pathol. 2003;27(1):110–20.
6. Sah RP, Pannala R, Chari ST, et al. Prevalence, diagnosis, and profile of autoimmune pancreatitis presenting with features of acute or chronic pancreatitis. Clin Gastroenterol Hepatol. 2010;8(1):91–6.
7. Weber SM, Cubukcu-Dimopulo O, Palesty JA, et al. Lymphoplasmacytic sclerosing pancreatitis: inflammatory mimic of pancreatic carcinoma. J Gastrointest Surg. 2003;7(1):129–37. discussion 137-9.
8. Chari ST, Takahashi N, Levy MJ, et al. A diagnostic strategy to distinguish autoimmune pancreatitis from pancreatic cancer. Clin Gastroenterol Hepatol. 2009;7(10):1097–103.
9. Park DH, Kim M-H, Chari ST. Recent advances in autoimmune pancreatitis. Gut. 2009;58(12):1680–9.
10. Chari ST, Longnecker DS, Klöppel G. The diagnosis of autoimmune pancreatitis: a Western perspective. Pancreas. 2009;38(8):846–8.
11. Iida Y, Onitsuka A, Katagiri Y. Immunoglobulin G4-related sclerosing cholangitis without pancreatic involvement. Dig Surg. 2009;26(2):117–8.
12. Webster GJM, Pereira SP, Chapman RW. Autoimmune pancreatitis/IgG4-associated cholangitis and primary sclerosing cholangitis–overlapping or separate diseases? J Hepatol. 2009;51(2):398–402.

13. Kobayashi T, Teruya M, Shimizu S. Immunoglobulin G4-associated cholangitis. Surgery. 2010;147(5):748–9.
14. Otsuki M, Chung JB, Okazaki K, et al. Asian diagnostic criteria for autoimmune pancreatitis: consensus of the Japan-Korea symposium on autoimmune pancreatitis. J Gastroenterol. 2008;43(6):403–8.
15. Frulloni L, Scattolini C, Falconi M, et al. Autoimmune pancreatitis: differences between the focal and diffuse forms in 87 patients. Am J Gastroenterol. 2009;104(9):2288–94.
16. Hamano H, Kawa S, Horiuchi A, et al. High serum IgG4 concentrations in patients with sclerosing pancreatitis. N Eng J Med. 2001;344(10):732–8.
17. Morselli-Labate AM, Pezzilli R. Usefulness of serum IgG4 in the diagnosis and follow up of autoimmune pancreatitis: a systematic literature review and meta-analysis. J Gastroenterol Hepatol. 2009;24(1):15–36.
18. Volmar KE, Vollmer RT, Routbort MJ, Creager AJ. Pancreatic and bile duct brushing cytology in 1000 cases: review of findings and comparison of preparation methods. Cancer. 2006;108(4):231–8.
19. Thomas T, Kaye PV, Ragunath K, Aithal G. Efficacy, safety, and predictive factors for a positive yield of EUS-guided Trucut biopsy: a large tertiary referral center experience. Am J Gastroenterol. 2009;104(3):584–91.
20. Chandan VS, Iacobuzio-Donahue C, Abraham SC. Patchy distribution of pathologic abnormalities in autoimmune pancreatitis: implications for preoperative diagnosis. Am J Surg Pathol. 2008;32(12): 1762–9.
21. Moon S-H, Kim M-H, Park DH, et al. Is a 2-week steroid trial after initial negative investigation for malignancy useful in differentiating autoimmune pancreatitis from pancreatic cancer? A prospective outcome study. Gut. 2008;57(12):1704–12.
22. Zamboni G, Capelli P, Scarpa A, et al. Nonneoplastic mimickers of pancreatic neoplasms. Arch Pathol Lab Med. 2009;133(3):439–53.
23. Schnelldorfer T, Lewin DN, Adams DB. Long-term results after surgery for autoimmune sclerosing pancreatitis. J Gastrointest Surg. 2007;11(1):56–8.

# 11 Approach to Therapy

Phil A. Hart and Suresh T. Chari

## Introduction

Autoimmune pancreatitis (AIP) and IgG4-associated cholangitis (IAC) are part of a systemic fibro-inflammatory disease that can involve multiple organs which characteristically have a lymphoplasmacytic infiltrate with abundant IgG4-positive cells. The term IgG4-related disease (IgG4-RD) has been proposed by consensus as the umbrella term to describe this multiorgan disease [1]. The target of therapy in IgG4-RD is the inflammatory process which is exquisitely sensitive to steroids, in contrast to the fibrosis which can often lead to damage and even destruction of the involved organ.

## Definitions of Treatment Outcomes

When discussing treatment in AIP, it is important to use specific terms that help identify treatment goals and responses.

*Remission*: Refers to the resolution of various aspects of the disease process. Remission can be as follows:

(a) Symptomatic: Refers to resolution of presenting symptoms, for example, jaundice or abdominal pain. This occurs promptly following start of therapy.
(b) Biochemical: Normalization of liver test abnormalities due to biliary stricture; this is an important indicator of disease remission in IAC.
(c) Serologic: Associated with normalization of serum IgG4. This is not always achieved and it does not correlate with radiologic remission.
(d) Radiologic: Resolution or stable improvement in imaging abnormalities.
(e) Histologic: Implies complete absence of the inflammatory component. This is almost never confirmed in clinical practice due to the ability to follow the preceding less invasive markers of disease activity. Moreover, the patchy nature of disease makes it difficult to conclusively prove histologic remission.

*Recrudescence*: Refers to flare of the disease which is not yet in remission, for example, during steroid taper.

*Relapse*: Recurrence of disease after complete remission. Relapse can be as follows:

(a) Symptomatic: For example, recurrence of jaundice. Abdominal pain in the absence of other objective evidence of relapse is not a common feature of the disease.
(b) Biochemical: Rise of liver test abnormalities >2–3× upper limit of normal suggests biliary relapse, even before jaundice develops.
(c) Serologic: While elevation of serum IgG4 levels often precedes or accompanies relapses, it can also occur without evidence

P.A. Hart, MD (✉) • S.T. Chari, MD
Division of Gastroenterology and Hepatology, Internal Medicine, Mayo Clinic College of Medicine, 200 First Street SW, Rochester, MN 55905, USA
e-mail: hart.philip@mayo.edu

M.J. Levy and S.T. Chari (eds.), *Autoimmune (IgG4-related) Pancreatitis and Cholangitis*, DOI 10.1007/978-1-4419-6430-4_11, of relapse. Relapses can also be seronegative, that is, without accompanying elevation in serum IgG4. So, serum IgG4 elevation alone should not be considered disease relapse.

(d) Radiologic: Development of new imaging abnormalities signifies true relapse. This may occur in an organ not previously known to be affected.

(e) Histologic: True disease relapse shows evidence of inflammation in the involved organ.

## Principles of Management of AIP and IAC

Patients may present either acutely (e.g., with obstructive jaundice) or in the late or post-acute phase of disease, many months after initial onset of symptoms. The disease is treated if symptomatic or is active, as assessed by persistent or worsening radiographic or biochemical parameters. There is no benefit to treating burnt-out disease (e.g., an atrophic pancreas). The initial goal of therapy is to induce remission, which refers to the treatment of acute symptomatic and radiologic manifestations of AIP with the goal of achieving disease control. Induction treatment frequently requires adjuvant therapy due to either disease- or treatment-related complications. Maintenance of disease remission refers to the prevention of subsequent disease relapse with maintenance therapy.

## Induction of Remission

Remission may occur spontaneously or with steroids (steroid-induced remission), keeping in mind that in AIP, fibrosis-induced glandular and ductal distortion may prevent complete restitution of the gland to normal architecture (and hence normal appearance on imaging).

### Management of the Acute Presentation of AIP

Currently steroids are the only proven approach for inducing disease remission in AIP. Our understanding of the effects of steroid treatment in the acute phase of AIP is evolving. The benefits of steroid therapy are as follows:

(a) *Quick Response*: The use of steroids brings about remission consistently and more quickly than if no treatment were given. Steroids rapidly relieve disease-related symptoms (abdominal pain, obstructive jaundice). If diagnosis is certain, biliary stenting can be avoided as jaundice is promptly relieved by steroids, and cholangitis is rare if the biliary tree has not been contaminated by instrumentation.

(b) *Induction of Remission*: Concomitant with amelioration of symptoms, an improvement in radiologic abnormalities is also seen with treatment (Figs. 11.1 and 11.2). The disease can be brought into remission with more prolonged use of steroids.

(c) *Confirmation of Diagnosis*: If there is any doubt about the diagnosis, the rapid response to steroids is reassuring and confirms the diagnosis. This includes resolution of pancreatic changes (ductal abnormalities, enlargement or mass) and of extrapancreatic manifestations (biliary strictures, retroperitoneal fibrosis, etc.). However, since AIP is associated with intense fibrosis, many radiologic changes (e.g., ductal changes, retroperitoneal fibrosis) may improve only partially or in some cases remain unchanged after treatment.

Steroids should be offered to all AIP patients with active disease; however, there is no role for steroids in patients who present in the post-acute phase with pancreatic atrophy unless they have extrapancreatic disease requiring therapy.

### Steroid Regimen for Induction of Remission

There is no consensus on steroid regimen and duration of treatment in AIP. Starting doses range from 30 to 40 mg in most studies [2–6]. These doses are effective in the majority of patients; however, it is not known whether lower doses (10–20 mg) would also be effective. Starting doses are typically given for 3–4 weeks followed

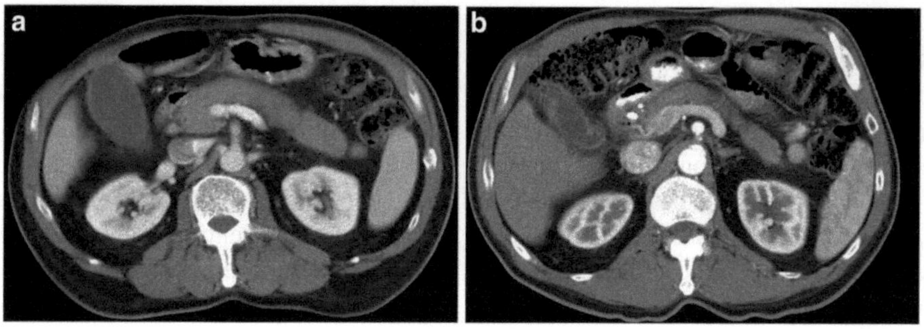


**Fig. 11.1** *Panel A* demonstrates the classic diffuse pancreatic enlargement with a faint hyperenhancing rim. *Panel B* demonstrates resolution of the pancreatic swelling after 1 month of treatment with prednisone

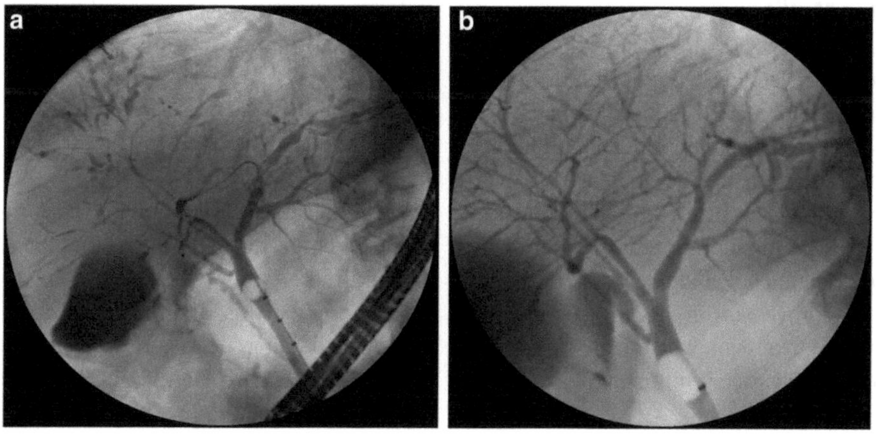


**Fig. 11.2** Evidence of intra- and extrahepatic biliary ductal stricturing was demonstrated at the time of a baseline ERCP to evaluate obstructive jaundice (*panel A*). In the presence of evidence of chronic pancreatitis and serum IgG4 level elevated greater than two times the upper limit of normal, this patient was treated with prednisone. After a 12-week course of prednisone, there was resolution of their IgG4-associated cholangitis (*panel B*)

by a taper of varying duration. We have used prednisone 40 mg daily for 4 weeks followed by taper of 5 mg per week (total of 11 weeks of therapy) [2]. Response is typically rapid with significant radiologic improvement at 2–3 weeks [7]. In patients who experience a complete radiologic response, normalization of imaging findings typically occurs at 4–6 weeks [7].

## Diagnostic Steroid Trials

Response to steroid treatment is one of the diagnostic criteria for many diagnostic classifications, including the HISORt criteria [2]. A diagnostic steroid trial refers to the use of a brief 2-week steroid course with the intent of meeting this criterion to secure the diagnosis of AIP. A typical scenario in which this is considered would be the patient presenting with a pancreatic mass that is negative on fine-needle aspiration for malignancy and with some other collateral evidence for AIP. Caution is advised prior to considering a diagnostic trial and close follow-up with repeat imaging to ensure improvement is essential. One study showed that no patients with pancreatic cancer had a radiographic response to steroids and CA 19–9 levels continued to increase during the diagnostic trial, in contrast to the patients with AIP, suggesting that in cases where malignancy has been ruled out, this is a reasonable option [8].

## Adjuvant Therapy

Adjuvant therapy is frequently needed for the management of complications either related to steroid treatment (e.g., diabetes mellitus) or directly related to the disease (e.g., obstructive jaundice, steatorrhea) or steroid treatment. Occasionally other organ involvement mandates intervention (e.g., ureteral stenting for retroperitoneal fibrosis-induced hydronephrosis).

### Diabetes Mellitus

A common problem during induction treatment is either the onset of steroid-induced diabetes mellitus or aggravation of premorbid diabetes mellitus. Prior to starting treatment, patients should be provided with a clear plan regarding the need for vigilant glucose monitoring and titration of their antidiabetic regimen. Paradoxically, some patients will have improvement in their glycemic control during steroid treatment, which is felt to represent resolution of endocrine insufficiency.

### Obstructive Jaundice

Patients presenting with obstructive jaundice typically require endoscopic retrograde cholangiogram with or without pancreatogram. In patients with a bilirubin >3 mg/dL, it is our practice to dilate any apparent biliary strictures, perform a biliary sphincterotomy, and place a plastic biliary stent to improve biliary drainage during initial treatment. The stents typically remain in place until endoscopic follow-up 6–8 weeks after initiation of steroids. Stenting is not routinely performed for patients with known IAC who develop a biliary relapse, unless they do not rapidly respond to reinitiation of steroids.

### Exocrine Insufficiency

Pancreatic exocrine insufficiency is uncommon in patients at the time of presentation; however, it can become problematic as the disease burns out. A large multicenter Japanese study showed that 58 of 300 (20 %) patients with radiographic follow-up had pancreatic atrophy following their initial treatment, although the frequency of steatorrhea was not reported [9]. For patients presenting with steatorrhea, it is typically steroid responsive, so we do not start enzyme supplementation immediately. However, for those with persistent steatorrhea, following steroid treatment supplementation may be necessary. For older patients with a longer duration of disease, the pancreatic atrophy can be progressive and the need for supplementation may develop.

## Patient Follow-up

The initial goal of follow-up is to ensure sustained clinical remission and, if any remaining doubt, to ensure there is no evidence of malignancy. Our most commonly used follow-up protocol involves repeat laboratory tests and imaging 4–6 weeks after commencing steroid therapy. If a biliary stent was placed at presentation for biliary strictures, stent removal is possible 6–8 weeks after starting steroids in the majority of patients (unpublished data).

The subsequent goals of follow-up are monitoring for treatment-related complications, disease relapse, and either endocrine or exocrine pancreatic dysfunction. To identify relapses early periodic follow-up of patients who have initially responded to treatment is recommended. In the study by Hirano et al., imaging was performed every 6 months with laboratory testing every 3–6 months to assess for relapse [4]. Our follow-up protocol is largely based on the organ involved. In patients with biliary strictures, we repeat laboratory testing (liver enzymes, serum IgG4) every 12 weeks for the first 1–2 years. In patients without biliary disease, assessment for recurrence is more difficult and we have monitored patients for recurrent symptoms, and only then do we consider imaging. These practices will likely be refined as more data on long-term outcomes become available.

## Prevention of Disease Relapses

Do all patients need maintenance therapy to prevent disease relapse? Interestingly, the fact that there is a high relapse rate (30–50 %) has led to development to different approaches to management. The high frequency of relapses has led many Japanese investigators to maintain patients on low-dose daily prednisolone (2.5–10 mg) over the long term [5]. In this approach, patients are tapered down to 5–10 mg/day of prednisolone and maintained at this dose for 18–36 months. We have viewed the fact that >50 % of patients do not relapse after initial therapy as a reason to avoid unnecessary exposure to long-term steroids in all patients. Instead, our approach has been to withdraw steroids after 11–12 weeks of therapy and only use maintenance therapy after the first or second relapse of disease.

Although patients universally have a quick and dramatic initial response to steroid treatment, anywhere from 15 % to 60 % of patients will develop disease relapse either after steroid treatment is complete or during the steroid taper [9–13]. Factors contributing to the variable relapse rates include differences in the proportion of surgically treated patients (who are less likely to relapse), type 1 vs. type 2 disease, and overall length of follow-up.

Identification of risk factors for relapse may help us determine the high-risk patients who would benefit from maintenance therapy upfront and allow short-term therapy in lower-risk patients who may not need long-term treatment. The strongest and most consistent predictor of having an initial disease relapse is the presence of proximal biliary tract disease [11, 12, 14]. Diffuse pancreatic enlargement was also associated with disease relapse, but the effect size was small [11]. Studies are conflicted about whether or not lack of serum IgG4 normalization after steroid treatment predicts relapse [9, 12]. The most common locations of relapse are the biliary tree and pancreas [9, 11].

## Treatment of Disease Relapses

At present, there are three options for treatment of a patient with relapsing AIP: (1) repeat a course of steroids, then either taper off or continue low-dose steroids when the disease is in remission; (2) repeat a course of steroids, taper off when the disease is in remission, and start an immunomodulator for maintenance treatment; or (3) treat with rituximab. Each of these options currently seems viable based on preliminary data; however, the choice of long-term therapy for maintenance of remission needs further studies with larger numbers of patients to assess the risk/benefit ratio of each approach. The duration of use of maintenance therapy is also unknown and needs further study.

### Steroids Alone

Kamisawa et al. reported in their large multicenter Japanese series that steroid re-treatment was effective for reinducing remission in 123 (98 %) of 126 patients who relapsed; however, no further details regarding follow-up were available. Steroids have the strongest body of evidence supporting their use in treatment of AIP, are cost-effective, and are readily accessible. However, the major drawback of this strategy is that many patients cannot tolerate high-dose steroids due to side effects, or their disease is unable to be maintained in remission without dependence on high doses of steroids. For patients who do tolerate the steroids and can be successfully weaned, some have considered an additional attempt at maintenance treatment with a low dose; however, there is no literature to guide this decision.

### Steroids plus Immunomodulators

Instead of using long-term low-dose steroids, we have opted to give high-dose steroids, then use immunomodulatory medications for maintenance of remission in patients who relapse. In our experience, azathioprine (2 mg/kg/day) or mycophenolate mofetil (750–1,000 mg twice daily) appears to be equally effective in maintaining remission (100 %, median follow-up 6 months) after relapse in a small number ($n=7$) of patients [14]. Subsequently, groups from the

United States and the United Kingdom have also presented their experience with azathioprine for patients with relapsing AIP. Raina et al. reported a 100 % response rate in 10 patients, two of which had a relapse after azathioprine was discontinued [15]. In the third series, there was a similar high initial response with only one patient having an extrapancreatic relapse while on azathioprine (1 mg/kg/day) (median follow-up 14 months) [12]. In sum, although the cumulative experience is small, preliminary data suggest adding immunomodulators to steroids may be one option for weaning steroids in steroid-dependent patients and may potentially be useful as maintenance treatment for preventing future relapse, but this needs confirmation in larger studies.

### Rituximab

The use of rituximab has been described in a small number of patients with refractory disease. This is a monoclonal CD20 antibody that works by causing rapid B-cell depletion. The rationale for its use comes from the high proportion of CD20-positive B cells in the inflammatory infiltrate in AIP. Similar infiltrates have been seen in patients with orbital pseudolymphoma, a condition which is known to be responsive to infliximab [16]. Our initial report involved a patient with autoimmune pancreatitis and biliary strictures refractory to multiple courses of steroids, treatment with an immunomodulator, and endoscopic interventions [16]. He had a favorable response with removal of his biliary stents. More recently, Khosroshahi et al. reported treating 10 patients with IgG4-RD with rituximab [17]. While the majority of these patients were treated for systemic symptoms (e.g., orbital disease, sialadenitis), one patient had AIP with IAC and another had isolated IAC. Both of these patients responded to their two-dose protocol, although the patient with AIP/IAC developed a disease relapse 6 months later requiring re-treatment. Our standard protocol, which borrows the dosing schedule from studies on lymphoma, consists of administering 375 mg/m$^2$ intravenously for 4 consecutive weeks following by infusions every 3 months for the following 2 years. Whether or not giving maintenance doses compared to the shorter 2-dose protocol is justified will become more evident with longer follow-up. Due to the high cost of rituximab therapy, this should be reserved for refractory patients until additional studies investigating the effectiveness of rituximab in the AIP/IAC population have been completed.

## Treatment-Related Complications

### Steroids

The most frequent treatment-related complications that arise in the management of AIP are those related to steroids. Although it has never been systematically assessed in this population, in our experience over 50 % of patients develop some steroid-related side effect, usually minor. Almost half of these patients (25 % of all treated with steroids) developed hyperglycemia requiring either addition of increased doses of insulin or premature tapering of prednisone to compensate (unpublished data). Less frequently observed problems, but just as serious, include perturbation of previously controlled depression and/or anxiety disorders. Otherwise, concerns have been raised regarding the long-term side effects that result from cumulative steroid exposure. In their multicenter study, Kamisawa et al. reported ten patients developed osteoporosis (eight with immediate complications of compression fractures or avascular necrosis of the hip) [9]. It is likely these numbers underestimate the true frequency of side effects given the relatively short duration of follow-up and the possibility of underreporting due to management of complications by general physicians during disease remission.

### Immunomodulators

There were no serious side effects reported in any of the series using immunomodulators; however, similar to steroids immunomodulatory drugs have significant side effects. Azathioprine can result in allergic reactions, nausea, bone marrow suppression (2–5 %), hepatotoxicity (2 %), increased risk of infections, and rarely pancreatitis [18]. Significant side effects leading to drug discontinuation occur in approximately 10–30 % of patients [18]. Mycophenolate mofetil also has significant adverse effects including headache (30–50 %), diarrhea (up to 30 %), peripheral edema (20 %), hypertension, leukopenia, and increased risk of infection [19]. Both drugs also appear to have a slightly increased long-term risk of lymphoma [19].

### Rituximab

In general, treatment with rituximab is safe and well tolerated. The most common adverse events are acute infusional reactions producing flu-like symptoms and less commonly hypotension, bronchospasm, or pruritus [20]. These cytokine-mediated side effects are most common during the first infusion and typically abate with discontinuation of the infusion and supportive measures. Reactivation of viral hepatitis B and C has been reported and should be screened for prior to initiation of treatment [20]. The majority of late adverse events are a consequence of interstitial pneumonitis [21].

## Areas of Uncertainty/Future Study

Almost 10 years after the increase in recognition of AIP, there is still much to learn regarding the treatment of this condition. One of the major challenges in understanding how to treat these patients is that various studies included a heterogeneous group of patients based on various diagnostic schemes. Recently, an international consensus for the diagnostic criteria for autoimmune pancreatitis has been achieved, which will help clinically by ensuring patients are diagnosed correctly, and from a research perspective by standardization of terms [22]. Many questions remain:

*Do steroids alter the natural history of this disease, and more specifically does treatment prevent the development of organ dysfunction?*

The Hirano study showed a lower incidence of relapse in steroid-treated patients receiving low-dose maintenance prednisolone compared to those not receiving steroids at all [4]. It remains unclear if patients treated with short courses of steroids without maintenance therapy would also have lower relapse rates than untreated patients. If this were so, it may justify treating asymptomatic patients with short courses of steroids to prevent long-term disease complications. It appears that progression to pancreatic atrophy occurs in approximately one-third of AIP patients. We have also seen progression to cirrhosis in patients with biliary disease. Treatment of acute flares is often necessary to alleviate acute disease complications; however, it is unclear whether steroid treatment prevents or decreases the likelihood of disease progression.

*What is the clinical significance of isolated serologic relapse?*

Isolated serum IgG4 elevation is a common and often confusing clinical scenario. Serum IgG4 levels fall with steroid treatment, even if the IgG4 elevation is not a consequence of autoimmune pancreatitis [3]. In most cases, the IgG4 levels will return to normal after treatment. In one study, the failure of IgG4 levels to normalize after steroids was associated with a higher rate of relapse (30 %) compared to patients who normalized their IgG4 levels (10 %) [9]. However, this association was not seen in a later study [12]. If additional evidence confirms these patients are more likely to progress to clinical relapse, it would be more compelling, but at the present we do not restart treatment for isolated serologic relapse, but rather follow these patients expectantly.

*Should patients with type 2 AIP be treated differently than type 1 patients?*

There are ongoing discussions regarding whether or not these are variants of one disease or two separate diseases. In symptomatic patients, steroids are highly effective. However, a considerable proportion of patients with type 2 AIP are asymptomatic at the time of diagnosis, either because their initial presentation was acute pancreatitis which has since resolved or because the diagnosis was incidental. These patients overall

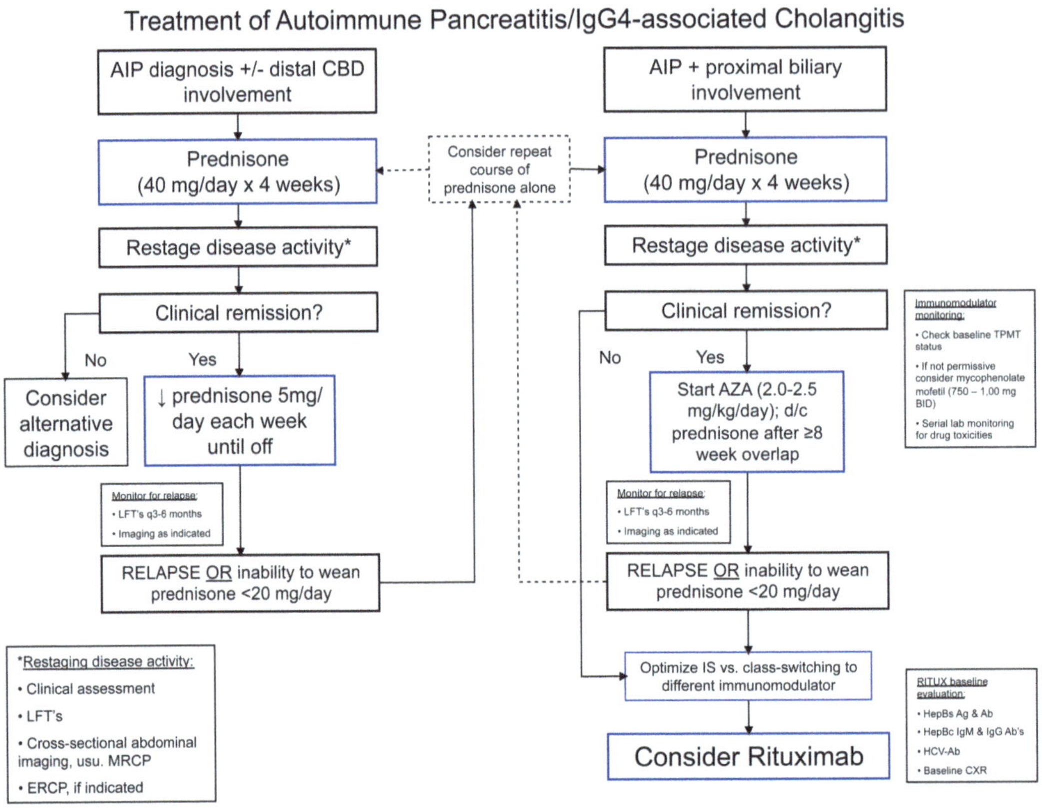


**Fig. 11.3** Mayo Clinic treatment algorithm for management of disease relapses for patients with autoimmune pancreatitis

have incredibly low rates of disease relapse, so maintenance therapy is not justified and the goal of induction therapy is not to decrease risk of relapse, but rather to control the acute symptoms [11, 23, 24]. Whether or not treating asymptomatic patients prevents or minimizes future organ dysfunction is unclear.

*Do different manifestations of IgG4-related disease have different disease courses?*

IgG4-related disease can involve multiple organs (pancreas, bile duct, retroperitoneum, kidneys, lungs, salivary glands). It is unclear if relapse rates and long-term prognosis differ with various manifestations of the disease. If so, then the mode and duration of treatment may need to be tailored based on the involved organs.

## Conclusion

Autoimmune pancreatitis and IgG4-associated cholangitis are diseases characterized by a dramatic symptomatic, biochemical, serologic, and radiographic response to steroid treatment. There is a wide variation in the dose and duration of steroid administration, and although there are no direct comparisons, response rates are universally high. Disease relapses in the biliary tree and pancreas are common occurring in up to half of all patients. The strategy of treating disease relapses and the role of maintenance therapy with steroids, immunomodulators, and/or rituximab are evolving. A summary of our current approach to treating relapsing AIP and IAC is shown in Fig. 11.3.

## References


1. Umehara H, Okazaki K, Masaki Y, Kawano M, Yamamoto M, Saeki T, Matsui S, Sumida T, Mimori T, Tanaka Y, Tsubota K, Yoshino T, Kawa S, Suzuki R, Takegami T, Tomosugi N, Kurose N, Ishigaki Y, Azumi A, Kojima M, Nakamura S, Inoue D. A novel clinical entity, IgG4-related disease (IgG4RD): general concept and details. Mod Rheumatol. 2012;22:1–14.
2. Chari ST, Smyrk TC, Levy MJ, Topazian MD, Takahashi N, Zhang L, Clain JE, Pearson RK, Petersen BT, Vege SS, Farnell MB. Diagnosis of autoimmune pancreatitis: the Mayo Clinic experience. Clin Gastroenterol Hepatol. 2006;4:1010–6. quiz 934.
3. Hamano H, Kawa S, Horiuchi A, Unno H, Furuya N, Akamatsu T, Fukushima M, Nikaido T, Nakayama K, Usuda N, Kiyosawa K. High serum IgG4 concentrations in patients with sclerosing pancreatitis. N Eng J Med. 2001;344:732–8.
4. Hirano K, Tada M, Isayama H, Yagioka H, Sasaki T, Kogure H, Nakai Y, Sasahira N, Tsujino T, Yoshida H, Kawabe T, Omata M. Long-term prognosis of autoimmune pancreatitis with and without corticosteroid treatment. Gut. 2007;56:1719–24.
5. Kamisawa T, Yoshiike M, Egawa N, Nakajima H, Tsuruta K, Okamoto A. Treating patients with autoimmune pancreatitis: results from a long-term follow-up study. Pancreatology. 2005;5:234–8. discussion 238–40.
6. Nishino T, Toki F, Oyama H, Oi I, Kobayashi M, Takasaki K, Shiratori K. Biliary tract involvement in autoimmune pancreatitis. Pancreas. 2005;30:76–82.
7. Kamisawa T, Egawa N, Nakajima H, Tsuruta K, Okamoto A. Morphological changes after steroid therapy in autoimmune pancreatitis. Scand J Gastroenterol. 2004;39:1154–8.
8. Moon SH, Kim MH, Park DH, Hwang CY, Park SJ, Lee SS, Seo DW, Lee SK. Is a 2-week steroid trial after initial negative investigation for malignancy useful in differentiating autoimmune pancreatitis from pancreatic cancer? A prospective outcome study. Gut. 2008;57:1704–12.
9. Kamisawa T, Shimosegawa T, Okazaki K, Nishino T, Watanabe H, Kanno A, Okumura F, Nishikawa T, Kobayashi K, Ichiya T, Takatori H, Yamakita K, Kubota K, Hamano H, Okamura K, Hirano K, Ito T, Ko SB, Omata M. Standard steroid treatment for autoimmune pancreatitis. Gut. 2009;58:1504–7.
10. Ryu JK, Chung JB, Park SW, Lee JK, Lee KT, Lee WJ, Moon JH, Cho KB, Kang DW, Hwang JH, Yoo KS, Yoo BM, Lee DH, Kim HK, Moon YS, Lee J, Lee HS, Choi HS, Lee SK, Kim YT, Kim CD, Kim SJ, Hahm JS, Yoon YB. Review of 67 patients with autoimmune pancreatitis in Korea: a multicenter nationwide study. Pancreas. 2008;37:377–85.
11. Sah RP, Chari ST, Pannala R, Sugumar A, Clain JE, Levy MJ, Pearson RK, Smyrk TC, Petersen BT, Topazian MD, Takahashi N, Farnell MB, Vege SS. Differences in clinical profile and relapse rate of type 1 versus type 2 autoimmune pancreatitis. Gastroenterology. 2010;139:140–8. quiz e12–3.
12. Sandanayake NS, Church NI, Chapman MH, Johnson GJ, Dhar DK, Amin Z, Deheragoda MG, Novelli M, Winstanley A, Rodriguez-Justo M, Hatfield AR, Pereira SP, Webster GJ. Presentation and management of post-treatment relapse in autoimmune pancreatitis/immunoglobulin G4-associated cholangitis. Clin Gastroenterol Hepatol. 2009;7:1089–96.
13. Zamboni G, Luttges J, Capelli P, Frulloni L, Cavallini G, Pederzoli P, Leins A, Longnecker D, Kloppel G. Histopathological features of diagnostic and clinical relevance in autoimmune pancreatitis: a study on 53 resection specimens and 9 biopsy specimens. Virchows Arch. 2004;445:552–63.
14. Ghazale A, Chari ST, Zhang L, Smyrk TC, Takahashi N, Levy MJ, Topazian MD, Clain JE, Pearson RK, Petersen BT, Vege SS, Lindor K, Farnell MB. Immunoglobulin G4-associated cholangitis: clinical profile and response to therapy. Gastroenterology. 2008;134:706–15.
15. Raina A, Yadav D, Krasinskas AM, McGrath KM, Khalid A, Sanders M, Whitcomb DC, Slivka A. Evaluation and management of autoimmune pancreatitis: experience at a large US center. Am J Gastroenterol. 2009;104:2295–306.
16. Topazian M, Witzig TE, Smyrk TC, Pulido JS, Levy MJ, Kamath PS, Chari ST. Rituximab therapy for refractory biliary strictures in immunoglobulin G4-associated cholangitis. Clin Gastroenterol Hepatol. 2008;6:364–6.
17. Khosroshahi A, Carruthers MN, Deshpande V, Unizony S, Bloch DB, Stone JH. Rituximab for the treatment of IgG4-related disease: lessons from 10 consecutive patients. Medicine. 2012;91:57–66.
18. Su C, Lichtenstein GR. Treatment of inflammatory bowel disease with azathioprine and 6-mercaptopurine. Gastroenterol Clin North Am. 2004;33:209–34, viii.
19. Wang K, Zhang H, Li Y, Wei Q, Li H, Yang Y, Lu Y. Safety of mycophenolate mofetil versus azathioprine in renal transplantation: a systematic review. Transplant Proc. 2004;36:2068–70.
20. Kimby E. Tolerability and safety of rituximab (MabThera). Cancer Treat Rev. 2005;31:456–73.
21. Ram R, Ben-Bassat I, Shpilberg O, Polliack A, Raanani P. The late adverse events of rituximab therapy–rare but there! Leuk Lymphoma. 2009;50:1083–95.
22. Shimosegawa T, Chari ST, Frulloni L, Kamisawa T, Kawa S, Mino-Kenudson M, Kim MH, Kloppel G, Lerch MM, Lohr M, Notohara K, Okazaki K, Schneider A, Zhang L. International consensus diagnostic criteria for autoimmune pancreatitis: guidelines of the International Association of Pancreatology. Pancreas. 2011;40:352–8.
23. Deshpande V, Gupta R, Sainani N, Sahani DV, Virk R, Ferrone C, Khosroshahi A, Stone JH, Lauwers GY. Subclassification of autoimmune pancreatitis: a histologic classification with clinical significance. Am J Surg Pathol. 2011;35:26–35.

24. Kamisawa T, Chari ST, Giday SA, Kim MH, Chung JB, Lee KT, Werner J, Bergmann F, Lerch MM, Mayerle J, Pickartz T, Lohr M, Schneider A, Frulloni L, Webster GJ, Reddy DN, Liao WC, Wang HP, Okazaki K, Shimosegawa T, Kloeppel G, Go VL. Clinical profile of autoimmune pancreatitis and its histological subtypes: an international multicenter survey. Pancreas. 2011;40:809–14.

# Part II

# IgG4-Related Sclerosing Cholangitis

# Secondary Sclerosing Cholangitis

# 12

Gideon M. Hirschfield

## Abbreviations

| | |
|---|---|
| ERCP | Endoscopic retrograde cholangiopancreatography |
| MRCP | Magnetic resonance cholangiopancreatography |
| PSC | Primary sclerosing cholangitis |
| SSC | Secondary sclerosing cholangitis |

## Introduction

'Sclerosing cholangitis (SC)' is the term applied to a distinct group of bile duct cholangiopathies that are evident radiologically and/or pathologically and which are usually accompanied by cholestatic liver biochemistry [1, 2]. Histologically an inflammatory and obliterative biliary fibrosis occurs which leads to bile duct strictures, which predispose patients to bacterial cholangitis, secondary biliary cirrhosis, liver failure and malignancy.

The first description of sclerosing cholangitis dates to Delbet in 1924, and it is only over the last 30–40 years that greater insights into this group of diseases have been gained [3, 4]. These have resulted in a clearer distinction between primary and secondary disease. SC is now seen to represent a spectrum of chronic biliary diseases that are characterised either as having an unknown aetiology, albeit with clear association with inflammatory bowel disease (i.e. primary sclerosing cholangitis), or as the consequence of identifiable insults to the biliary tree (i.e. secondary). The interest in secondary sclerosing cholangitis (SSC) comes not just from the individual patient perspective but from the drive to better understand primary disease, for which there remains a lamentable lack of treatment other than transplantation.

A multifocal biliary stricturing process usually characterises SSC. Although small duct disease alone is possible, making a secure diagnosis becomes more challenging in this scenario. It has an array of aetiologies (Table 12.1) consequent to known pathogenic processes or injury such as obstruction of the bile ducts due to malignancy or stones; operative, toxic or ischemic injury; bacterial infections; or congenital abnormalities [5, 6]. It also includes IgG4-related autoimmune pancreatitis, which is extensively discussed elsewhere in this book. This chapter provides an overview of secondary sclerosing cholangitis, without necessarily being exhaustive as regards every reported potential aetiology, but with the aim of highlighting important themes.

G.M. Hirschfield, MB, BChir, Ph.D., FRCP (✉)
Centre for Liver Research, NIHR Biomedical Research Unit, University of Birmingham, Institute of Biomedical Research, Birmingham, United Kingdom, B15 2TT
e-mail: g.hirschfield@bham.ac.uk

M.J. Levy and S.T. Chari (eds.), *Autoimmune (IgG4-related) Pancreatitis and Cholangitis*,
DOI 10.1007/978-1-4419-6430-4_12, 

**Table 12.1** Secondary causes of sclerosing cholangitis[a]

| Mechanism | Examples | | |
|---|---|---|---|
| Infection | AIDS cholangiopathy/papillary stenosis | Recurrent pyogenic cholangitis/ oriental cholangiopathy | Systemic fungal infection<br>Schistosomiasis |
| Vascular | Hepatic artery thrombosis/ischemia reperfusion/preservation injury | Portal biliopathy/hereditary haemorrhagic telangiectasia | 'ICU' syndrome |
| Toxic | Intra-arterial chemotherapy, e.g. intra-arterial floxuridine | Formaldehyde administered to treat a hydatid cyst | |
| Immunologic | IgG4 autoimmune sclerosing vcholangitis | Eosinophilic cholangitis | |
| Obstructive | Cholangiocarcinoma | Choledocholithiasis/chronic pancreatitis | Diffuse intrahepatic metastasis |
| Infiltrative | Histiocytosis X | Mast cell cholangiopathy | Amyloidosis/sarcoidosis |
| Traumatic | Surgical biliary trauma | | |
| Congenital | Carolis/choledochal cyst | MDR3 mutations | Cystic fibrosis |

[a]Some aetiologies mechanistically overlap; some aetiologies may not be true sclerosing cholangitis, but give a radiological picture that is easily mistaken for SC

## Clinical Presentation and Epidemiology

There is no reliable epidemiologic data for SSC, as there is no way to track its incidence or prevalence, given presently inadequate diagnostic codes [7]. Clinic descriptions are liable to referral bias based on whether it is a medical, surgical or endoscopic practice, whilst case reports in the literature have similar issues. Broadly nevertheless it remains an uncommon biliary disease, seemingly less so than PSC. In one retrospective 10-year review (1992–2002) from the Mayo Clinic [8], there were 31 cases of SSC identified, as compared to over 1,000 cases of PSC. Fifty-eight percent of these patients were men, and the mean age at diagnosis was 57 years. In this case series, the most common causes of SSC were surgical trauma during cholecystectomy (42 %) and choledocholithiasis (39 %). Additional documented aetiologies of SSC were recurrent pancreatitis and abdominal injury. In an ambulatory, secondary and tertiary non-transplant hepatology practice in Canada just under 20 % of patients had a secondary aetiology for sclerosing cholangitis, predominantly autoimmune pancreatitis (Table 12.2). Once again, a referral bias may however be evident.

**Table 12.2** Aetiologies of sclerosing cholangitis in an ambulatory general liver clinic setting (data based on Alswat K et al. Am J Gastroenterol. 2012;107:56–63)

| Characteristic | Summary |
|---|---|
| Number of patients | $n=168$ |
| Gender | Female: 82 (49 %) |
| | Male: 86 (51 %) |
| Age at diagnosis (years) | 38 +/−14.2 |
| Ethnicity | Caucasian: 116 (69 %) |
| | Other: 52 (31 %) |
| Disease classification | Large duct: 106 (63 %) |
| | Small duct: 14 (8 %) |
| | AIH/PSC: 18 (11 %) |
| | Secondary: 30 (18 %) |
| Secondary aetiologies | AIP/SC: 14 (8 %) |
| | Biliary stones: 5 (3 %) |
| | Portal vein thrombosis: 4 (2 %) |
| | Kasai: 3 (2 %) |
| | Misc: 4 (2 %) |

SSC patients present clinically in a wide variety of ways, from asymptomatic incidental presentations all the way through to presentation with cholangitis or end-stage liver disease. Patient evaluation must clearly be personalised given the array of secondary aetiologies, and it is most important to carefully listen to the patient's history when determining investigations, rather than investigating everyone in the same way. Generally having diagnosed a patient with a large duct cholangiopathy by MRCP or ERCP, most clinicians routinely ensure patency of the portal vein by ultrasonography, extend imaging to include the pancreas and other abdominal organs, measure IgG4 levels and actively screen for colonic disease (including with colonic biopsies even if endoscopically the mucosa appears normal) as a minimum. Investigations beyond this must be tailored to the patient as it is not usual to subsequently identify a secondary aetiology for SC that is not strongly suggested from either the patient history or facets of the carefully reviewed imaging, blood work or histology.

## Pathophysiologic Themes

The presence of such a variety of secondary causes that can mimic the histological and radiological features of primary sclerosing cholangitis (including autoimmunity, ischemia, infection and toxins) suggests commonality in certain final pathways associated with biliary injury [9, 10]. Greater appreciation of these processes may aid understanding of primary disease and facilitate the development of new treatments. The fundamental injury is not to hepatocytes but rather to medium- and large-sized bile ducts with cholangiography often demonstrating intra- and/or extrahepatic bile ducts with localised or multifocal strictures and intervening segments of normal or dilated ducts. Histologically concentric periductal fibrosis ('onion-skinning') occurs that progresses to narrowing and obliteration of small bile ducts. Across disease aetiologies there is initial damage to portal bile ducts with associated portal/periportal changes (inflammation, ductular reaction) and resultant secondary parenchymal changes. The cholangiocytes demonstrate reactive features including expression of adhesion molecules, inflammatory and profibrogenetic cytokines and receptors, as well as growth factors stimulating extracellular matrix production, accumulation and proliferation of periductal myofibroblasts.

The pathogenesis of PSC duct lesions is of course uncertain, but one concept proposes an immunologic attack on components of the subepithelial (periductal) mesenchyme leading to progressive periductal fibrosis and subsequent interruption of fluid and nutrient exchange between the peribiliary capillary plexus and the biliary epithelium. The end product would be ischemic duct injury/loss and interestingly mechanistically ischemic cholangiopathy is probably the most understood of all secondary aetiologies, given that bile ducts are supplied with blood exclusively via hepatic arteries [11, 12]. Depending on the nature, localisation and relative speed of vascular change, ischemic cholangiopathy may present as acute formation of biliary casts, bile duct necrosis or chronic disease with sclerosing cholangitis. Whereas the extrahepatic biliary system has a good vascular supply (from two parallel running arteries to the common bile duct fed by branch vessels, e.g. the retroduodenal artery, gastroduodenal artery, left and right hepatic artery), the intrahepatic ducts are supplied by a nonaxial network of small arteries forming a plexus of arterioles, venules and capillaries within the peribiliary adventitia with a second plexus within the biliary wall primarily composed of capillaries ('peribiliary capillary plexus') derived only from the right and left hepatic artery. These are therefore functional end arteries making intrahepatic bile ducts vulnerable to ischemic events, given that other than peripherally, portal venous blood does not contribute to biliary tree blood supply. Ischemic bile duct injury occurs if the small hepatic arteries or the peribiliary vascular plexus are damaged, or if all arterial blood supply is interrupted, for example, in a transplanted liver with hepatic artery thrombosis. This latter scenario is unique as the liver allograft is devoid of a collateral arterial circulation, especially early post transplantation. Indeed liver transplantation has aptly highlighted the sensitivity of biliary epithelium to a wide variety of vascular insults. Biliary strictures in liver transplant recipients can relate to a combination of large hepatic artery occlusion (e.g. surgical reconstruction or sepsis/bile leak) and/or damage to small arteries and the peribiliary plexus (e.g. preservation injury, ischemia–reperfusion, rejection, ABO incompatibility, CMV infection) [13–15].

The strong association between PSC and colitis has also furthered the possibility that penetration of infectious or toxic agents through an inflamed, and 'leaky', colon into the portal system may be important in precipitating biliary inflammation. In secondary sclerosing cholangitis, recurrent infection either as a primary or secondary event is often important, and mechanistically infectious aetiologies also provide a more readily understandable pathway to biliary damage, with recurrent direct inflammatory cholangitis resulting in a fibrosing cholangiopathy. The syndrome of immunodeficiency-related aetiologies demonstrates how cholangitis when recurrent, persistent and not easily eradicated can result in SC [16]. In such patients a variety of organisms, including *Cryptosporidium*, *Microsporidium* and *Cytomegalovirus*, have been isolated from the bile. It may also be the case that a virus such as HIV directly interferes with innate responses to biliary infection—the HIV-1 Tat protein, for example, is reported to suppress cholangiocyte toll-like receptor 4 expression and defence against *Cryptosporidium parvum* [17]. Given these associations there have been attempts to culture potential culprit pathogens in cohorts of patients with established PSC, but these have failed to show any specific infection associated with disease. However, newer genomic/microbiome technologies may in time discover previously unidentified bacterial (or viral) species relevant to pathogenesis.

The close connection between PSC and inflammatory bowel disease also suggests that adaptive and innate immune responses can generate chronic and progressive tissue-specific (biliary) inflammatory responses with production of injurious proinflammatory cytokines [18]. Pathogenesis of duct injury may relate to activation of innate immune responses through special pattern recognition receptors that detect conserved microbial structures known as *pathogen-associated molecular patterns* including toll-like receptors that can activate innate immune responses, mediated by activated macrophages, dendritic cells and natural killer cells. The subsequent peribiliary recruitment of gut-primed T cells may mediate further bile duct injury. Clearly IgG4-associated cholangitis demonstrates the potential role for immune-mediated injury in large bile duct cholangiopathy aptly.

Some rare inherited diseases are also mechanistically insightful in both man and experimental models. In mice it is possible to recapitulate features of sclerosing cholangitis by introducing a deletion in the *Mdr2* gene, the product of which is an important biliary transporter [19, 20]. This canalicular phospholipid flippase (Mdr2/MDR3) normally mediates biliary excretion of phospholipids, allowing the formation of mixed micelles with bile acids and cholesterol, which protect the bile duct epithelium from the detergent properties of bile acids. *Mdr2* knockout mice are not capable of excreting phospholipids into bile and spontaneously develop bile duct injury with macroscopic and microscopic features closely resembling sclerosing cholangitis. Impairment of MDR3 ultimately leads to a lithogenic and toxic bile milieu. The bile ducts have disrupted tight junctions and basement membranes, bile acid leakage into portal tracts, induction of a portal inflammatory infiltrate and activation of proinflammatory and profibrogenic cytokines. This results in activation of periductal myofibroblasts, leading to periductal fibrosis, separating the peribiliary plexus from bile duct epithelial cells resulting in atrophy and loss of the bile duct epithelium. In man, ABCB4 deficiency, or low phospholipid-associated cholelithiasis, is characterised by symptomatic cholelithiasis at a young age (<40 years), recurrence of biliary symptoms despite cholecystectomy and recurrent intra- and extrahepatic biliary stones, with secondary sclerosing cholangitis sometimes encountered [21]. Even rarer causes of sclerosing cholangitis can be further used to highlight important cellular themes. Therefore, the fact that claudin-1 gene mutations are found in neonatal sclerosing cholangitis, in association with ichthyosis, implicates deficiencies in tight junction function as relevant [22]. In the liver, tight junctions separate bile flow from plasma and are composed of strands of claudins and occludin. In this syndrome it is speculated that cholestasis is due to the absence of claudin-1, leading to increased paracellular permeability and to hepatocyte and bile duct injuries secondary to paracellular bile regurgitation.

## Infections and Secondary Sclerosing Cholangitis

Although robust epidemiologic data is lacking, recurrent infection is a prominent cause of secondary sclerosing cholangitis and is encountered in a number of settings: persistent biliary obstruction, post-biliary surgery/manipulation, recurrent biliary stones and immunodeficiency states. Whilst atypical infections (e.g. cryptosporidiosis) are reported because of clinical interest, it seems most likely that the more common scenario of recurrent bacterial cholangitis related to fixed anatomical defects is more relevant for the majority. Nevertheless atypical infections in immunocompromised hosts are important. In children with primary immunodeficiency and liver disease, clinical evidence of liver disease was documented in ~ one in four patients with abnormal liver biochemistry [23]. Of these, sclerosing cholangitis was diagnosed in 60 %, based on radiological and histological criteria. Infection with *Cryptosporidium parvum* was proven in about 2/3rds of those with SC. Prior to effective HIV therapy, HIV/AIDS cholangiopathy was also relatively frequently seen. Biliary involvement in this setting includes papillary stenosis and sclerosing cholangitis, and cholangiographic abnormalities can regress if effective antiviral therapy is given [24]. Infection of the biliary or duodenal epithelium is the primary cause of ductal abnormalities in AIDS cholangiopathy with infectious agents including *Cryptosporidia* [25], *Isospora belli* [26] and CMV [27, 28].

Among the many pathogens identified, *Cryptosporidium* species are the most common identifiable aetiology [29, 30]. These are a family of protozoan parasites that may be contracted through infected animals or from contaminated food and water. When the encysted *C. parvum* are ingested, sporozoites are released from the exocyst, after exposure to the low pH of the stomach and proximal duodenal digestive enzymes. Sporozoites have a lectin on their surface that mediates adherence to intestinal epithelial cells. Sporozoites disrupt the microvilli and enter the cytoplasm leading to diarrhoea and can also migrate up the biliary tree to infect biliary epithelial cells. Acalculous cholecystitis and/or sclerosing cholangitis may then develop. Of 82 HIV-infected patients exposed to *Cryptosporidia* in a waterborne outbreak, the development of abdominal pain associated with biliary tract disease occurred in 29 % of cases and was confirmed by cholangiography in 40 % [31]. If undetected by blood or stool cultures, the next most common organisms are *Microsporidia* species. Other recognised infections include *cytomegalovirus, Enterocytozoon bieneusi, Septata intestinalis, Mycobacterium avium–intracellulare, Isospora belli* and possibly a direct effect of HIV infection itself as alluded to above. As many as 50 % of patients with AIDS cholangiopathy may still have no identifiable opportunistic infection. Malignancies such as lymphoma and Kaposi sarcoma can also been associated with cholangitis but rarely present as a cholangiopathy, and if imaging identifies an isolated CBD stricture, particular suspicion to excluding primary lymphoma or pancreatic disease should be made.

Treatment is directed at identified pathogens and should be guided by infectious disease specialists, as well as to the physical biliary tree changes, and when effective can lead to resolution of biliary changes. Antimicrobial therapy against *Cryptosporidia* species with trimethoprim–sulphamethoxazole is indicated, especially if patients have diarrheal symptoms, whilst effective treatment against *Microsporidia* species remains elusive. Ganciclovir for CMV and multidrug regimens against *M. avium–intracellulare* can also be given as indicated whilst albendazole for infection with *S. intestinalis* has been shown to result in symptom improvement when present. Symptomatic patients likely require interventional therapy as well and endoscopic sphincterotomy has been shown to relieve pain and biliary obstruction in patients with papillary stenosis, whilst balloon dilatation or stent placement may be needed to manage biliary strictures.

Oriental cholangiohepatitis (otherwise known as recurrent pyogenic cholangitis and Oriental cholangitis) is the name given to a disease defined by intrabiliary pigment stone formation that occurs equally in men and women [32]. The biliary obstruction that results leads to localised stricturing and recurrent cholangitis and a markedly abnormal biliary tree with extrahepatic and intrahepatic ductal dilatation and focal areas of intrahepatic stricturing/fibrosis. The common clinical presentation is that of right upper quadrant pain, recurrent fevers and jaundice. It is a secondary cause of sclerosing cholangitis, which, whilst once considered an exclusive problem for those who live or who have lived in Southeast Asia, is now recognised as occurring worldwide. Cholangiography can demonstrate multiple strictures of both the intrahepatic and extrahepatic biliary tree, with the bile ducts filled with sludge and stones. When analysed, the bile is purulent and laden with debris composed of bile pigment, desquamated epithelial cells, bacteria and pus. The initial insult is thought usually to be caused by hepatobiliary infestation with *Clonorchis sinensis* (liver fluke), although other infections with *Ascaris lumbricoides*, *Fasciola hepatica*, *Opisthorchis sinensis* and *Entamoeba* have been implicated [33]. The fluke seems to act as a nidus for stone formation, either directly or by causing strictures. Transient portal bacteraemia is thought to also introduce bacteria into the biliary ducts, and this perpetuates cyclical infection and stone formation. Management is either through endoscopic/radiological clearance of the biliary tree or more commonly through surgery: cholecystectomy and improved biliary drainage with either Roux-en-Y choledochojejunostomy or choledochoduodenostomy; partial hepatectomy may be required for localised disease [34].

## Vascular Aetiologies

As described above the vascular supply to the biliary tree predisposes it to vascular injury and the development of secondary ischemic cholangiopathy. This is commonly a result of specific loss of blood supply from damage to the hepatic artery, particularly after transplantation. More global vascular insults can also be relevant (e.g. the cholangiopathy seen with severe ischemia–reperfusion injury or in patients with widespread shunting in hereditary haemorrhagic telangiectasia, Fig. 12.1). Sclerosing cholangitis in critically ill patients, including those with severe burns, is an entity describing a severe biliary disease with

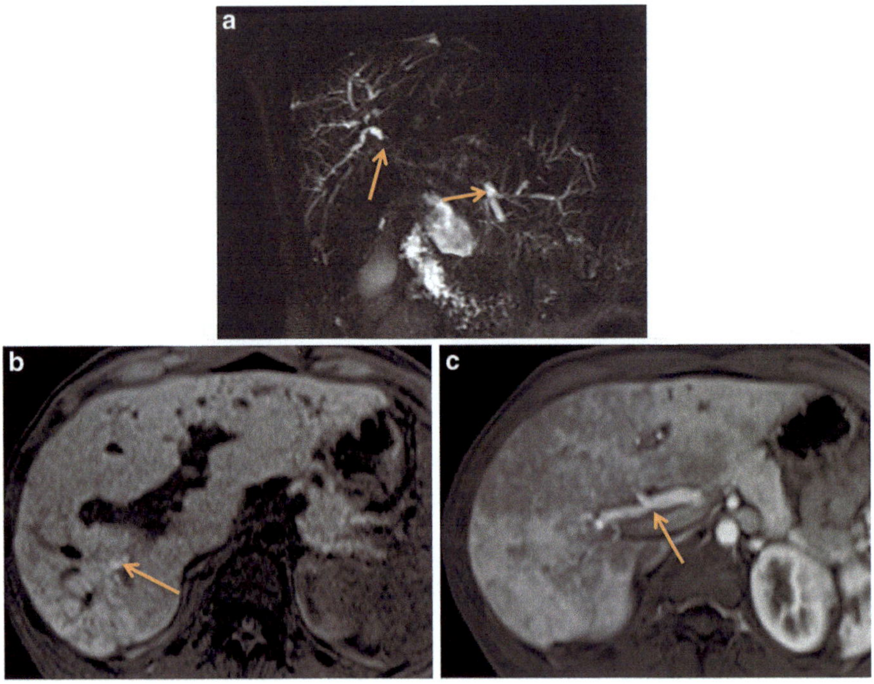


**Fig. 12.1** Secondary sclerosing cholangitis secondary to ischemia in hereditary haemorrhagic telangiectasia. (**a**) Coronal thick slab MRCP image depicting segmental dilatation of bile ducts with multifocal strictures (*arrows*). (**b**) *Left image*: Axial T1 weighted precontrast image shows atrophy of the right lobe with high signal stone in the right posterior bile duct typical of biliary necrosis. (**c**) *Right image*: Axial arterial phase image shows a markedly enlarged hepatic artery (*arrow*) and heterogeneously enhancing liver parenchyma, both due to arteriovenous shunts in the liver

progression to liver cirrhosis that is seen in critically ill patients on the ICU, who previously likely did not survive their critical traumatic or septic illnesses. The mechanisms leading to this form of cholangiopathy with stricture formation and complete obliteration of bile ducts are unknown, but ischemic injury of the biliary tree with the formation of biliary casts and subsequent ongoing biliary infection due to multiresistant bacteria seem likely to be major pathogenic mechanisms [35–37].

## Portal Biliopathy

'Portal biliopathy' is the term applied to biliary changes seen in patients with chronic portal vein thrombosis, in which there is common bile duct obstruction caused by extrinsic compression of the ducts from large venous collaterals at the porta hepatis (Fig. 12.2) [38]. Worldwide it is not an infrequent problem given the many infective aetiologies of portal vein thrombosis, resultant from a portal pyemia, or the sequelae of missed appendicitis. Often the thrombosis seems to have occurred, frequently silently, when young, but patients tend to present in adulthood. Mechanical protrusion of the paracholedochal veins (venous plexus of Petren) in the lumen of the bile duct and a secondary ischemic vascular bile duct injury are believed relevant to pathophysiology [26].

Partial or complete bile duct obstruction is common and patients are frequently symptomatic, although cholangitis seems to be a late manifestation. Good Doppler interrogation of the portal venous circulation is needed, and this can be challenging to interpret with extensive cavernous transformation, the Doppler signal of the cavernoma not infrequently being initially misinterpreted as portal venous flow. Cross-sectional imaging with appropriate contrast CT studies can help. Cholangiography normally shows most abnormalities to be in the common bile duct and includes wall irregularities, localised saccular dilatation and filling defects suggesting common bile duct calculi. Strictures of the common hepatic ducts, as well as mild intrahepatic duct irregularities, can also be seen. Therapeutic strategies are generally for those symptomatic patients who have developed choledocholithiasis and obstructive jaundice and are usually endoscopy based. The presence of extensive venous collaterals increases the risk of intervention, requiring appropriate caution from the

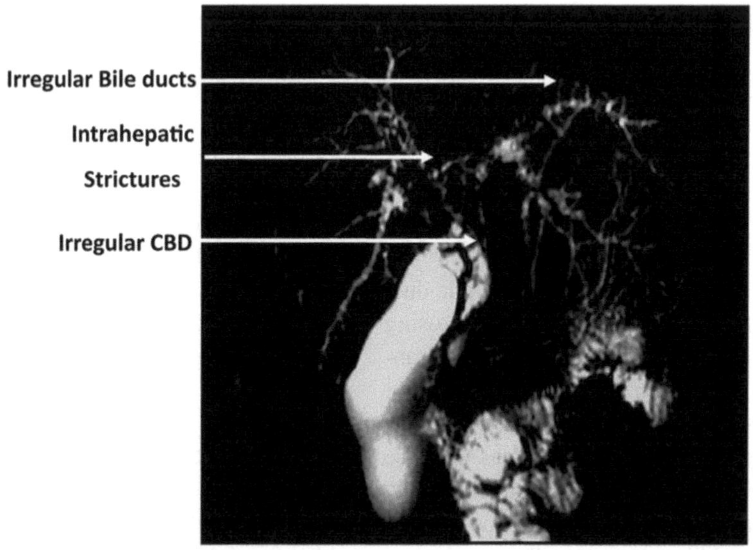


**Fig. 12.2** Typical MR findings in portal biliopathy

endoscopist, hemobilia being more likely iatrogenic than spontaneously occurring. Obstructive jaundice can arise from a dominant stricture or other anatomic bile duct defects in the absence of common bile duct stones but not due to choledochal varices alone. Surgery is best avoided where possible, but portosystemic shunts or transplant has been used occasionally [39].

## Toxic Aetiologies

A well-recognised and not surprising cause of secondary sclerosing cholangitis is related to hepatic artery infusion with the chemotherapy agent floxuridine (FUDR) [40, 41]. Involvement of the common hepatic duct bifurcation with sparing of the CBD is characteristic, and this relates to the arterial supply of extrahepatic bile ducts being derived primarily from the gastroduodenal arcade, which is often excluded from hepatic artery infusion. Ischemia, rather than direct FUDR toxicity to biliary epithelium, appears to be the underlying mechanism of action. The clinical picture closely resembles PSC but usually can be managed by discontinuation of infusion and, in some cases, percutaneous transhepatic drainage or ERCP. The injection of 20 % formaldehyde with sodium chloride or ethanol for the treatment of hydatid disease has also been associated with SSC [42]. Direct sclerosant-type effects on biliary epithelia are the proposed mechanism of action.

## Gallstones, Pancreatitis and Secondary Sclerosing Cholangitis

Chronic pancreatitis can lead to benign bile duct strictures that may appear similar to sclerosing cholangitis [43, 44]. In acute pancreatitis transient partial obstruction of the distal common bile duct caused by inflammation and oedema is not an infrequent occurrence, whereas in those with chronic pancreatitis, a distal bile duct obstruction caused by inflammation and pancreatic parenchymal fibrosis occurs. These strictures involve the entire intrapancreatic segment of the common bile duct and are associated with dilatation of the entire proximal biliary tree. Benign strictures of the bile duct can also result from the chronic inflammation associated with gallstones in either the gallbladder or common bile duct. Bile duct strictures caused by cholelithiasis are usually associated with a narrowing at the level of the common hepatic duct caused by a stone impacted in the infundibulum of the gallbladder.

The vast majority of iatrogenic bile duct injuries occur during laparoscopic cholecystectomy, most commonly being when a portion of the common bile duct is resected with the gallbladder [45]. Bile duct injuries are often not recognised at the time of surgery and may present weeks later with sepsis or jaundice. Late complications, including biloma formation and biliary stricture, may occur. The incidence of bile duct injury with open cholecystectomy is estimated at <0.2 %, which includes minor duct (of Luschka) injuries. Initial reports of bile duct injury from laparoscopic cholecystectomy in up to 2 % of cases have now fallen to the same frequencies as expected after open cholecystectomy.

Autoimmune pancreatitis (AIP) is now a well-described multisystem inflammatory disease with a variety of clinical manifestations that include acute or chronic pancreatitis, biliary or pancreatic strictures and/or pancreatic lesions [46]. The typical magnetic resonance characteristics of AIP include focal or diffuse enlargement of the pancreas (mass-forming type), absence of parenchymal atrophy or dilatation proximal to the site of stenosis, absence of peripancreatic spread, clear demarcation of the culprit lesion and the presence of a peripancreatic rim. The predominant feature on cholangiopancreatography may be that of a diffusely or segmentally irregular and narrow main pancreatic duct (i.e. the duct-stenotic type). In addition, strictures of the distal bile ducts may be evident (Fig. 12.3). This steroid responsive disease is described in greater detail elsewhere.

## Eosinophilic Cholangitis

Eosinophilic infiltrates of the portal triads with or without peripheral eosinophilia usually suggest a parasitic, fungal or drug-induced disease. There

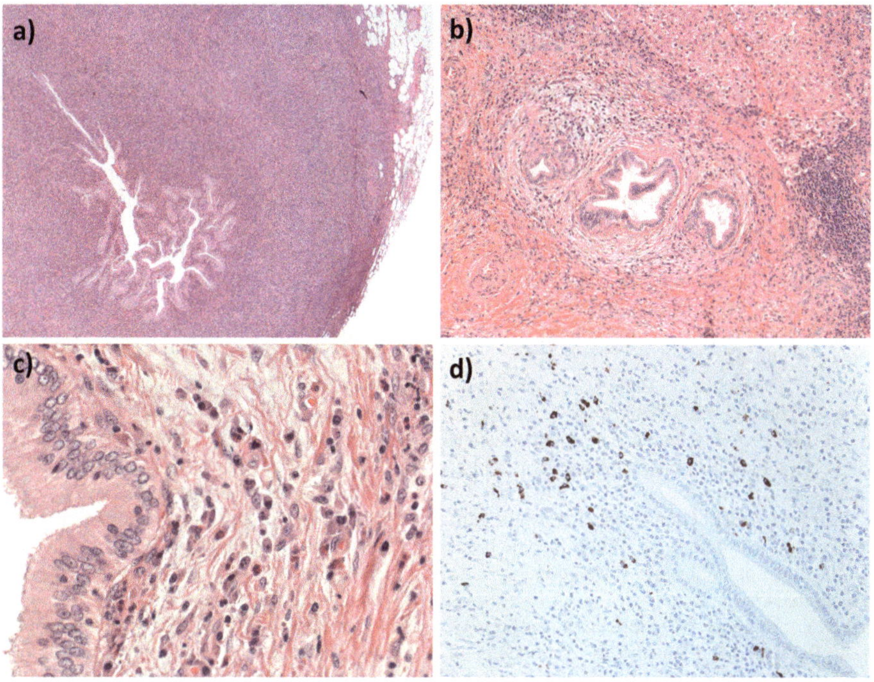


**Fig. 12.3** Histological features of IgG4-associated cholangitis. (**a**) Extrahepatic bile duct with dense transmural mononuclear infiltrate, HE stain, ×50. (**b**) Intrahepatic bile ducts with chronic inflammation and periductal oedema, HE stain, ×100. (**c**) Portal area with plasma cell infiltrate around bile duct, HE stain, ×400. (**d**) Numerous IgG4-positive plasma cells in bile duct wall, IgG4 immunostain, ×200 (Image courtesy of Dr S Fischer, Pathology, University Health Network, Toronto)

are however reports of primary eosinophilic cholangitis in the literature with marked eosinophilic infiltration of the hepatobiliary tree, including development of a secondary sclerosing cholangiopathy [47]. This is rare as a primary process but it is telling perhaps mechanistically that not infrequently patients with colitis and PSC are noted to have eosinophilia of unknown significance [48].

## Conclusion

Sclerosing cholangitis is a disease with a broad spectrum of aetiologies. It has the potential to lead to important clinical outcomes, including recurrent cholangitis, liver cirrhosis and a need for transplant. The variety of secondary aetiologies has highlighted a number of important biologic pathways that lead to large bile duct injury. These pathways may prove of importance in the future as new therapies for primary disease are tested.

## References

1. LaRusso NF, Shneider BL, Black D, Gores GJ, James SP, Doo E, Hoofnagle JH. Primary sclerosing cholangitis: summary of a workshop. Hepatology. 2006;44:746–64.
2. Chapman R, Fevery J, Kalloo A, Nagorney DM, Boberg KM, Shneider B, Gores GJ. Diagnosis and management of primary sclerosing cholangitis. Hepatology. 2010;51:660–78.
3. Sherlock S. Chronic cholangitides: aetiology, diagnosis, and treatment. Br Med J. 1968;3:515–21.
4. Tinckler L. Primary sclerosing cholangitis. Postgrad Med J. 1971;47:666–70.
5. Abdalian R, Heathcote EJ. Sclerosing cholangitis: a focus on secondary causes. Hepatology. 2006;44:1063–74.
6. Ruemmele P, Hofstaedter F, Gelbmann CM. Secondary sclerosing cholangitis. Nat Rev Gastroenterol Hepatol. 2009;6:287–95.
7. Lazaridis KN. Sclerosing cholangitis epidemiology and etiology. J Gastrointest Surg. 2008;12:417–9.
8. Gossard AA, Angulo P, Lindor KD. Secondary sclerosing cholangitis: a comparison to primary sclerosing cholangitis. Am J Gastroenterol. 2005;100:1330–3.
9. Weismuller TJ, Wedemeyer J, Kubicka S, Strassburg CP, Manns MP. The challenges in primary sclerosing

cholangitis–aetiopathogenesis, autoimmunity, management and malignancy. J Hepatol. 2008;48 Suppl 1:S38–57.
10. Bowlus CL. Cutting Edge Issues in Primary Sclerosing Cholangitis. Clin Rev Allergy Immunol. 2011;41: 139–50.
11. Deltenre P, Valla DC. Ischemic cholangiopathy. Semin Liver Dis. 2008;28:235–46.
12. Strazzabosco M, Fabris L. Functional anatomy of normal bile ducts. Anat Rec (Hoboken). 2008;291:653–60.
13. Buis CI, Hoekstra H, Verdonk RC, Porte RJ. Causes and consequences of ischemic-type biliary lesions after liver transplantation. J Hepatobiliary Pancreat Surg. 2006;13:517–24.
14. Heidenhain C, Pratschke J, Puhl G, Neumann U, Pascher A, Veltzke-Schlieker W, Neuhaus P. Incidence of and risk factors for ischemic-type biliary lesions following orthotopic liver transplantation. Transpl Int. 2010;23:14–22.
15. Adeyi O, Fischer SE, Guindi M. Liver allograft pathology: approach to interpretation of needle biopsies with clinicopathological correlation. J Clin Pathol. 2010;63:47–74.
16. De Angelis C, Mangone M, Bianchi M, Saracco G, Repici A, Rizzetto M, Pellicano R. An update on AIDS-related cholangiopathy. Minerva Gastroenterol Dietol. 2009;55:79–82.
17. O'Hara SP, Small AJ, Gajdos GB, Badley AD, Chen XM, Larusso NF. HIV-1 Tat protein suppresses cholangiocyte toll-like receptor 4 expression and defense against Cryptosporidium parvum. J Infect Dis. 2009;199:1195–204.
18. Aron JH, Bowlus CL. The immunobiology of primary sclerosing cholangitis. Semin Immunopathol. 2009;31:383–97.
19. Fickert P, Fuchsbichler A, Wagner M, Zollner G, Kaser A, Tilg H, Krause R, Lammert F, Langner C, Zatloukal K, Marschall HU, Denk H, Trauner M. Regurgitation of bile acids from leaky bile ducts causes sclerosing cholangitis in Mdr2 (Abcb4) knockout mice. Gastroenterology. 2004;127:261–74.
20. Mair M, Zollner G, Schneller D, Musteanu M, Fickert P, Gumhold J, Schuster C, Fuchsbichler A, Bilban M, Tauber S, Esterbauer H, Kenner L, Poli V, Blaas L, Kornfeld JW, Casanova E, Mikulits W, Trauner M, Eferl R. Signal transducer and activator of transcription 3 protects from liver injury and fibrosis in a mouse model of sclerosing cholangitis. Gastroenterology. 2010;138:2499–508.
21. Rosmorduc O, Poupon R. Low phospholipid associated cholelithiasis: association with mutation in the MDR3/ABCB4 gene. Orphanet J Rare Dis. 2007;2:29.
22. Hadj-Rabia S, Baala L, Vabres P, Hamel-Teillac D, Jacquemin E, Fabre M, Lyonnet S, De Prost Y, Munnich A, Hadchouel M, Smahi A. Claudin-1 gene mutations in neonatal sclerosing cholangitis associated with ichthyosis: a tight junction disease. Gastroenterology. 2004;127:1386–90.
23. Rodrigues F, Davies EG, Harrison P, McLauchlin J, Karani J, Portmann B, Jones A, Veys P, Mieli-Vergani G, Hadzic N. Liver disease in children with primary immunodeficiencies. J Pediatr. 2004;145:333–9.
24. Bilgin M, Balci NC, Erdogan A, Momtahen AJ, Alkaade S, Rau WS. Hepatobiliary and pancreatic MRI and MRCP findings in patients with HIV infection. AJR Am J Roentgenol. 2008;191:228–32.
25. Chen XM, LaRusso NF. Cryptosporidiosis and the pathogenesis of AIDS-cholangiopathy. Semin Liver Dis. 2002;22:277–89.
26. Walser EM, Runyan BR, Heckman MG, Bridges MD, Willingham DL, Paz-Fumagalli R, Nguyen JH. Extrahepatic portal biliopathy: proposed etiology on the basis of anatomic and clinical features. Radiology. 2011;258:146–53.
27. Bouche H, Housset C, Dumont JL, Carnot F, Menu Y, Aveline B, Belghiti J, Boboc B, Erlinger S, Berthelot P, et al. AIDS-related cholangitis: diagnostic features and course in 15 patients. J Hepatol. 1993;17:34–9.
28. Pol S, Romana CA, Richard S, Amouyal P, Desportes-Livage I, Carnot F, Pays JF, Berthelot P. Microsporidia infection in patients with the human immunodeficiency virus and unexplained cholangitis. N Engl J Med. 1993;328:95–9.
29. Chen XM, LaRusso NF. Mechanisms of attachment and internalization of Cryptosporidium parvum to biliary and intestinal epithelial cells. Gastroenterology. 2000;118:368–79.
30. Chen XM, Keithly JS, Paya CV, LaRusso NF. Cryptosporidiosis. N Engl J Med. 2002;346:1723–31.
31. Vakil NB, Schwartz SM, Buggy BP, Brummitt CF, Kherellah M, Letzer DM, Gilson IH, Jones PG. Biliary cryptosporidiosis in HIV-infected people after the waterborne outbreak of cryptosporidiosis in Milwaukee. N Engl J Med. 1996;334:19–23.
32. Tsui WM, Chan YK, Wong CT, Lo YF, Yeung YW, Lee YW. Hepatolithiasis and the syndrome of recurrent pyogenic cholangitis: clinical, radiologic, and pathologic features. Semin Liver Dis. 2011;31:33–48.
33. Marcos LA, Terashima A, Gotuzzo E. Update on hepatobiliary flukes: fascioliasis, opisthorchiasis and clonorchiasis. Curr Opin Infect Dis. 2008;21:523–30.
34. Cheon YK, Cho YD, Moon JH, Lee JS, Shim CS. Evaluation of long-term results and recurrent factors after operative and nonoperative treatment for hepatolithiasis. Surgery. 2009;146:843–53.
35. Jaeger C, Mayer G, Henrich R, Gossner L, Rabenstein T, May A, Guenter E, Ell C. Secondary sclerosing cholangitis after long-term treatment in an intensive care unit: clinical presentation, endoscopic findings, treatment, and follow-up. Endoscopy. 2006;38: 730–4.
36. Gelbmann CM, Rummele P, Wimmer M, Hofstadter F, Gohlmann B, Endlicher E, Kullmann F, Langgartner J, Scholmerich J. Ischemic-like cholangiopathy with secondary sclerosing cholangitis in critically ill patients. Am J Gastroenterol. 2007;102:1221–9.
37. Esposito I, Kubisova A, Stiehl A, Kulaksiz H, Schirmacher P. Secondary sclerosing cholangitis after intensive care unit treatment: clues to the

histopathological differential diagnosis. Virchows Arch. 2008;453:339–45.
38. Dhiman RK, Behera A, Chawla YK, Dilawari JB, Suri S. Portal hypertensive biliopathy. Gut. 2007;56:1001–8.
39. Oo YH, Olliff S, Haydon G, Thorburn D. Symptomatic portal biliopathy: a single centre experience from the UK. Eur J Gastroenterol Hepatol. 2009;21:206–13.
40. Barnett KT, Malafa MP. Complications of hepatic artery infusion: a review of 4580 reported cases. Int J Gastrointest Cancer. 2001;30:147–60.
41. Alazmi WM, McHenry L, Watkins JL, Fogel EL, Schmidt S, Sherman S, Lehman GL. Chemotherapy-induced sclerosing cholangitis: long-term response to endoscopic therapy. J Clin Gastroenterol. 2006;40:353–7.
42. Tsimoyiannis EC, Grantzis E, Moutesidou K, Lekkas ET. Secondary sclerosing cholangitis: after injection of formaldehyde into hydatid cysts in the liver. Eur J Surg. 1995;161:299–300.
43. Vijungco JD, Prinz RA. Management of biliary and duodenal complications of chronic pancreatitis. World J Surg. 2003;27:1258–70.
44. Abdallah AA, Krige JE, Bornman PC. Biliary tract obstruction in chronic pancreatitis. HPB (Oxford). 2007;9:421–8.
45. Wu YV, Linehan DC. Bile duct injuries in the era of laparoscopic cholecystectomies. Surg Clin North Am. 2010;90:787–802.
46. Sugumar A, Chari ST. Diagnosis and treatment of autoimmune pancreatitis. Curr Opin Gastroenterol. 2010;26:513–8.
47. Tenner S, Roston A, Lichtenstein D, Brooks D, Herlihy E, Carr-Locke D. Eosinophilic cholangiopathy. Gastrointest Endosc. 1997;45:307–9.
48. Horiuchi K, Kakizaki S, Kosone T, Ichikawa T, Sato K, Takagi H, Mori M, Sakurai S, Fukusato T. Marked eosinophilia as the first manifestation of sclerosing cholangitis. Intern Med. 2009;48:1377–82.

# 13 Histologic Features

Lizhi Zhang and Vikram Deshpande

## Introduction and Outline

Autoimmune pancreatitis is a fibroinflammatory disease of the pancreas. In a seminal and apparently serendipitous discovery, Harmano and coworkers detected elevated levels of serum IgG4 in patients with autoimmune pancreatitis [1]. Subsequent to this discovery, serum and tissue IgG4 rapidly emerged as robust biomarkers of autoimmune pancreatitis. In 2003, Kamisava proposed a systemic form of "autoimmune pancreatitis," and this hypothesis was to a large extent based on the presence of elevated numbers of IgG4 plasma cells at extrapancreatic sites of the disease [2]. Over the next decade, this systemic form of IgG4-related disease has been shown to involve virtually every organ system [3]. The nomenclature of this multiorgan disease is in flux, and a number of competing terms have been used including IgG4-related sclerosing disease, IgG4-associated autoimmune disease, hyper-IgG4 disease, IgG4-related systemic sclerosing disease, and IgG4-related systemic disease (IgG4-RSD) – the last term will be used in this chapter [4].

L. Zhang, M.D.
Department of Laboratory and Anatomic Pathology, Mayo Clinic, Hilton 10, 200 1st ST., SW, Rochester, MN 55905, USA
e-mail: zhang.lizhi@mayo.edu

V. Deshpande, M.D. (✉)
Department of Pathology, Massachusetts General Hospital, 55 Fruit Street, Boston, MA 02114, USA
e-mail: vdeshpande@partners.org

Two variants of autoimmune pancreatitis are now widely recognized: type 1 and type 2, with only the former variant being consistently, but not always, associated with elevated serum and tissue levels of IgG4 [5, 6]. In fact, type 2 disease is virtually confined to the pancreas, and hence this chapter will focus on the pathology of type 1 autoimmune pancreatitis and its involvement of the hepatobiliary tree. The preferred designation for this hepatobiliary involvement by IgG4-related disease is IgG4-related sclerosing cholangitis (ISC) [7].

Morphologically, ISC may involve both the extrahepatic and the intrahepatic portions of the bile duct with extrahepatic ISC being much more common than intrahepatic disease. In fact, Whipple resections from patients with type 1 autoimmune pancreatitis almost universally show diffuse involvement of the resected portion of the bile duct. A smaller percentage of cases show involvement of both regions of the bile duct [7]. This chapter will initially discuss the intrahepatic manifestations followed by a description of the extrahepatic disease, with the implicit understanding that simultaneous involvement of both sites is relatively common. Similar to other forms of IgG4-RSD, some patients present with hepatic tumefactive lesions. Finally, we will also describe gallbladder involvement by IgG4-RSD. Examination of the gallbladder may provide a powerful diagnostic tool for distinguishing ISC from its closest mimics, primary sclerosing cholangitis (PSC) and cholangiocarcinoma.

M.J. Levy and S.T. Chari (eds.), *Autoimmune (IgG4-related) Pancreatitis and Cholangitis*,
DOI 10.1007/978-1-4419-6430-4_13, © Springer Science+Business Media New York 2013

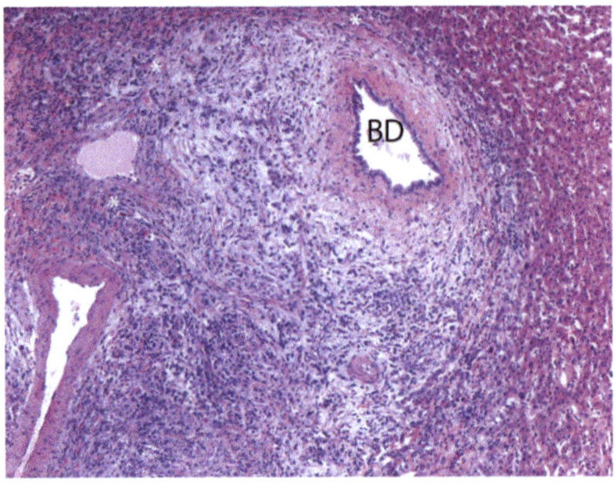


**Fig. 13.1** IgG4-associated cholangitis. This wedge biopsy shows a portal-based inflammatory nodule. The inflammation tends to spare the bile duct (BD)

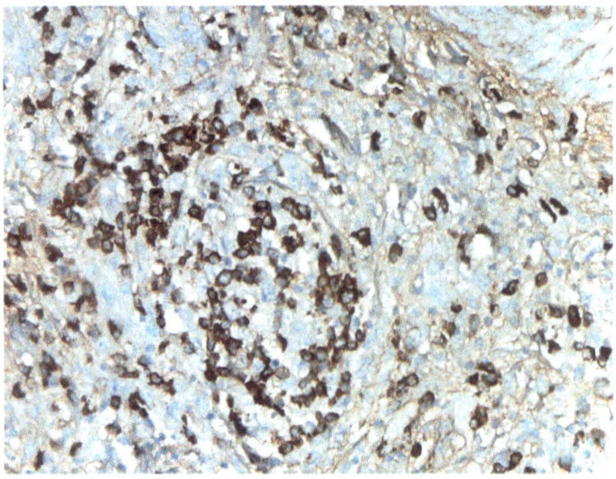

**Fig. 13.2** An IgG4 immunoperoxidase stain on the case illustrated in Fig. 13.1. Note the large numbers of IgG4-positive plasma cells

## Pathology of Intrahepatic ISC

This form of ISC may mimic PSC. In most instances, the diagnosis of ISC is preceded by pancreatic involvement, i.e., autoimmune pancreatitis, and only rarely may precede clinically inapparent pancreatic involvement. Most patients present with obstructive jaundice [7]. On cholangiogram, both intra- and extrahepatic strictures may be present [7, 8].

### Histology

Histologically, the presence of portal-based inflammatory nodules is highly characteristic of ISC (Fig. 13.1) [9]. The inflammatory nodules are composed of lymphocytes, plasma cells, and eosinophils, admixed with fibroblasts. Although obliterative phlebitis, an almost obligate feature of autoimmune pancreatitis, is not seen in peripheral liver biopsies, a perivenular accentuation in portal tracts is often present. This histologic appearance is remarkably similar to other forms of IgG4-RSD. In fact, the histologic appearance within the stromal nodules is virtually identical to the interlobular stroma of type 1 autoimmune pancreatitis and the stroma of salivary glands involved by autoimmune pancreatitis [5, 10]. The peripheral bile ducts may show histologic evidence of injury, but accentuation of the inflammation around the duct is rarely seen. Although more commonly seen in PSC and often used as a diagnostic feature of PSC, periductal onion skin-type fibrosis is occasionally seen in ISC as well and hence cannot help distinguish PSC from ISC. Sections from the hilar region of the liver, however, may show both obliterative phlebitis and inflammation of large caliber bile ducts.

The key to arriving at the correct diagnosis is a tissue stain for IgG4. Liver biopsy in ISC shows elevated numbers of IgG4-positive plasma cells (Fig. 13.2). In one series, 70 % of biopsies from ISC cases showed >5 IgG4-positive plasma cells per HPF, while in PSC, IgG4-positive plasma cells were either absent or fewer than 5 per HPF [5, 11]. It should be noted that there are marked variations between microscopes with regard to the size of one HPF. A recently published study highlights this issue [12]: although these authors found that cases with ISC had significantly ($p=0.0002$) higher IgG4-bearing plasma cells, the mean number of such cells was only 2.2 per HPF [12]. Although only a relatively small number of cases have been evaluated, IgG4-positive plasma cells have not been observed in liver biopsies from patients with chronic viral hepatitis and primary biliary cirrhosis [13]. IgG4-positive plasma cells have been identified in a subset of cases of autoimmune hepatitis [14].

**Table 13.1** Comparison of clinical and histologic features of IAC and PSC

| | IgG4-associated cholangitis | Primary sclerosing cholangitis |
|---|---|---|
| Age | Predominantly older (mean age 63) | Younger (mean age 39) |
| Sex | Male predominance | Male predominance |
| IBD | Occasional | Very common |
| Pancreas involvement | Most cases | Occasional |
| ERCP | Extrahepatic involved; intrahepatic strictures less common | Both extrahepatic and intrahepatic biliary strictures |
| Histology and immunohistochemistry | Inflammatory portal-based nodules and IgG4-positive plasma cells | Variable portal-based inflammation, periductal fibrosis |
| | | IgG4 plasma cells – typically rare to absent in biopsy material |

Furthermore, 23 % of explant livers from patients with PSC showed IgG4-positive plasma cells [15]. Interestingly, when compared with cases without IgG4-positive plasma cells, those with elevated IgG4 cells had a more aggressive clinical course [15]. Thus, without the appropriate morphological features (i.e., inflammatory nodules), the significance of occasional IgG4-positive cells remains uncertain. An IgG4 to IgG ratio may help improve the specificity of this biomarker; however, a diagnostic cutoff for this variable has not been established.

## Differential Diagnosis

Clinically and pathologically ISC may mimic PSC. This distinction has significant therapeutic implications since unlike PSC, ISC is a steroid-responsive disease. The presence of pancreatic disease that is compatible with autoimmune pancreatitis would strongly support a diagnosis of ISC. The presence of IgG4-positive cells, portal inflammation dominated by plasma cells, and inflammatory nodules are histologic clues that assist in distinguishing ISC from PSC (Table 13.1). Nonetheless, it should be emphasized that these histologic features may not be seen in every liver biopsy. Furthermore, although significant numbers of IgG4-positive plasma cells (defined as >10/HPF) are seldom seen in needle biopsies from PSC cases, one of the authors (VD) has noted the presence of significant numbers of IgG4-positive plasma cells in two patients with PSC arising in the background of ulcerative colitis (the colonic biopsies from these patients also demonstrated an elevated number of IgG4-positive plasma cells). The histologic diagnosis of ISC should not be based solely on the presence of elevated IgG4 cells: correlation with the clinical and imaging features and corroborating histologic features is an absolute requirement.

## Extrahepatic Bile Duct Involvement

The overall rate of extrahepatic bile duct involvement in autoimmune pancreatitis type 1 is 71–100 % [7, 9, 16–20] and represents the most commonly involved extrapancreatic site in autoimmune pancreatitis. ISC can present either as bile duct wall thickening with dense lymphoplasmacytic infiltration and marked interstitial fibrosis resulting in bile duct stricture or as mass-forming lesion in the hilum mimicking extrahepatic cholangiocarcinoma (Fig. 13.3). Isolated ISC, i.e., biliary disease not associated with autoimmune pancreatitis, can also occur. ISC without autoimmune pancreatitis has similar histopathological features as ISC arising in the setting of autoimmune pancreatitis.

## Histology

Microscopically, ISC has similar morphological changes as seen in type 1 autoimmune

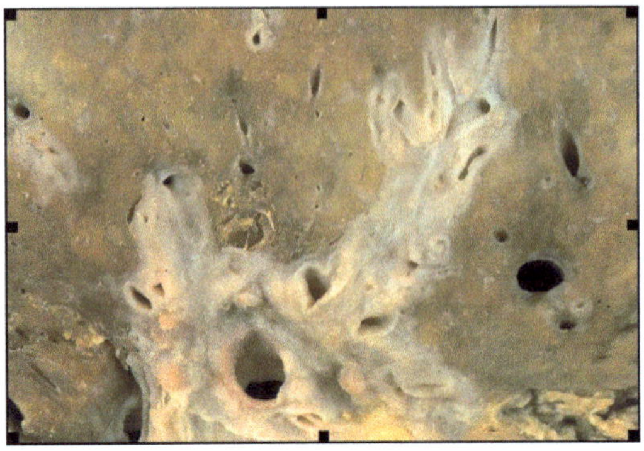

**Fig. 13.3** Extrahepatic biliary tract involvement by ISC. Note the hepatic hilar fibrosis, bile duct thickening, and stricture formation

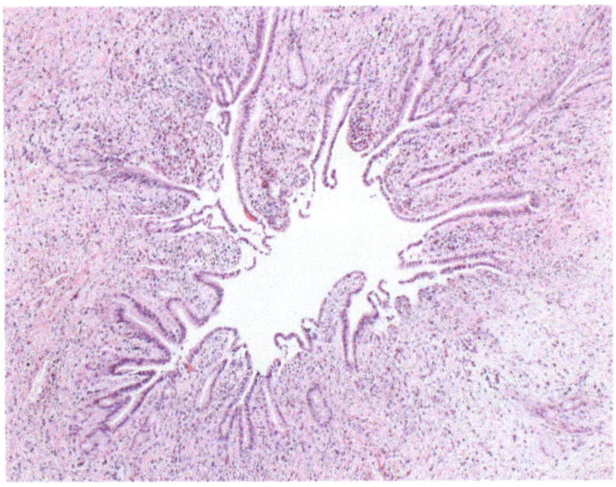

**Fig. 13.4** IgG4-associated cholangitis. The liver shows periductal lymphoplasmacytic infiltrate and fibrosis with stellate narrowing of bile duct

pancreatitis. The characteristic features include transmural lymphoplasmacytic infiltration, marked fibrosis with storiform pattern, and obliterative phlebitis. The lymphoplasmacytic infiltration is transmural and extends to involve the periductal connective tissue and peribiliary glands. The lymphoplasmacytic infiltrate tends to localize beneath the bile duct epithelium but only rarely infiltrates the epithelium to cause epithelial damage (Fig. 13.4). The dense lymphoplasmacytic infiltrate involves the intrapancreatic common bile duct and lower half of common bile duct, but it may extend proximally to extrapancreatic common bile ducts and hepatic ducts. The lumen of the bile duct is narrowed by periductal

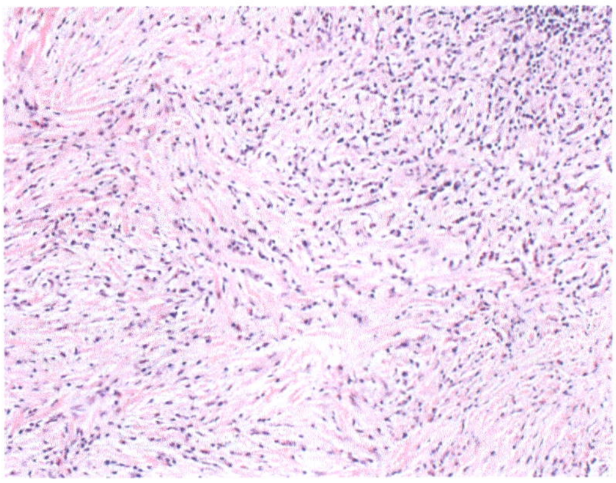

**Fig. 13.5** IgG4-assocaited cholangitis with storiform fibrosis. Inflammatory cells intermixed with fibroblasts and short swirling collagen fibers producing a storiform pattern

inflammation and fibrosis. Prominent lymphoid aggregates and follicles in the periductal connective tissue can be seen in some cases, but this is a nonspecific feature.

Eosinophils are present in most cases. Small-sized epithelioid granulomas without necrosis within the wall of common bile ducts may be seen [21]. A small number of neutrophils can be seen occasionally, but abscess formation with/without tissue necrosis is not present.

The periductal fibrosis shows a storiform pattern similar to that described in autoimmune pancreatitis. The fibrosis also contains high numbers of lymphocytes and plasma cells intermixed with fibroblasts and short swirling collagen fibers which produces a storiform pattern (Fig. 13.5). This inflammed stroma is essentially identical to the reaction seen at other organ sites involved by IgG4-RSD. A tumefactive appearance with effacement of tissue architecture may be seen in severe cases.

Obliterative phlebitis is pathognomonic for ISC as it is in autoimmune pancreatitis type 1. The inflammation typically begins at the periphery of venous walls (perivenulitis), spreading through the wall as the lesion progresses. Fully developed lesion (obliterative phlebitis) is characterized by obstruction of the lumen and destruction of the wall by dense lymphoplasmacytic infiltration (Fig. 13.6). These venous lesions are located adjacent to arteries and show a round

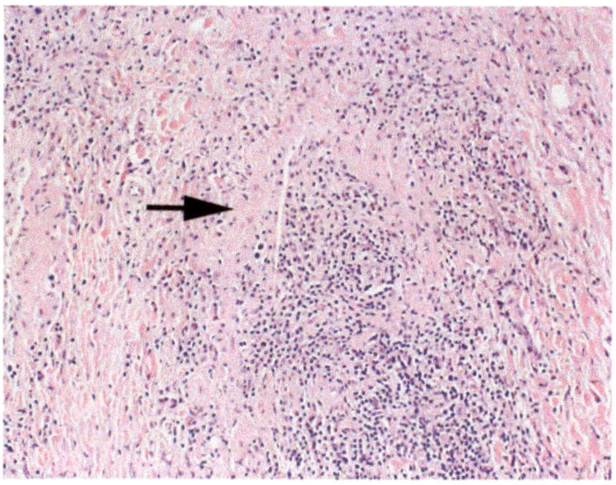

**Fig. 13.6** IgG4-associated cholangitis. Obliterative phlebitis characterized by organized obstruction of veins with wall destruction by dense lymphoplasmacytic infiltration (*arrow*)

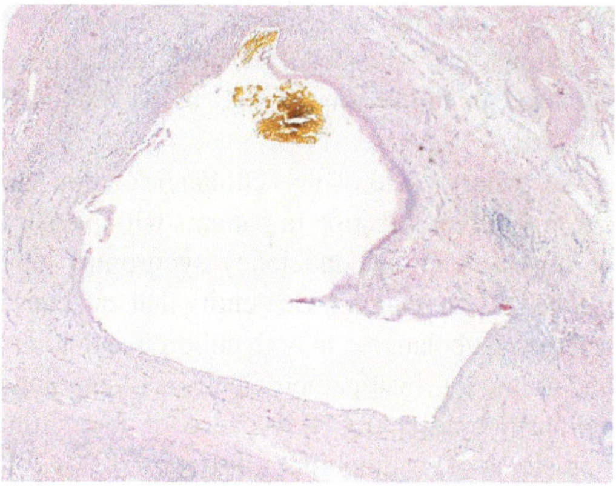

**Fig. 13.7** Primary sclerosing cholangitis. Inflamed biliary epithelium with edema ulceration and periductal lamellated fibrosis. Note that the inflammatory infiltrate is significantly less than seen in ISC (compare with Fig. 13.4)

to oval outline with accentuation of the lymphoplasmacytic infiltration at the periphery of the lesion. An elastic Van Gieson stain may uncover subtle forms of obliterative phlebitis.

## IgG4 Immunostain

Moderate (>10 cells/HPF) or severe (>30 cells/HPF) increase in IgG4+ plasma cell infiltrate is a useful diagnostic tool for ISC, although it is not entirely specific [22, 23, 24]. Nearly 90 % ISC show moderately increased IgG4+ plasma cell infiltrates [7]. But increased IgG4 immunostaining can occur in resected specimens in about 25 % of primary sclerosing cholangitis (PSC) as well as 20 % of cholangiocarcinoma patients [15].

## Differential Diagnosis

The two diseases to consider in the differential diagnosis are PSC and cholangiocarcinoma. Histologically, the extrahepatic bile ducts in PSC are thickened by fibrosis and moderate to marked lymphoplasmacytic infiltrate intermixed with eosinophils and neutrophils. But unlike ISC, where the transmural lymphoplasmacytic infiltration spares the biliary lining epithelium, the surface epithelium in PSC is often inflamed with edema, sloughing, erosion, and neutrophilic infiltration. Furthermore, the inflammation in PSC is concentrated around the periluminal portion of the bile duct with only mild inflammatory changes in the outer layer of the bile duct. The periductal reaction in PSC differs from the storiform fibrosis seen in ISC: fibrosis in PSC is composed of dense collagen with a well-organized laminated pattern and lesser numbers of inflammatory cells (Fig. 13.7). Obliterative phlebitis is not seen in PSC cases [15, 21].

The diagnosis of ISC on routine intraductal forceps biopsy specimens can be challenging. The superficial nature of the sample, tissue fragmentations, and crushing artifact limit the pathologist's ability to appreciate storiform fibrosis or obliterative phlebitis. Under these circumstances, a definitive diagnosis of ISC is seldom possible on a small biopsy specimen, although even limited information gleaned from a biopsy when viewed in conjunction with clinical and imaging features can provide meaningful information. It should be noted that the sensitivity of brush cytology and intraductal forceps biopsy for bile duct carcinoma is relatively low. Fluorescence in situ hybridization (FISH) test on cytology specimen can also be helpful for the detection of malignancy in biliary tract strictures, but false-positive FISH results have occurred in the setting of ISC as well as AIP [25, 26].

Secondary sclerosing cholangitis due to chronic biliary infection in patients with primary or acquired immunodeficiency syndromes may mimic ISC on imaging. One entity that can cause sclerosing cholangitis in both children and adults and mimic ISC histopathologically is Langerhans cell histiocytosis (LCH) because of interstitial fibrosis and eosinophilic infiltration [27, 28]. LCH usually lacks the dense lymphoplasmacytic infiltration of ISC. Langerhans cells have abundant eosinophilic cytoplasm and grooved nuclei with indented nuclear membranes. Immunoreactivity of Langerhans cells to CD1a and S100 can confirm the diagnosis of LCH.

## IgG4-Associated Inflammatory Pseudotumor

IgG4-associated inflammatory pseudotumors may present as a solitary peripheral liver nodule or as a tumoral lesion in the porta hepatis (Fig. 13.8). While sclerosing cholangitis is invariably noted in cases with hilar disease, sclerosing cholangitis may not be present in cases with a peripheral nodule.

### Histology

A recent study [29] described two types of inflammatory pseudotumors involving liver and bile ducts: fibrohistiocytic and lymphoplasmacytic. The lymphoplasmacytic type is believed to represent an IgG4-related disease, while the evidence linking the former entity to IgG4 is less robust. The fibrohistiocytic inflammatory pseudotumors typically show xanthogranulomatous inflammation, multinucleated giant cells, and neutrophilic infiltration and mostly occur in the peripheral hepatic parenchyma. In addition, the fibrohistiocytic type does not show obliterative phlebitis, cholangitis with periductal fibrosis, and increased IgG4-positive plasma cells: these being features typical of the lymphoplasmacytic variant.

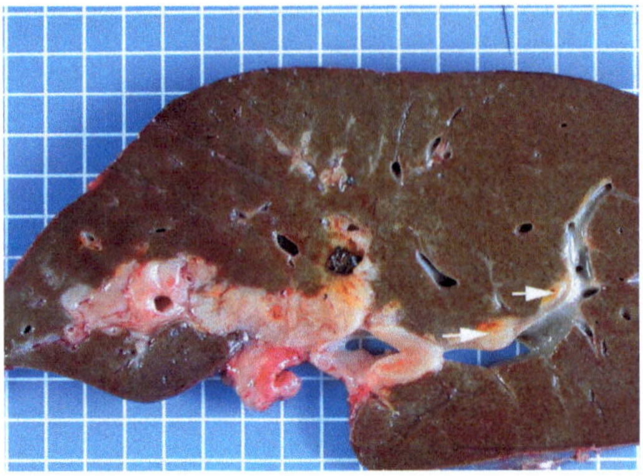

**Fig. 13.8** A hepatectomy performed with the presume diagnosis of cholangiocarcinoma. The fleshy hilar mass mimics malignancy. Also note the peripheral liver nodules (*arrows*) (Source: Image from IgG4-associated cholangitis: a comparative histological and immunophenotypic study with primary sclerosing cholangitis on liver biopsy material)

### Differential Diagnosis

The primary clinical and radiologic differential diagnosis in these cases is cholangiocarcinoma and metastatic carcinoma. Histologically, with a generous biopsy sample, a cholangiocarcinoma can readily be excluded. It should be noted that a cholangiocarcinoma may rarely show a brisk peritumoral lymphoplasmacytic infiltrate, and this feature could mimic IgG4-associated inflammatory pseudotumor.

Another diagnostic possibility on a biopsy sample showing a fibroinflammatory infiltrate is an inflammatory myofibroblastic tumor. However, IgG4-associated inflammatory pseudotumor shows significantly higher numbers of IgG4-positive plasma cells and higher IgG4 to IgG ratios [30]. In one series, all 22 cases showed IgG4 to IgG ratios of >30 %, while all 16 cases of inflammatory myofibroblastic tumor showed ratios less than 30 % [30]. Furthermore, ALK expression is restricted to inflammatory myofibroblastic tumor, although the stain is positive in only 50 % of cases [31]. Other entities in the differential diagnosis of

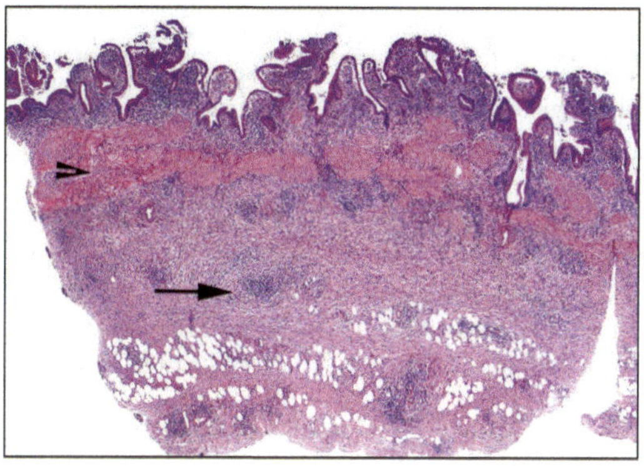

**Fig. 13.9** Gallbladder from a patient with type 1 autoimmune pancreatitis. The wall of the gallbladder is markedly thickened by a lymphoplasmacytic infiltrate. The inflammatory pathology (*arrow*) is predominantly located beyond the muscularis propria (*arrowhead*)

an IgG4-associated pseudotumor include follicular dendritic cell tumor and interdigitating dendritic cell tumor [31].

## Gallbladder Disease in Autoimmune Pancreatitis

It should come as no surprise that IgG4-RSD may also involve the cystic duct and gallbladder. However, unlike other forms of cholecystitis, gallbladder involvement by this disease is generally asymptomatic. Nonetheless, 53 % of cases in one series showed a thickened gallbladder on imaging [32].

Histologically, in our experience, gallbladders with a predominantly extramural pattern of inflammation (Fig. 13.9), inflammatory nodules, and phlebitis are strongly associated with autoimmune pancreatitis [33]. Half (11 of 22) of the autoimmune pancreatitis-associated gallbladders we studied showed at least one of these three patterns of involvement [33]. Furthermore, the presence of >10 IgG4+ plasma cells/HPF and/or an IgG4/IgG ratio of >0.5 within the gallbladder was indicative of autoimmune pancreatitis. Histologic evaluation of the gallbladder, when available, can be of value in two situations: (1) gallbladders with autoimmune pancreatitis-like morphology, these findings could raise the possibility or support the clinical impression of autoimmune pancreatitis, and (2) in individuals with sclerosing cholangitis, this histologic appearance would raise the possibility of ISC. Nonetheless, although histologic evaluation of the gallbladder emerges as a potential diagnostic resource in autoimmune pancreatitis, this data is best viewed in conjunction with other relevant clinical, serologic, and imaging features.

## Conclusion

The morphological picture of ISC is essentially similar to other forms of IgG4-RSD: storiform fibroinflammatory stroma, obliterative phlebitis, and elevated numbers of IgG4-positive plasma cells. Biopsies from the ampulla, bile ducts, and liver when combined with a tissue IgG4 immunoperoxidase stain may provide accurate tissue diagnosis (Table 13.2). We would urge caution on relying solely on an IgG4 immunoperoxidase stain since elevated numbers of IgG4-positive plasma cells may rarely be seen in malignancy.

## Key Points

- ISC is usually associated with autoimmune pancreatitis type 1.
- The disease can affect the extrahepatic and/or the intrahepatic portion of the bile duct or form a tumefactive lesion.
- Key morphological features include the following: transmural lymphoplasmacytic infiltration, marked interstitial fibrosis with storiform pattern, obliterative phlebitis, and increased IgG4-positive plasma cells.
- Biopsies from the liver, bile duct, and ampulla when viewed in conjunction with a IgG4 immunoperoxidase stain may help support a diagnosis of ISC.
- The differential diagnosis primarily includes PSC and cholangiocarcinoma.

**Table 13.2** Key histologic features and IgG4 cut points

| | Biopsy | Key histologic findings | IgG4 suggested cut points for diagnosis |
|---|---|---|---|
| Intrahepatic disease | Liver biopsy – wedge or needle[a] | Portal-based inflammatory nodules | >10/HPF |
| Extrahepatic disease | Bile duct/ampullary biopsy | Bile duct – storiform fibrosis, obliterative phlebitis[b] | Bile duct – >10/HPF |
| | | Ampulla – lymphoplasmacytic inflammation (nonspecific histologic finding) | Ampulla – >10/HPF (41/66 cases of IAC/AIP showed >10 IgG4cell/HFP)30–32 |
| IgG4-associated pseudotumor | Liver or hilar mass | Lymphoplasmacytic inflammation, storiform fibrosis | >50 HPF; ALK – negative |

[a]A liver biopsy is more likely to show elevated numbers of IgG4-positive plasma cells in individuals with intrahepatic strictures
[b]Seldom seen in biopsy samples

## References


1. Hamano H, Kawa S, Horiuchi A, et al. High serum IgG4 concentrations in patients with sclerosing pancreatitis. N Engl J Med. 2001;344:732–8.
2. Kamisawa T, Funata N, Hayashi Y, et al. A new clinicopathological entity of IgG4-related autoimmune disease. J Gastroenterol. 2003;38:982–4.
3. Khosroshahi A, Stone JH. A clinical overview of IgG4-related systemic disease. Curr Opin Rheumatol. 2011;23:57–66.
4. Cheuk W, Chan JK. IgG4-related sclerosing disease: a critical appraisal of an evolving clinicopathologic entity. Adv Anat Pathol. 2010;17:303–32.
5. Deshpande V, Gupta R, Sainani N, et al. Subclassification of autoimmune pancreatitis: a histologic classification with clinical significance. Am J Surg Pathol. 2011;35:26–35.
6. Sah RP, Chari ST, Pannala R, et al. Differences in clinical profile and relapse rate of type 1 versus type 2 autoimmune pancreatitis. Gastroenterology. 2010;139:140–8. quiz e12-3.
7. Ghazale A, Chari ST, Zhang L, et al. Immunoglobulin G4-associated cholangitis: clinical profile and response to therapy. Gastroenterology. 2008; 134:w706–15.
8. Nakazawa T, Ohara H, Sano H, et al. Cholangiography can discriminate sclerosing cholangitis with autoimmune pancreatitis from primary sclerosing cholangitis. Gastrointest Endosc. 2004;60:937–44.
9. Deshpande V, Sainani NI, Chung RT, et al. IgG4-associated cholangitis: a comparative histological and immunophenotypic study with primary sclerosing cholangitis on liver biopsy material. Mod Pathol. 2009;22:1287–95.
10. Zhang L, Notohara K, Levy MJ, Chari ST, Smyrk TC. IgG4-positive plasma cell infiltration in the diagnosis of autoimmune pancreatitis. Mod Pathol. 2007; 20:23–8.
11. Naitoh I, Zen Y, Nakazawa T, et al. Small bile duct involvement in IgG4-related sclerosing cholangitis: liver biopsy and cholangiography correlation. J Gastroenterol. 2011;46:269–76.
12. Nishino T, Oyama H, Hashimoto E, et al. Clinicopathological differentiation between sclerosing cholangitis with autoimmune pancreatitis and primary sclerosing cholangitis. J Gastroenterol. 2007; 42:550–9.
13. Umemura T, Zen Y, Hamano H, Kawa S, Nakanuma Y, Kiyosawa K. Immunoglobin G4-hepatopathy: association of immunoglobin G4-bearing plasma cells in liver with autoimmune pancreatitis. Hepatology. 2007;46:463–71.
14. Chung H, Watanabe T, Kudo M, Maenishi O, Wakatsuki Y, Chiba T. Identification and characterization of IgG4-associated autoimmune hepatitis. Liver Int. 2010;30:222–31.
15. Zhang L, Lewis JT, Abraham SC, et al. IgG4+ plasma cell infiltrates in liver explants with primary sclerosing cholangitis. Am J Surg Pathol. 2010;34:88–94.
16. Nishino T, Toki F, Oyama H, et al. Biliary tract involvement in autoimmune pancreatitis. Pancreas. 2005;30:76–82.
17. Kamisawa T, Tu Y, Egawa N, Nakajima H, Tsuruta K, Okamoto A. Involvement of pancreatic and bile ducts in autoimmune pancreatitis. World J Gastroenterol. 2006;12:612–4.
18. Hamano H, Arakura N, Muraki T, Ozaki Y, Kiyosawa K, Kawa S. Prevalence and distribution of extrapancreatic lesions complicating autoimmune pancreatitis. J Gastroenterol. 2006;41:1197–205.
19. Ghazale A, Chari S. Is autoimmune pancreatitis a risk factor for pancreatic cancer? Pancreas. 2007;35:376.
20. Kamisawa T, Egawa N, Nakajima H. Autoimmune pancreatitis is a systemic autoimmune disease. Am J Gastroenterol. 2003;98:2811–2.
21. Zen Y, Harada K, Sasaki M, et al. IgG4-related sclerosing cholangitis with and without hepatic inflammatory pseudotumor, and sclerosing

pancreatitis-associated sclerosing cholangitis: do they belong to a spectrum of sclerosing pancreatitis? Am J Surg Pathol. 2004;28:1193–203.
22. Kubota K, Kato S, Akiyama T, et al. Differentiating sclerosing cholangitis caused by autoimmune pancreatitis and primary sclerosing cholangitis according to endoscopic duodenal papillary features. Gastrointest Endosc. 2008;68:1204–8.
23. Kamisawa T, Tu Y, Egawa N, Tsuruta K, Okamoto A. A new diagnostic endoscopic tool for autoimmune pancreatitis. Gastrointest Endosc. 2008; 68:358–61.
24. Kawakami H, Zen Y, Kuwatani M, et al. IgG4-related sclerosing cholangitis and autoimmune pancreatitis: histological assessment of biopsies from Vater's ampulla and the bile duct. J Gastroenterol Hepatol. 2010;25:1648–55.
25. Kipp BR, Stadheim LM, Halling SA, et al. A comparison of routine cytology and fluorescence in situ hybridization for the detection of malignant bile duct strictures. Am J Gastroenterol. 2004;99:1675–81.
26. Fritcher EG, Kipp BR, Halling KC, et al. A multivariable model using advanced cytologic methods for the evaluation of indeterminate pancreatobiliary strictures. Gastroenterology. 2009;136:2180–6.
27. Jaffe R. Liver involvement in the histiocytic disorders of childhood. Pediatr Dev Pathol. 2004;7:214–25.
28. Gey T, Bergoin C, Just N, et al. [Langerhans cell histiocytosis and sclerosing cholangitis in adults]. Rev Mal Respir. 2004;21:997–1000.
29. Zen Y, Fujii T, Sato Y, Masuda S, Nakanuma Y. Pathological classification of hepatic inflammatory pseudotumor with respect to IgG4-related disease. Mod Pathol. 2007;20:884–94.
30. Yamamoto H, Yamaguchi H, Aishima S, et al. Inflammatory myofibroblastic tumor versus IgG4-related sclerosing disease and inflammatory pseudotumor: a comparative clinicopathologic study. Am J Surg Pathol. 2009;33:1330–40.
31. Gleason BC, Hornick JL. Inflammatory myofibroblastic tumours: where are we now? J Clin Pathol. 2008;61:428–37.
32. Kamisawa T, Tu Y, Nakajima H, et al. Sclerosing cholecystitis associated with autoimmune pancreatitis. World J Gastroenterol. 2006;12:3736–9.
33. Wang W-L, Farris AB, Lauwers GY, et al. Autoimmune pancreatitis-related cholecystitis: a morphologically and immunologically distinctive form of lymphoplasmacytic sclerosing cholecystitis. Histopathology 2009;54:829–36.

# CT and MRI Features

# 14

Ali D. Karaosmanoglu, Naoki Takahashi,
and Dushyant V. Sahani

## Introduction and Short Review of Autoimmune Pancreatitis

Autoimmune pancreatitis (AIP) is a recently defined clinical entity with unique clinical and histological features. AIP was described as "lymphoplasmacytic sclerosing pancreatitis with cholangitis" by Kawaguchi et al. in 1991. The term "AIP" was introduced in 1995 by Yoshida et al., and since then it has been the most common term used to describe this clinicopathologic entity. Two types of AIP are now recognized. Original reports pertained almost exclusively to type 1 AIP that accounts for nearly all patients in Asia and is termed "lymphoplasmacytic sclerosing pancreatitis (LPSP)." The hallmark histological features of type 1 AIP include infiltration of the pancreatic periductal areas with lymphocytes, plasma cells, and fibrosis and by obliterative phlebitis. The more recently described type 2 AIP, termed "idiopathic duct-centric pancreatitis (IDCP)," while uncommon in Asia, accounts for a large percentage of Western patients with AIP. The pathognomonic histological feature of type 2 AIP is the finding of granulocytic epithelial lesions with consequent destruction of the pancreatic duct epithelium (1). The remainder of this chapter focuses on the clinical, radiologic, and histological manifestations of IgG4-related sclerosing cholangitis (IgG4-SC) in patients with type 1 AIP.

Antinuclear antibodies (ANAs) and other autoantibodies are frequently detected in the serum samples of patients with AIP. More than 90 % of patients have high serum IgG levels, particularly IgG4. In addition, IgG4+ plasma cells are often histologically detected in the tissue samples from the pancreas and other affected organs (2, 3).

Imaging plays a crucial role in the diagnosis and follow-up of these patients. Characteristic imaging findings include diffuse pancreatic enlargement, so-called sausage-like appearance, and an enhancing band-like peripancreatic rim with or without mild peripancreatic stranding (4). AIP sometimes manifests with focal pancreatic enlargement and a mass-like lesion that may be difficult to differentiate from a pancreatic neoplasm. Pancreatic duct dilatation is absent in most patients with AIP, in contrast to pancreatic neoplasia. However, in a minority of patients, mild pancreatic duct dilatation may be associated with focal narrowing of the main pancreatic duct. Published studies showed that the caliber of the main pancreatic duct proximal to the stricture is smaller in patients with AIP (<4 mm in 67 % of the patients and 4–6 mm in 33 %) than in those with pancreatic ductal adenocarcinoma (<4 mm in 4 %, 4–6 mm in 22 %, and >6 mm in 74 %) (5–8).

A.D. Karaosmanoglu, M.D. • D.V. Sahani, MD (✉)
Department of Radiology, Massachusetts General Hospital (ADK, DS), 55 Fruit Street, Boston, MA 02114, USA
e-mail: AKARAOSMANOGLU@partners.org; dsahani@partners.org

N. Takahashi, M.D.
Department of Radiology, Mayo Clinic, 200 First Street SW, Rochester, MN 55905, USA
e-mail: takahashi.naoki@mayo.edu

M.J. Levy and S.T. Chari (eds.), *Autoimmune (IgG4-related) Pancreatitis and Cholangitis*,
DOI 10.1007/978-1-4419-6430-4_14, 

## Extrapancreatic Features of AIP

Several extrapancreatic disorders may be associated with AIP. Lacrimal and salivary gland lesions, hilar lymphadenopathy, retroperitoneal fibrosis, tubulointerstitial nephritis, and sclerosing cholangitis have all been reported with varying frequencies and clinical outcomes (9). Among the extrapancreatic organ features, biliary tract involvement is the most common, with a reported frequency of 33–90 % (8, 10, 11). These extrapancreatic features may present concurrently or remotely in time from the diagnosis of AIP, and they show favorable clinical and radiographic response to steroid therapy (9). At times, it may be difficult to differentiate other organ involvement from inherent diseases of the affected organs. Conversely, the recognition of extrapancreatic manifestations may aid in the diagnosis of AIP.

## IgG4-Related Sclerosing Cholangitis (IgG4-SC)

### Introduction

IgG4-SC is the most common extrapancreatic manifestation and may affect the intra- and/or extrahepatic bile ducts (12). Jaundice is the most common presenting symptom and is reported in 70–80 % of the patients in some series (13). Histological features of IgG4-SC include diffuse bile duct wall and gallbladder infiltration with CD3-positive T lymphocytes, plasma cells, and often fibrosis. CD4- and CD8-positive lymphocytes are also abundant on the pathologic specimens. The plasma cells are also predominantly IgG4 or IgG1 positive rather than IgG2- or IgG3-positive cells (14). Cholestasis and hyperbilirubinemia in AIP patients most often result from either parenchymal inflammation and/or fibrosis within the pancreatic head, secondarily obstructing the bile duct or as a direct result of IgG4-SC. The histological findings in the pancreas and the biliary system support the notion that AIP does not represent solely a pancreatic disorder, rather one component of a multiorgan disorder.

### Symptomatology and Basic Pathophysiology

The diagnosis of IgG4-SC is typically established in patients 50–60 years of age (15). Obstructive jaundice is the most common presenting feature (8, 10, 11) and results primarily from stenosis of the distal extrahepatic bile duct in 80 % of the patients (16) versus stenoses of the hilar and intrahepatic bile ducts in fewer than 10 % of patients (16). Approximately 35 % of patients complain of abdominal pain and weight loss is also a common feature (17, 18).

There is a link to other autoimmune diseases, with Sjögren's the most common. The presence of both disorders is termed "systemic exocrinopathy" (18). While the association of AIP and IgG4-SC with inflammatory bowel disease (IBD) has been suggested (19, 20), the causality and association has been questioned by others (21–23). The diagnosis of IgG4-SC is often suggested by the finding of increased levels of serum bilirubin and IgG4 levels and the presence of classic imaging findings.

IgG4-SC most often affects the extrahepatic bile ducts but may also involve the intrahepatic bile ducts or present with diffuse biliary disease (12). Distal extrahepatic bile duct (intrapancreatic) involvement must be distinguished from pancreatic malignancies, which can also be confused with AIP-related pseudotumors due to overlapping clinical, imaging, and laboratory findings (4). Visualization of the pancreatic duct throughout the mass-like pseudotumor, i.e., duct penetrating sign, and less significant dilatation of the downstream pancreatic duct may help indicate the presence of AIP pseudotumors rather than a pancreatic neoplasia (4, 24, 25).

The major underlying pathology leading to biliary stenosis is massive bile duct wall thickening due to lymphoplasmacytic infiltration and myofibroblasts proliferation that results in fibrosis (26). Interestingly, the epithelial cells lining the bile ducts are spared, in contrast to primary sclerosing cholangitis, and the pathologic changes are almost exclusively detected within deeper layers of the bile duct wall (26). This process may result in biliary cirrhosis and even the need for liver transplantation (27).

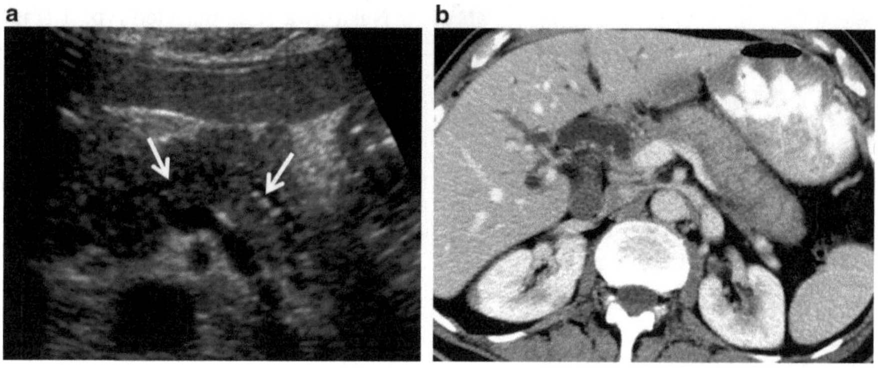


**Fig. 14.1** A 43-year-old man presenting with jaundice and mild abdominal pain. (**a**) Transabdominal US image demonstrates the mildly distended main pancreatic duct with multiple strictures (*arrows*), a common finding in AIP. (**b**) CT images did not demonstrate the mild ductal dilatation seen on transabdominal US. Note diffuse dilatation in extra- and intrahepatic biliary systems on CT

## Ultrasound Findings

Although transabdominal ultrasound (TUS) findings are nonspecific, in selected patients they may help the diagnosis of IgG4-SC. Biliary stenosis is observed in approximately 88 % of patients (15), mostly confined to the distal extrahepatic bile duct (16) (Fig. 14.1). The length of the narrowing is reported to be 10–40 mm (mean 30 mm) with smooth tapering in 83 % versus abrupt narrowing in 17 % of patients (10). Intrahepatic ductal dilatation may also be detected in the minority of the patients. TUS often reveals the typically smooth and circumferential bile duct wall thickening associated with IgG4-SC. TUS may also detect the underlying cause of biliary obstruction, such as intraductal stones, or a mass involving the hepatic hilum or pancreatic head.

The role of intraductal ultrasound (IDUS) in the assessment of bile duct wall thickening has also been studied in detail (28). Although technically challenging and invasive, IDUS may be useful in selected patients. Hyodo N. et al. (28) demonstrated diffuse bile duct wall thickening in the corresponding stenotic segments detected during endoscopic retrograde cholangiography (ERC). Wall thickening within non-stenotic segments of the bile duct is a common feature but may also develop secondary to the presence of an indwelling stent. The use of ultrasound contrast allows visualization of bile duct wall enhancement, which resolves following steroid treatment. The bile duct wall thickening detected with IDUS could not be visualized with conventional TUS in the same study.

## Computed Tomography (CT) and Magnetic Resonance Imaging (MRI)

The use of cross-sectional imaging (CT or MRI) is key to the diagnosis of IgG4-SC. The degree of biliary obstruction is generally more severe for intrapancreatic bile duct strictures (8, 11). The stricture typically appears smoothly tapered with minimal secondary upstream dilatation (19, 28) (Figs. 14.2 and 14.3). Coronal images ideally demonstrate the bile duct stricture, associated wall thickening, and increased enhancement manifest of the underlying infiltrate with inflammation and fibrosis (Fig. 14.4) (5, 10, 29, 30). However, the presence of an indwelling stent may obscure cross-sectional imaging due to reactive changes and pneumobilia (Fig. 14.5) (8). Enlarged lymph nodes, measuring up to 3 cm in their shortest dimension (mean 14 mm), had been reported with IgG4-SC and may range in number from two to ten (mean, 4.5). MRI findings are similar to those for CT. There are few data concerning the role of MRCP in the diagnosis of IgG4-SC (Figs. 14.6 and 14.7).

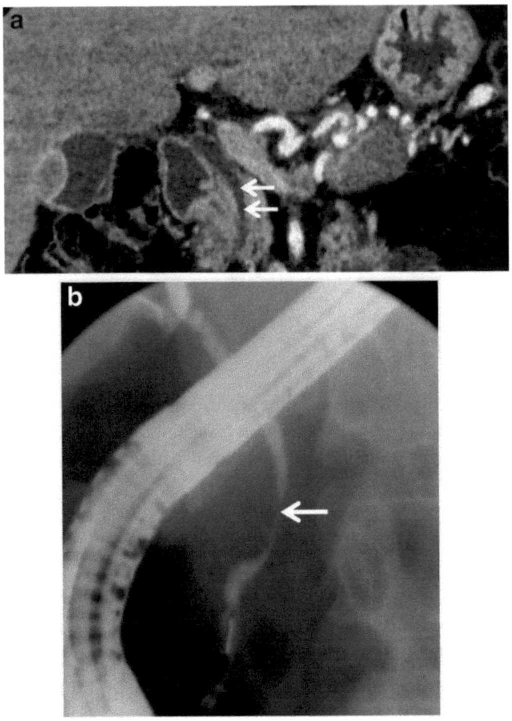


**Fig. 14.2** A 55-year-old woman with new onset jaundice. (**a**) Coronal CT demonstrates severe stenosis of the intrahepatic portion of the common bile duct (*arrows*). (**b**) Corresponding ERCP confirmed the CT findings (*arrow*)

## Cholangiography

Cholangiography performed either percutaneously in antegrade fashion or retrograde via ERCP is the most reliable imaging modality for the endoluminal evaluation of the biliary system. As for CT and MRI, the most common cholangiographic finding is distal extrahepatic bile duct stenosis (31). However, sclerosing changes of the intrahepatic and hilar biliary ducts are more often reported at cholangiography, affecting as many as 50 % of patients (31). Nakazawa et al. have categorized the cholangiographic findings of IgG4-SC into four subgroups:

Type 1: Stenoses only in the distal extrahepatic bile duct

Type 2: Multiple stenoses in extra- and intrahepatic biliary system

Type 3: Stenoses detected in hilar region distal extrahepatic bile duct

Type 4: Stenoses only in the hilar region

Nakazawa et al. detected type 1 (Fig. 14.8) as the most common subgroup followed by type 2 with types 3 and 4 less often, but equally detected (31). They also reported that a long-segment stricture, a long-segment stricture with pre-stenotic dilatation, and a stricture of the distal extrahepatic bile duct were characteristic, but nonspecific features of IgG4-SC (Fig. 14.9). Conversely, patients with PSC more often demonstrated biliary band-like short-segment strictures, a beaded or pruned-tree appearance, or diverticulum-like formations in the biliary tree. A shaggy-appearing biliary system and hilar strictures were noted in a few IgG4-SC and PSC patients. The authors also noted that the presence of concomitant pancreatic changes may serve as a clue to IgG4-SC, due to their uncommon occurrence with PSC. Comparative cholangiographic findings of IgG4-SC and PSC are listed in Table 14.1.

## Differential Diagnosis of IgG4-SC

(A) Pancreatic Cancer

It is important to consider pancreatic cancer (PC) when evaluating patients with suspected IgG4-SC, because of the similar clinical and radiographic features, different treatment strategies, and impact on prognosis following delayed diagnosis. IgG4-SC and PC are diagnosed at a similar age in patients often presenting with vague abdominal pain, cholestasis, and obstructive jaundice. However, the abdominal pain associated with PC tends to be more severe, persistent, and progressive compared to IgG4-SC (9). A serum CA 19–9 level >150 IU/L is reported to significantly correlate with PC in contrast to elevated IgG4 levels that predict AIP (32). However, elevated IgG4 levels are reported in about 10 % of PC patients, which is particularly important given the far greater occurrence of PC compared to AIP. The clinical findings for IgG4-SC and PC are outlined in Table 14.2.

On cross-sectional imaging, PC most often appears as a hypodense or T1 hypointense mass associated with upstream main pancreatic duct dilatation and parenchymal atrophy. While

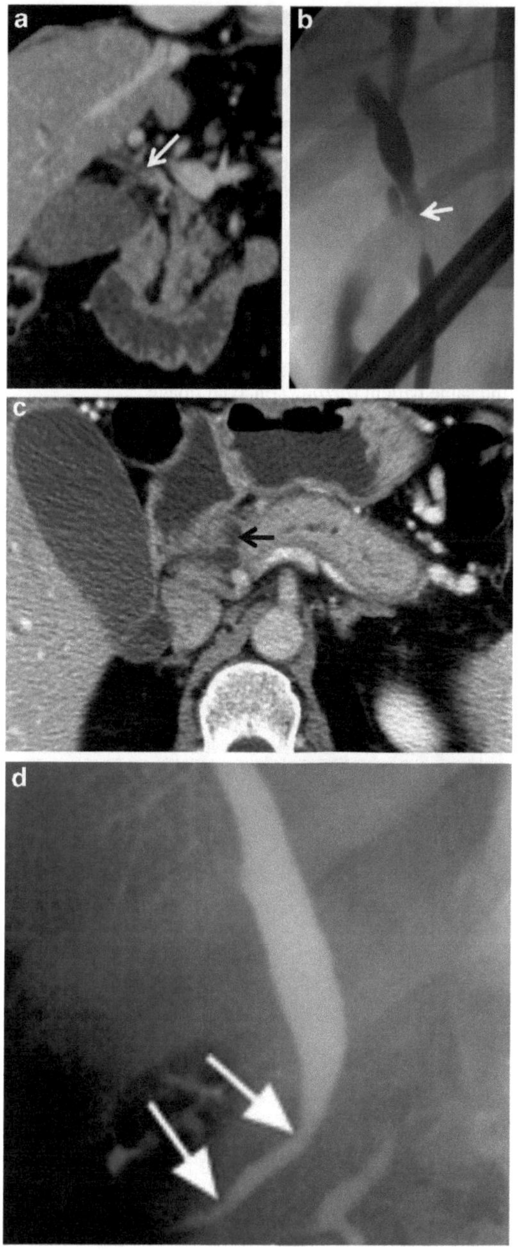


**Fig. 14.3** A 53-year-old man with newly diagnosed AIP. (**a**) Abrupt stenosis of the mid extrahepatic bile duct with proximal dilatation (*arrow*). Also note the contrast enhancement of the bile duct wall. (**b**) ERCP confirmed the CT findings (*arrow*). CT (**c**) and ERCP (**d**) images of a different patient with tapered distal biliary stenosis. Arrows in Fig. 14.3c–d denote the stenotic distal bile duct segment

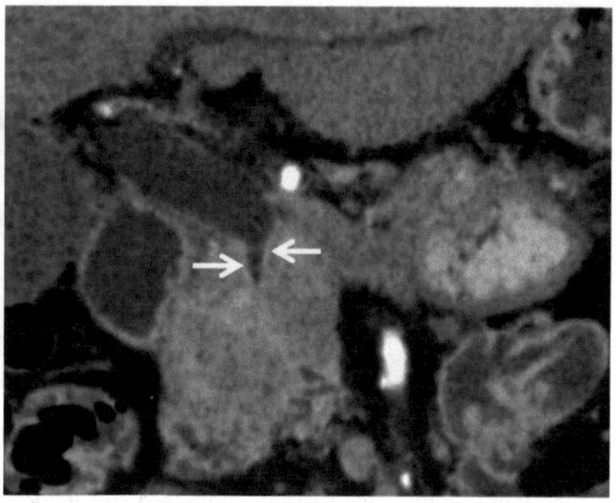

**Fig. 14.4** A 51-year-old woman presenting with severe jaundice and abdominal pain. Coronal CT demonstrates severe stenosis of the distal intrapancreatic bile duct with significant wall enhancement (*arrows*)

vascular invasion is indicative of PC, as many as 15 % of AIP patients have inflammatory changes that falsely suggest vascular invasion. In a report from Japan, 32 % of the patients with AIP had a focal pancreatic abnormality that was located in the pancreatic head in 85 % of patients, which is also the most common site for PC (33).

Features that favor the diagnosis of AIP over PC include an elevated IgG4 level (in particular >2xULN), a smoothly tapered pancreatic duct, less severe upstream pancreatic duct dilatation, coexisting features of IgG4-SC, or other extrapancreatic manifestations. On the contrary, PC is more likely with elevated serum CA 19-9, abrupt pancreatic duct cutoff, vascular invasion (especially arterial) (Figs. 14.10 and 14.11), and parenchymal atrophy (8, 34).

Abdominal CT distinguishes AIP from PC in 92.5 % of patients according to one report (35). However, current diagnostic algorithms do not rely on imaging alone. Endoscopic ultrasound- or CT- or TUS-guided percutaneous pancreatic biopsy may be necessary in some patients to confirm the diagnosis.

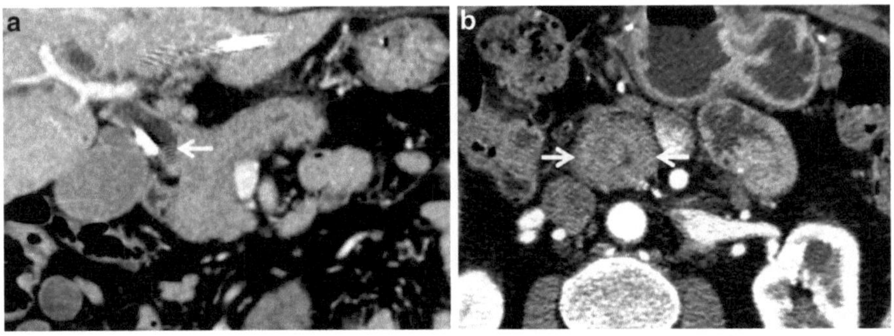


**Fig. 14.5** A 46-year-old woman with AIP. (**a**) Coronal CT images demonstrate contrast enhancement in the wall of the stenosed bile duct (*arrow*). Note the stent-induced artifact. (**b**) Diffuse enlargement of the pancreatic head in the same patient (*arrows*) on axial image

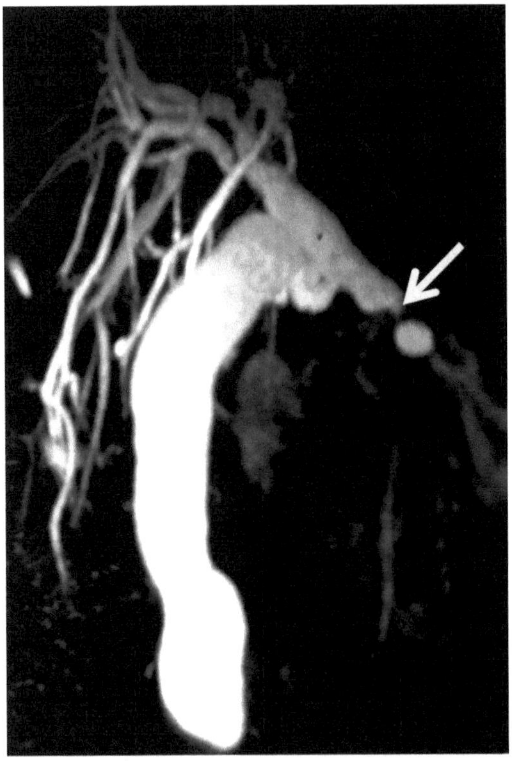

**Fig. 14.6** MRCP image of a 55-year-old patient with AIP. Severe distal biliary stenosis is well outlined on MRCP (*arrow*). Note pronounced upstream dilatation and gallbladder hydrops

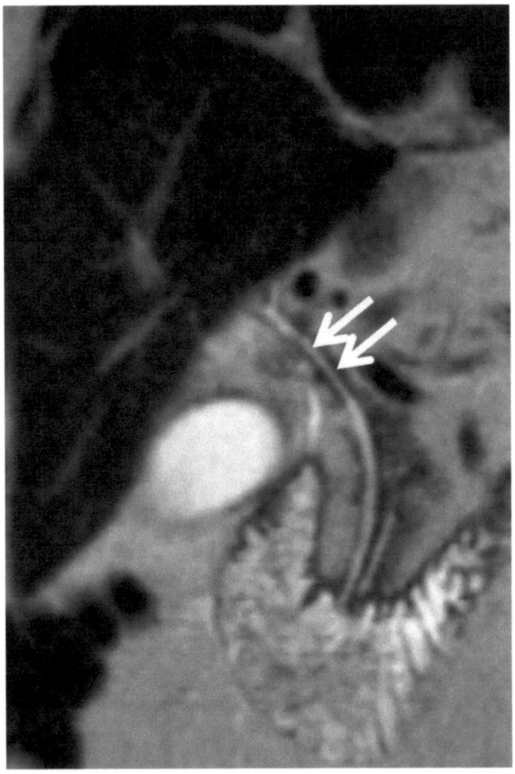

**Fig. 14.7** Coronal T2-weighted image of a 59-year-old patient demonstrates diffuse hypointense wall thickening predominantly in upper third of extrahepatic bile duct (*arrows*) and mild stenosis

(B) Primary Sclerosing Cholangitis

The clinical and imaging features of PSC often closely mimic those of IgG4-SC. PSC is a fibrosclerotic disease of the biliary tree, characterized by diffuse stricturing of the intra- and/or extrahepatic bile ducts (36). The presence of anti-neutrophil cytoplasmic antibody (pANCA) in the serum of 70–80 % of PSC patients supports the notion that PSC is an immunological disorder (37, 38). The disease is usually progressive, generally

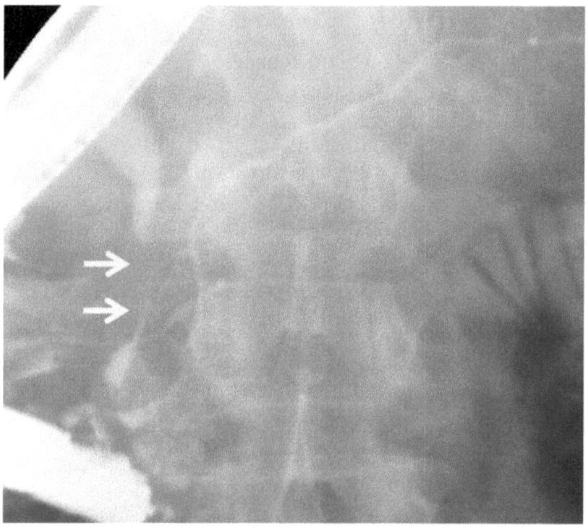

**Fig. 14.8** A 53-year-old man with AIP. ERCP demonstrates severe stenosis (*arrows*) in the lower third of the extrahepatic bile duct

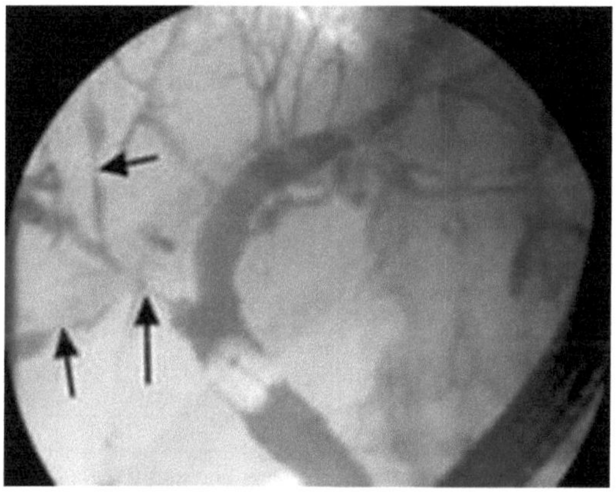

**Fig. 14.9** A 54-year-old-woman with multiple intrahepatic long-segment strictures (*arrows*) with associated upstream biliary dilatation typical of IgG4-SC involvement. Also note the severe stenosis of the right hepatic duct extending to the hilar region

unresponsive to current treatment options, with resulting transplantation or death occurring a mean of 12–18 years after the diagnosis (38). PSC and IgG4-SC are diagnosed more commonly in males with a two to one predominance over female patients (39). While the age at diagnosis varies, IgG4-SC patients tend to be older than patients with PSC (40). Obstructive jaundice, while common in IgG4-SC, is infrequent with PSC (39), highlighted by the findings of one study that reported the abrupt onset of obstructive jaundice in 75 % of the patients with AIP, in contrast to 4 % of the patients with PSC (23). Although hypergammaglobulinemia is detected in both, increased serum levels of IgG4 is more typical of IgG4-SC (23). Clinical findings for IgG4-SC and PSC are compared in Table 14.3.

**Table 14.1** Cholangiographic differences between IgG4-SC and PSC

| | IgG4-SC | PSC |
|---|---|---|
| *Band-like stricture* | – | + |
| *Beaded appearance* | – | + |
| *Pruned-tree appearance* | – | + |
| *Diverticulum-like formations* | – | + |
| *Long stenosis* | + | Uncommon |
| *Segmental stricture* | + | Uncommon |
| *Long stricture with pre-stenotic dilatation* | + | Uncommon |
| *Shaggy appearance* | + | + |
| *Hilar stricture* | + | + |
| *Distal CBD stricture* | Extremely common | Uncommon |
| *Pancreatic abnormalities* | Extremely common | Uncommon |

*AIP-SC* autoimmune pancreatitis-associated sclerosing cholangitis, *IgG4-SC* IgG4-related sclerosing cholangitis, *PSC* primary sclerosing cholangitis

The presence of inflammatory bowel disease, while common for PSC, is infrequent for type 1 AIP and IgG4-SC (39). The presence of cholangiocarcinoma (CCA) also strongly suggests underlying PSC.

When imaging patients with a putative diagnosis of PSC or IgG4-SC, the pancreas should be carefully inspected. Any pancreatic enlargement, minimal peripancreatic stranding, or main pancreatic duct irregularity should raise suspicion for IgG4-SC rather than PSC. The presence of bile duct wall thickening may suggest IgG4-SC, but care must be taken to also consider the influence of an indwelling stent or underlying CCA in this setting. The favorable response to steroid therapy strongly suggests IgG4-SC as compared to PSC that rarely responds to steroids and other immunosuppressive medications (41).

(C) Recurrent Pyogenic Cholangitis

Also referred to as oriental cholangiohepatitis, recurrent pyogenic cholangitis (RPC) is

**Table 14.2** Important points for differentiating IgG4-SC from pancreatic cancer

| | AIP and *IgG4-SC* | Pancreatic cancer |
|---|---|---|
| *Abdominal pain* | + (mild to moderate) | + (moderate to severe) |
| *Biliary obstruction* | + | + |
| *Main pancreatic duct dilatation* | + (mild, <6 mm in almost 100 %) | + (moderate to severe, >6 mm in 74 %) |
| *Lymphadenopathy* | + | + |
| *Venous invasion* | Very rare | Common |
| *Arterial invasion* | Never reported | Common |
| *IgG4 positivity* | Extremely common (81 %) | Rare (10 %) |
| *Ca 19–9 level* | <150 IU/L | >150 IU/L |
| *Pancreatic atrophy* | Uncommon at diagnosis | Downstream atrophy common |

*AIP* autoimmune pancreatitis, *IgG4-SC* IgG4-related sclerosing cholangitis

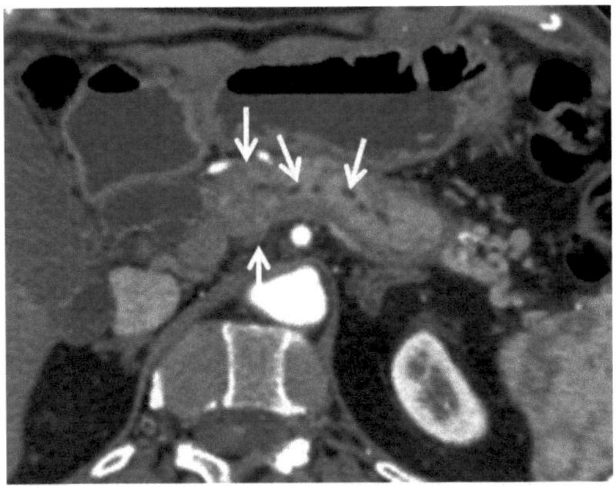

**Fig. 14.10** A 55-year-old man with typical features of AIP. Note mild main pancreatic duct dilatation (*arrowheads*) and fibroblastic pseudotumor at the pancreatic head (*arrows*). The pancreas looks swollen instead of atrophic seen in pancreatic cancer. The main pancreatic duct dilatation is not pronounced as in pancreatic cancer

**Table 14.3** Important clinical points for differentiating *IgG4-SC* from PSC

| | AIP-SC | PSC |
|---|---|---|
| *Patient age* | Elderly patients | Young adults to middle aged |
| *Gender* | Male predominance | Male predominance |
| *Presenting symptom* | Obstructive jaundice | Liver dysfunction |
| *IgG4 positivity* | + | – |
| *Location in biliary system* | Mostly extrahepatic | Mostly intrahepatic |
| *Treatment* | Strong steroid response | Almost no response |
| *Prognosis* | Favorable with treatment | Dismal even with treatment |
| *Need for liver transplant* | Extremely rare but reported | Standard treatment |

*IgG4-SC* IgG4-related sclerosing cholangitis, *PSC* primary sclerosing cholangitis

characterized by recurrent bouts of pyogenic cholangitis associated with biliary obstruction due to biliary strictures and/or pigmented stones (42) potentially related to microbial infection (43). The biliary segment most often involved in RPC is the lateral segment of the left lobe where multiple stones are typically found with cholangiography, cross-sectional imaging or MRCP. To the best of our knowledge, intrahepatic biliary stones have not been reported in patients with IgG4-SC, thereby potentially serving as another distinguishing feature.

(D) Cholangiocarcinoma

Cholangiocarcinomas are tumors of the biliary system that most often involve the hilar region (Klatskin tumor) but may also involve the intrahepatic and distal extrahepatic bile ducts (Fig. 14.12). The distinction of CCA and IgG4-SC is important given their disparate treatment and prognosis .The presentation of CCA is nonspecific and overlaps with that of IgG4-SC making clinical differentiation difficult. Similarly, the presence enlarged hilar or pancreatic lymph nodes is common to both CCA and IgG4-SC (10). The presence of

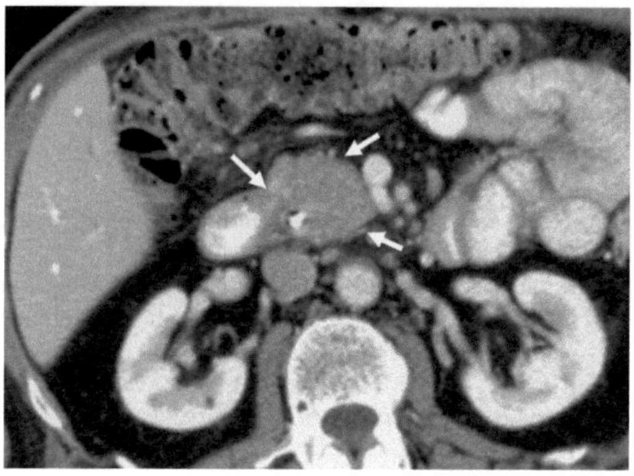

**Fig. 14.11** A 41-year-old man with AIP. Diffuse enlargement of the pancreatic head with a hardly appreciable hypodense mass-like lesion (*arrows*). Note that the perivascular planes are clear without any signs suggestive of malignant infiltration or invasion. The pancreas contours are also lobular without any evidence of spiculation

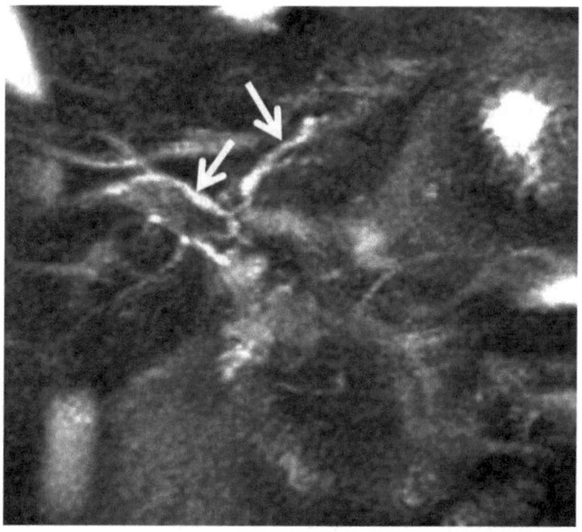

**Fig. 14.12** Multifocal dilatation in the left and right hepatic ducts (*arrows*). The imaging appearance may be suggestive of cholangiocarcinoma; however this patient has other organ involvement typically associated with IgG4-SC. Patient responded well to corticosteroid therapy

(E) Hepatic Inflammatory Pseudotumor

The association of hepatic inflammatory pseudotumor (HIP) and sclerosing cholangitis has been reported (26). More recently the association of HIP and IgG4-SC has been reported with histology demonstrating abundant IgG4-positive plasma cells (44) and steroid administration yielding a clinical and radiographic response (26).

## Gallbladder Involvement Associated with AIP or IgG4-SC

Gallbladder abnormalities are commonly associated with IgG4-SC, as in one report in which all 20 evaluated patients showed moderate or marked mucosal or transmural lymphoplasmacytic infiltration (45). In this report, the degree of gallbladder inflammation correlated well with extrahepatic bile duct lymphoplasmacytic infiltration (45).

Another study detected gallbladder wall thickening in 10/17 patients with IgG4-SC by TUS and/or CT, all 10 of whom also had extrahepatic bile duct strictures. Severe inflammation was detected in 75 % of the AIP patients who underwent resection and none of these patients demonstrated dysplasia or neoplasia. The authors proposed the term "sclerosing cholecystitis" for the chronically inflamed gallbladders in the setting of AIP (46). Histologically, abundant infiltration with IgG4-positive plasma cells was seen in the gallbladder and bile duct walls (46). The absence of dysplastic and neoplastic changes within the gallbladder of IgG4-SC patients is in contrast to that for PSC that is associated with malignant transformation (47).

## Key Points

- IgG4-SC is the most common associated extra-pancreatic abnormality in patients with AIP.
- The most commonly affected site in IgG4-SC is the distal (intrapancreatic) bile duct.
- ERP is currently the gold standard imaging modality for evaluating the biliary system with accumulating data supporting the role of MRCP.
- Biliary duct wall thickening and diffuse contrast uptake in cross are the most striking imaging findings on noninvasive (CT or MRI) imaging.
- PSC, cholangiocarcinoma, and pancreatic cancer often clinically and radiographically mimic IgG4-SC, and it is critical to distinguish these entities given their varied treatment and prognoses.

- There is no evidence of increased risk of biliary malignancy in IgG4-SC.
- The gallbladder may also be affected in IgG4-SC patients, manifested by diffuse wall thickening and lymphoplasmacytic infiltration.

## References


1. Kloppel G, Luttges J, Sipos B, et al. Autoimmune pancreatitis: pathological findings. JOP. 2005;6(1 suppl):97–101.
2. Hamano H, Kawa S, Horiuchi A, et al. High serum IgG4 concentrations in patients with sclerosing pancreatitis. N Engl J Med. 2001;344:732–8.
3. Kamisawa T, Funata N, Hayashi Y. Lymphoplasmacytic sclerosing pancreatitis is a pancreatic lesion of IgG4-related diseases (IgG4-RD). Am J Surg Pathol. 2004; 28:1114.
4. Okazaki K, Kawa S, Kamisawa T, et al. Japanese consensus guidelines for management of autoimmune pancreatitis: I. Concept and diagnosis of autoimmune pancreatitis. J Gastroenterol. 2010;45:249–65.
5. Yang DH, Kim KW, Kim TK, et al. Autoimmune pancreatitis: radiologic findings in 20 patients. Abdom Imaging. 2006;31:94–102.
6. Wakabayashi T, Kawaura Y, Satomura Y, et al. Clinical and imaging features of autoimmune pancreatitis with focal pancreatic swelling or mass formation: comparison with so-called tumor-forming pancreatitis and pancreatic carcinoma. Am J Gastroeterol. 2003; 98:2679–87.
7. Inoue K, Ohuchida J, Ohtsuka T, et al. Severe localized stenosis and marked dilatation of the main pancreatic duct are indicators of pancreatic cancer instead of chronic pancreatitis on endoscopic retrograde balloon pancreatography. Gastrointest Endosc. 2003;58:510–5.
8. Kawamoto S, Siegelman SS, Hruban RH, et al. Lymphoplasmacytic sclerosing pancreatitis (autoimmune pancreatitis): evaluation with multidetector CT. Radiographics. 2008;28:157–70.
9. Kawa S, Okazaki K, Kamisawa T, et al. Japanese consensus guidelines for management of autoimmune pancreatitis: II. Extrapancreatic lesions, differential diagnosis. J Gastroenterol. 2010;45:355–69.
10. Sahani DV, Kalva SP, Farrell J, et al. Autoimmune pancreatitis: imaging features. Radiology. 2004;233: 345–52.
11. Kamisawa T, Chen PY, Tu Y, et al. MRCP and MRI findings in 9 patients with autoimmune pancreatitis. World J Gastroenterol. 2006;12(18):2919–22.
12. Nishino T, Oyama H, Hashimoto E, et al. Clinicopathological differentiation between sclerosing cholangitis with autoimmune pancreatitis and primary sclerosing cholangitis. J Gastroenterol. 2007;42:550–9.
13. Okazaki K, Uchida K, Chiba T. Recent concept of autoimmune-related pancreatitis. J Gastroenterol. 2001;36:293–302.
14. Nishino T, Toki F, Oyama H, et al. Biliary tract involvement in autoimmune pancreatitis. Pancreas. 2005;30:76–82.
15. Detlefsen S, Drewes AM. Autoimmune pancreatitis. Scand J Gastroenterol. 2009;44:1391–407.
16. Kamisawa T, Anjiki H, Egawa N. Rapid changes in sclerosing cholangitis associated with autoimmune pancreatitis. Pancreas. 2009;38:601–2.
17. Kim KP, Kim MH, Song MH, et al. Autoimmune chronic pancreatitis. Am J Gastroenterol. 2004;99: 1605–16.
18. Kloppel G, Luttges J, Lohr M, et al. Autoimmune pancreatitis: pathological, clinical, and immunological features. Pancreas. 2003;27:14–9.
19. Pearson RK, Longnecker DS, Chari ST, et al. Controversies in clinical pancreatology: autoimmune pancreatitis-does it exist? Pancreas. 2003;27: 1–13.
20. Yoshida H, Tanaka S, Nagayama Y, et al. Autoimmune pancreatitis associated with ulcerative colitis (in Japanese). J Gastroenterol Imaging. 2002;4:66–74.
21. Notohara K, Burgart LJ, Yadav D, et al. Idiopathic chronic pancreatitis with periductal lymphoplasmacytic infiltration: clinicopathologic features of 35 cases. Am J Surg Pathol. 2003;27:1119–27.
22. Kamisawa T, Funata N, Hayashi Y, et al. Close relationship between auto-immune pancreatitis and multifocal fibrosis. Gut. 2003;52:683–7.
23. Nakazawa T, Ohara H, Sano H, et al. Clinical differences between primary sclerosing cholangitis and sclerosing cholangitis with autoimmune pancreatitis. Pancreas. 2005;30:20–5.
24. Yoshizaki K, Takeuchi K, Okuda K, et al. Abdominal ultrasonogram of autoimmune pancreatitis: five cases of pancreatic lesions accompanied by Sjogren syndrome. J Med Ultrason. 1999;26:1125–36.
25. Muraki T, Ozaki Y, Hamano H, et al. Ultrasonographic diagnosis of autoimmune pancreatitis. Biliary Tract Pancreas. 2005;26:711–6.
26. Nakanuma Y, Zen Y. Pathology and immunopathology of immunoglobulin G4-related sclerosing cholangitis: the latest addition to the sclerosing cholangitis family. Hepatol Res. 2007;37:S478–86.
27. Zamboni G, Luttges J, Capelli P, et al. Histopathological features of diagnostic and clinical relevance in autoimmune pancreatitis: a study on 53 resection specimens and 9 biopsy specimens. Virchows Arch. 2004;445:552–63.
28. Hyodo N, Hyodo T. Ultrasonographic evaluation in patients with autoimmune-related pancreatitis. J Gastroenterol. 2003;38:1155–61.
29. Kawamoto S, Siegelman SS, Hruban RH, et al. Lymphoplasmacytic sclerosing pancreatitis with obstructive jaundice: CT and pathology features. Am J Roentgenol. 2004;183(4):915–21.

30. Nikfarjam M, Muralidharan V, Christophi C, et al. Autoimmune pancreatitis. ANZ J Surg. 2002;72(6): 450–2.
31. Nakazawa T, Ohara H, Sano H, et al. Cholangiography can discriminate sclerosing cholangitis with autoimmune pancreatitis from primary sclerosing cholangitis. Gastrointest Endosc. 2004;60:937–44.
32. Sugumar A, Chari ST. Distinguishing pancreatic cancer from autoimmune pancreatitis: a comparison of two strategies. Clin Gastroenterol Hepatol. 2009;7(11 Suppl):59–62.
33. Kamisawa T, Okamoto A, Wakabayashi T, et al. Appropriate steroid therapy for autoimmune pancreatitis based on long-term outcome. Scand J Gastroenterol. 2008;43:609–13.
34. Kamisawa T, Egawa N, Nakajima H, et al. Clinical difficulties in the differentiation of autoimmune pancreatitis and pancreatic carcinoma. Am J Gastroenterol. 2003;98(12):2694–9.
35. Procacci C, Carbognin G, Biasiutti C, et al. Autoimmune pancreatitis: possibilities of CT characterization. Pancreatology. 2001;1(3):246–53.
36. Bjornsson E, Chapman RW. Sclerosing cholangitis. Curr Opin Gastroenterol. 2003;19:270–5.
37. Snook JA, Chapman RW, Fleming K, et al. Anti-neutrophil nuclear antibody in ulcerative colitis, Crohn's disease and primary sclerosing cholangitis. Clin Exp Immunol. 1989;76:30–3.
38. Webster GJM, Pereira SP, Chapman RW. Autoimmune pancreatitis/IgG4-associated cholangitis and primary sclerosing cholangitis-overlapping or separate diseases. J Hepatol. 2009;51:398–402.
39. Björnsson E, Chari ST, Smyrk TC, et al. Immunoglobulin G4 associated cholangitis: description of an emerging clinical entity based on review of the literature. Hepatology. 2007;45:1547–54.
40. Angulo P, Lindor KD. Primary sclerosing cholangitis. Hepatology. 1999;30:325–32.
41. Chen W, Gluud C. Glucocorticosteroids for primary sclerosing cholangitis. Cochrane Database Syst Rev. 2004;3, CD004036.
42. Menias CO, Surabhi VR, Prasad SR, et al. Mimics of cholangiocarcinoma: spectrum of disease. Radiographics. 2008;28:111–1129.
43. Park MS, Yu JS, Kim KW, et al. Recurrent pyogenic cholangitis: comparison between MR cholangiography and direct cholangiography. Radiology. 2001;220:677–82.
44. Zen Y, Harada K, Sasaki M, et al. IgG4-related sclerosing cholangitis with and without hepatic inflammatory pseudotumor, and sclerosing pancreatitis-associated sclerosing cholangitis: do they belong to a spectrum of sclerosing pancreatitis? Am J Surg Pathol. 2004;28:1193–203.
45. Abraham SC, Cruz-Correa M, Argani P, et al. lymphoplasmacytic chronic cholecystitis and biliary tract disease in patients lymphoplasmacytic sclerosing pancreatitis. Am J Surg Pathol. 2003;27:441–51.
46. Kamisawa T, Tu Y, Nakajima H, et al. Sclerosing cholecystitis associated with autoimmune pancreatitis. World J Gastroenterol. 2006;12(23): 3736–9.
47. Lewis JT, Talwalkar JA, Rosen CB, et al. Prevalence and risk factors for gallbladder neoplasia in patients with primary sclerosing cholangitis: evidence for a metaplasia-dysplasia-carcinoma sequence. Am J Surg Pathol. 2007;31:907–13.

# ERCP and EUS/IDUS Features

# 15

George Webster and Atsushi Irisawa

## Introduction

Endoscopic retrograde cholangiopancreatography (ERCP) is a useful, but not a mandatory, tool in the investigation or diagnosis of IgG4-related sclerosing cholangitis (IgG4-SC). As with other areas of pancreaticobiliary medicine, it has less of a solely diagnostic role than previously, and alternatives to its use should always be considered, mindful of the inherent risk, albeit low, of the procedure [1]. This is particularly relevant with respect to IgG4-SC, as the diagnosis may be definitively established on the basis of characteristic clinical, serological (e.g., serum IgG4), pathological, and radiological features [2]. Nevertheless, ERCP has three main roles in the patient with suspected IgG4-SC:

1. Definition of the biliary (+/− pancreatic) ductal system, which may advance the diagnosis
2. Tissue sampling, from both the pancreaticobiliary system and other areas of the upper GI tract, to confirm the diagnosis of IgG4-SC (and exclude malignancy)
3. Relief of jaundice and biliary obstruction

On the other hand, endoscopic ultrasound (EUS) and transpapillary intraductal ultrasonography (IDUS) during ERCP using mini-probe (20MHz) also provide important information for diagnosing IgG4-SC. Although it is difficult to make a definite diagnosis with EUS/IDUS image alone without tissue sampling, it assists in the diagnosis.

In this chapter, particular focus will be paid to the diagnostic information provided by cholangiography by ERCP and endosonographic image of EUS/IDUS, in patients with suspected IgG4-SC.

## ERCP

### Cholangiographic Features on ERCP

In IgG4-SC any part of the biliary tree may be involved [3], with proximal, hilar, or intrahepatic biliary stricturing reported in 49–82 % of cases [2, 4]. This is reflected in the site of biliary abnormality and stricturing found on ERCP. Jaundice is a presenting feature in >70 % of cases of IgG4-SC/AIP [3–5], usually due to stricturing of the distal, intrapancreatic portion of the bile duct. Nishino et al. reported stricturing of the biliary tree in 14/16 (88 %) patients with AIP, with the distal bile duct involved in 9/14 (64 %) [6]. Of 53 patients with IgG4-SC, Ghazale et al. reported that biliary strictures

G. Webster, B.Sc., M.D., FRCP (✉)
GI Services, University College London Hospitals, Ground Floor West 250 Euston Road, London NW1 2PG, UK
e-mail: george.webster@uclh.nhs.uk

A. Irisawa, M.D., Ph.D.
Department of Gastroenterology, Fukushima Medical University Aizu Medical Center, Aizuwakamatsu, Japan

M.J. Levy and S.T. Chari (eds.), *Autoimmune (IgG4-related) Pancreatitis and Cholangitis*,
DOI 10.1007/978-1-4419-6430-4_15, 

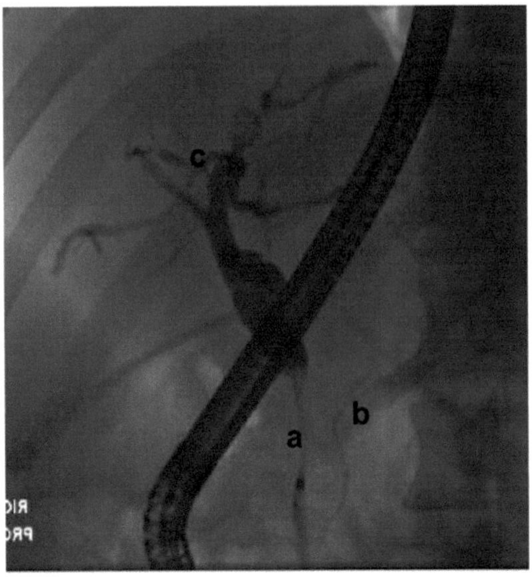


**Fig. 15.1** ERCP in a patient with IgG4-SC and AIP, showing a low bile duct stricture (**a**), diffusely narrowed main pancreatic duct (**b**), and intrahepatic duct strictures (**c**)

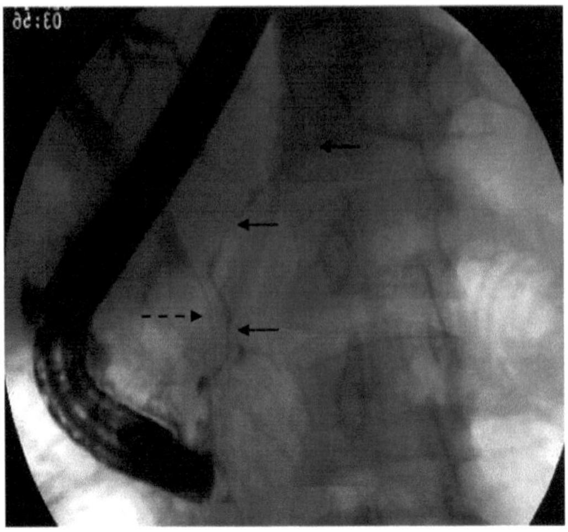

**Fig. 15.2** Pancreatogram in a patient with obstructive jaundice. Characteristic features of IgG4-SC/AIP are seen, including a stricture of the intrapancreatic portion of the bile duct (*broken arrow*), a diffusely narrowed main pancreatic duct, with multiple strictures (*bold arrow*), and no upstream pancreatic duct dilatation

were confined to the intrapancreatic bile duct in 51 % [2], and in a study from the UK, distal bile duct stricturing was found in 15/25 (60 %) AIP patients who had not undergone prior pancreaticobiliary surgery [4].

There do not appear to be cholangiographic features of a distal bile duct stricture in IgG4-SC which allow a clear distinction from other benign etiologies, or malignant disease, and this has contributed, in the setting of a pancreatic mass, to the assumption of pancreatic cancer. However, the finding of concomitant proximal biliary or pancreatic disease (mass or stricture) may offer a clue to the diagnosis of IgG4-SC/AIP (Fig. 15.1). A careful cholangiogram, sufficient to delineate the hilar and second order bile ducts, should be considered in such cases.

An important clue to the diagnosis of IgG4-SC may come from the appearance of the pancreatic duct at ERCP. As discussed, a distal bile duct stricture secondary to AIP may mimic pancreatic cancer. Several groups have assessed pancreatographic features that distinguish AIP from pancreatic cancer or other forms of chronic pancreatitis [7, 8]. Narrowing of the main pancreatic duct over >3 cm (or >1/3rd the duct length), multiple strictures, side branches arising from strictured main duct, and lack of upstream pancreatic duct dilatation all suggest a diagnosis of AIP [7, 8] (Fig. 15.2). Conversely, a short pancreatic duct stricture in the pancreatic head, adjacent to the distal bile duct stricture, and upstream main pancreatic duct dilatation of ≥4 mm [7], suggests pancreatic cancer rather than IgG4-SC/AIP. There is of course a balance to be struck in terms of the role of a pancreatogram. While a pancreatogram may provide useful diagnostic information, contrast injection (particularly with repeated injections) may induce pancreatitis [9]. We advocate pancreatography for suspected IgG4-SC/AIP when the diagnosis is not otherwise possible. A completely normal pancreatogram does not exclude the diagnosis of IgG4-SC. While 92 % of the IgG4-SC patients reported by Ghazale et al. [2] also had AIP, it is likely that the true frequency of AIP in patients with IgG4-SC is lower, as most previous reports have identified biliary disease (i.e., IgG4-SC) in patients with an established diagnosis of AIP.

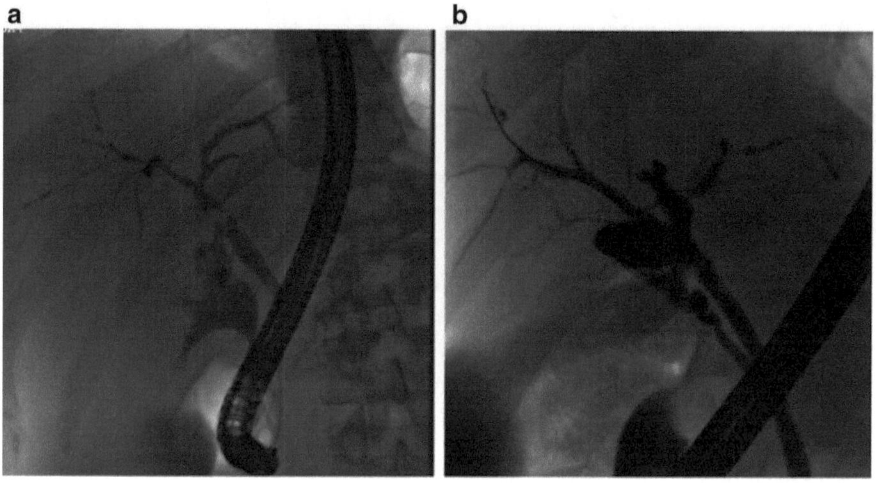

**Fig. 15.3** ERCs in two patients with obstructive jaundice and HISORt criteria confirming IgG4-SC. Both demonstrate diffuse intrahepatic biliary disease, with multiple long strictures, in the absence of obvious beading or significant dilatation

## Role of ERCP in the Differential Diagnosis of IgG4-SC

The two most important, and difficult, diseases to differentiate from IgG4-SC are primary sclerosing cholangitis (PSC) and cholangiocarcinoma (CCA). The focus here is on the appearances at ERCP that may present confusion, or allow distinction, as the full diagnostic parameters that may be applied clinically are addressed elsewhere.

IgG4-SC may mimic PSC, and the similarities and differences between the two diseases have become the subject of interest over the last few years [10–12]. A possible clinical or diagnostic overlap between IgG4-SC and PSC may also be suggested by serum IgG4 levels, with raised serum IgG4 levels demonstrated in 9–36 % of patients with PSC [11, 13], a much higher frequency than is seen in other types of pancreaticobiliary disease [13]. While a pancreatic mass is not a feature of classical PSC, pancreatic duct abnormalities have been reported in 7–15 % of patients [14]. Classical PSC is associated with inflammatory bowel disease (IBD) in 80 % of cases. While Japanese groups report minimal association between IgG4-SC and IBD, European groups have found IBD in >15 % of cases [4]. The presence of raised serum and tissue IgG4 [11, 15] in PSC, and the extent of disease overlap (in particular between IgG4-SC and IgG4+ PSC), is reviewed elsewhere. In view of the common presentation of IgG4-SC in the sixth/seventh decade, with obstructive jaundice and imaging often showing complex biliary stricturing and inflammatory mass lesions in the liver hilum, it is not surprising that the disease may be misdiagnosed as cholangiocarcinoma (CCA) [16–19]. In an important paper, Erdogan et al. showed that of 185 patients who had undergone surgery for presumed hilar cholangiocarcinoma, 32 (17 %) had benign disease, and of these nearly 50 % (15/32) had features of IgG4-SC [20].

Can ERCP help to distinguish IgG4-SC from PSC and CCA? Differences in biliary abnormality between IgG4-SC and PSC have been reported, including longer biliary strictures, associated distal bile duct stricturing in IgG4-SC (Figs. 15.1 and 15.3), and predominant band-like strictures with beading in PSC [5]. In a study by Oh et al. [21], 16 patients with hilar/intrahepatic strictures due to IgG4-SC were compared with patients with PSC and with CCA. Biliary imaging findings suggestive of IgG4-SC included multifocal biliary tree involvement ($n = 14$), concentric bile duct thickening with preserved luminal patency

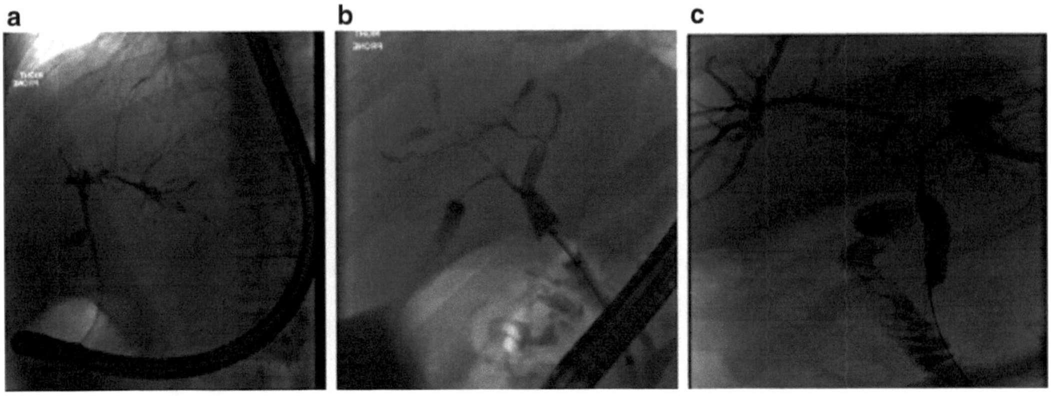

**Fig. 15.4** Representative ERCs of primary sclerosing cholangitis (**a**), IgG4-SC (**b**), and cholangiocarcinoma (**c**) used to assess the ability of observers to make a diagnosis of each disease, based on cholangiogram alone (From Kalaitzakis et al. [22])

($n=13$), and relatively mild proximal dilatation, despite prominent bile duct thickening ($n=11$). Patients with IgG4-SC were also characterized by marked improvement of biliary strictures after steroid therapy. In a recent international study, 17 clinicians with varying experience treating IgG4-SC from centers in the USA, Japan, and the UK were blinded to the correct diagnosis in 40 preselected ERCs of patients with IgG4-SC, PSC, and cholangiocarcinoma. The clinicians were asked to give the diagnosis and to identify key cholangiographic features [22] (Fig. 15.4). The overall specificity, sensitivity, and interobserver agreement for the diagnosis of IgG4-SC were 88 %, 45 %, and 0.18 %, respectively. High specificity for diagnosing IgG4-SC using ERC implies that while particular cholangiographic features may support the diagnosis, the poor sensitivity suggests that, based on ERC alone, many patients with IgG4-SC who might benefit from steroid therapy may be misdiagnosed with PSC or CCA. Misdiagnosis of IgG4-SC as CCA is well recognized [19, 23, 24], often resulting in erroneous surgery. The insertion of uncovered (and therefore usually unremovable) metal biliary stents in patients with presumed CCA [25] without pathological confirmation should be avoided, where the possibility of nonmalignant causes, such as IgG4-SC, exists [26, 27].

In conclusion, cholangiographic features may support a diagnosis of IgG4-SC, but definitively distinguishing IgG4-SC from other causes of benign and malignant disease, based on cholangiography alone, is difficult. However, at ERCP, the endoscopist has the potential to advance the diagnosis further, by means of tissue acquisition (Table 15.1).

## Tissue Acquisition

ERCP often provides important cholangiographic and pancreatographic diagnostic information and allows endoscopic therapy for dominant biliary strictures. ERCP also has a vital role in tissue acquisition. Because of the difficulty in diagnosing IgG4-SC, and excluding malignancy based upon imaging and/or serology (e.g., serum IgG4 levels), most include a tissue diagnosis into their diagnostic criteria [28].

It is important to exclude malignancy in patients with suspected IgG4-SC, many of whom are older and presenting with stricture-induced obstructive jaundice. Biliary brush cytology is mandatory in all patients at the time of ERCP. Brush cytology provides high diagnostic specificity for malignancy (98–100 %), but relatively low sensitivity (59–62 %) [29–31]. Brush cytology provides greater diagnostic yield for biliary strictures occurring secondary to CCA compared to those resulting from pancreatic cancer. In a series of 86 patients

**Table 15.1** Causes of biliary stricturing

| | |
|---|---|
| Pancreatic cancer[a] | Acute/chronic pancreatitis[a] |
| Cholangiocarcinoma | Lymphoma |
| Autoimmune pancreatitis[a] | Ampullary tumor/ stenosis[a] |
| Primary sclerosing cholangitis | Iatrogenic |
| IgG4-associated cholangitis | Stone disease |
| Sarcoidosis | Mirizzi's syndrome |
| *Clonorchis* infection | Ischemia |
| Metastatic disease | HIV cholangiopathy |
| Hepatocellular carcinoma | Tuberculosis |
| Hilar nodes | Gallbladder cancer |
| Peri-choledochal varices/cavernoma | |

[a]Predominant involvement of lower bile duct

with indeterminate biliary strictures, Glasbrenner et al. reported a sensitivity of 80% for CCA, but only 35.5% for pancreatic cancer [32]. In a series of 61 patients with PSC and dominant strictures, brush cytology reported as high-grade dysplasia/adenocarcinoma showed 73 % sensitivity, 95 % specificity, and an 85 % positive predictive value for CCA [33].

Published data on the role of biliary brush cytology in establishing the diagnosis of IgG4-SC/AIP are scanty, probably due to its low yield. Of 46 patients with proven IgG4-SC/AIP who have undergone ERCP at University College Hospital in London, the diagnosis could not be established in any patient with biliary brush cytology (GW, personal communication). Cytological analysis of EUS-guided fine needle aspirates was reported by Levy et al. to be insufficient for diagnosis in AIP among patients where the diagnosis was established by EUS-guided Trucut biopsy [34]. The role of endoscopic ultrasound is discussed separately [34, 35].

While brush cytology cannot diagnose IgG4-SC, the diagnosis may be established by ERCP or radiographically guided pinch biopsies taken from the biliary tree or papilla with identification of characteristic histological features, including an IgG4-positive lymphoplasmacytic infiltrate [19, 36] [37]. In a study of 23 patients with IgG4-SC, Naitoh et al. demonstrated a lymphoplasmacytic infiltrate in 17/17 (100 %) of patients undergoing intraductal biopsies at ERCP, although a diagnostically high IgG4-positive plasma cell infiltrate was seen in only 3/17 (18 %) cases [38]. They also report a useful role for intraductal ultrasound with circular-symmetric wall thickness, a smooth outer and inner margin, and a homogeneous internal echo within a biliary stricture strongly suggesting IgG4-SC, compared to cholangiocarcinoma ($p<0.01$). They also noted that a bile duct wall thickness of >0.8 mm in non-strictured regions strongly suggested IgG4-SC (sensitivity 95.0 %, specificity 90.9 %, accuracy 93.5 %) [38].

Peroral direct cholangioscopy allows visualization of the biliary mucosa and directed biopsies and is acquiring an emerging role in the assessment of biliary strictures [39] (Fig. 15.5a, b). It has been proposed as having a specific role in the assessment of strictures in patients with sclerosing cholangitis [40]. Although a high degree of accuracy in differentiating benign from malignant strictures through visualization alone has been reported [41], it is likely that the greatest utility arises from visually targeted biopsy. In a retrospective study of 134 patients undergoing peroral cholangioscopy and intraductal biopsy, Itoi et al. found a sensitivity of 99.0 %, specificity of 95.8 %, and positive predictive value of 99.0 % for malignancy [42]. We have diagnosed one patient with IgG4-SC, based on cholangiography and cholangioscopically directed Spybite™ biopsy (GW, personal communication. Figure 15.5c, d).

The systemic nature of many cases of IgG4-SC and the similar histological pattern of all involved tissues [43] provide the potential for diagnosis based on endoscopic biopsies from outside the biliary tree. An increased propensity for gastric ulceration has been reported in patients with IgG4-SC/AIP [44], and an IgG4-positive lymphoplasmacytic infiltrate may be found [45]. A specific search for gastric ulcers should be made at the time of ERCP for suspected IgG4-SC. Probably the most fruitful source of extrabiliary biopsies is from the duodenal papilla. In a small initial study, Kamisawa et al. demonstrated high levels of IgG4+ plasma cells (>10/high power film) in biopsies from the duodenal papilla in all 3 patients with AIP, compared with absent or low

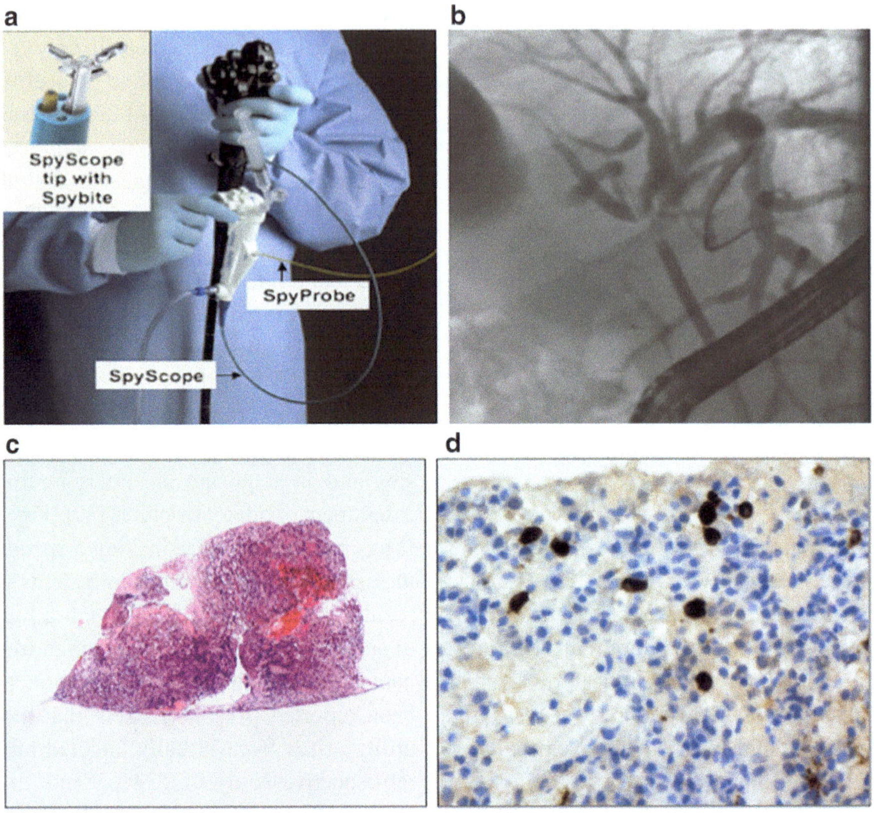


**Fig. 15.5** Peroral direct cholangioscopy, using Spyglass™ cholangioscope and Spybite™ biopsy forceps (**a**), allows visualization and directed biopsies in a patient with suspected IgG4-SC (**b**). Intraductal biopsies showed a fluoric lymphoplasmacytic infiltrate (**c**), with immunostaining demonstrating >10 IgG4+ plasma cells/high power film (**d**)

levels in controls [46], and these findings have been supported by a larger study from the same group, with an IgG4-positive infiltrate in 80 % of patients with AIP [47]. A ratio of IgG4+/IgG+ plasma cells within the ampulla of >0.10 provides a diagnostic sensitivity and specificity of 86% and 95 %, respectively, when compared to adenocarcinoma and other forms of chronic pancreatitis [48]. While the duodenal papilla may appear swollen endoscopically in IgG4-SC/AIP [49], characteristic histological findings may be found even if it appears endoscopically normal. Endoscopic biopsy of the duodenal papilla is straightforward and very low risk, and although evidence for characteristic findings has to date largely been derived from patients with AIP, rather than specifically those with IgG4-SC, it is our practice to take ampullary biopsies, and immunostain for the presence of an IgG4+ lymphoplasmacytic infiltrate, in any patient undergoing ERCP for suspected IgG4-SC.

## ERCP and Response to Treatment

There are no randomized placebo-controlled data regarding the therapy of IgG4-SC. Nevertheless, a response to steroids is a central component of the HISORt criteria for IgG4-SC [28], and cholangiographic improvement can be gratifying and occasionally dramatic. In addition to resolution of distal bile duct stricturing (often in association with resolution of the pancreatic enlargement associated with AIP), marked improvement may

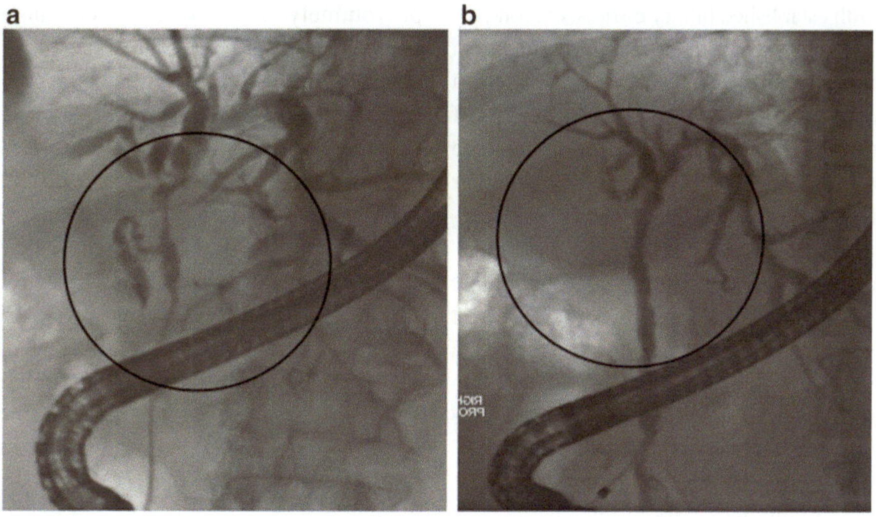


**Fig. 15.6** ERC in a patient with IgG4-SC and significant extrahepatic biliary stricturing (**a**). Considerable improvement is seen after 3 months of steroid therapy (**b**)

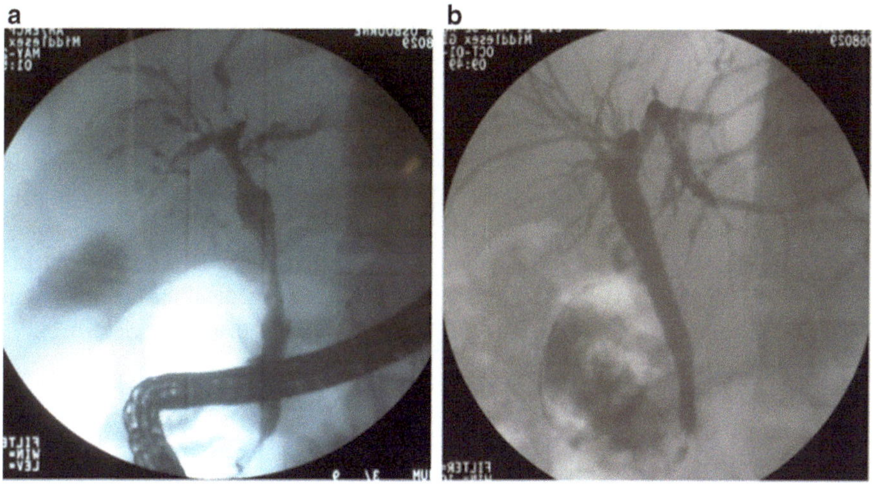


**Fig. 15.7** ERC in a patient with IgG4-SC and significant intrahepatic biliary stricturing (**a**). Considerable improvement is seen after steroid therapy (**b**)

be seen within the rest of the extrahepatic (Fig. 15.6a, b) and intrahepatic biliary tree (Fig. 15.7a, b). Although there is no consensus on steroid regimens, most groups from Japan, Europe, and the USA administer oral Prednisolone 30–40 mg daily [28, 50–52], and a clinical and cholangiographic improvement is usually seen within 4 weeks. It is unclear what factors determine a favorable response and hence which patients should be selected for treatment. Patients with recent-onset disease, with acute jaundice, and demonstrable change in imaging over a short period of time seem most likely to respond. This probably reflects the predominant inflammatory, rather than fibro-stenotic, nature of early disease. In contrast, long-standing, static disease, which has been present for years, appears to respond less well. Nevertheless, steroid therapy for patients with established biliary cirrhosis secondary to IgG4-SC may show marked improvement in liver synthetic function [4]. High levels of serum IgG4 may normalize as the disease activity of AIP settles, either spontaneously or in response to steroids [53]. It remains to be proven whether raised pretreatment serum IgG4 in IgG4-SC predicts a favorable response to steroids.

Just as a response to steroids is a diagnostic feature of IgG4-SC, resolution or significant improvement of dominant biliary strictures is a characteristic feature. In those patients who have required an initial ERCP (for biliary stenting) and been commenced on steroids, our practice is to repeat the ERCP after 6 weeks. Resolution of jaundice, marked improvement in liver function tests, and significant improvement/resolution of distal bile duct stricturing are characteristically seen. If this has not occurred and certainly if stricturing has worsened, an alternative diagnosis to IgG4-SC should be actively sought. It may be that not all patients presenting with biliary obstruction and a new diagnosis of IgG4-SC require an ERCP. If the diagnosis can be established promptly (e.g., on the basis of classical pancreaticobiliary imaging, a raised serum IgG4, and other organ involvement), then steroid therapy may be commenced without the inherent risks of ERCP. Nevertheless, close monitoring is essential, in view of the risks of biliary sepsis in the setting of steroid therapy and biliary obstruction. In those in whom ERCP is deemed necessary (for both diagnostic and therapeutic purposes), it is not clear how dominant biliary strictures should be managed. Although there is a move towards balloon dilatation, rather than endoscopic stenting, in the management of dominant strictures in PSC [54–56], it is our practice to use stent short term rather than perform balloon dilatation, in patients newly diagnosed with IgG4-SC. This is due to the rapidly reversible nature of stricturing, with steroids, particularly in those patients with recent-onset disease. In our own experience (GW, personal communication), 10F plastic stents spontaneously migrate from distal biliary strictures within 6 weeks in >60% of patients following the introduction of steroids, again reflecting the steroid response. ERCP should not be routinely used to assess cholangiographic response to treatment, unless there is a specific need for intervention (e.g., stent change).

Clinical relapse may occur after an initial course of steroids for AIP, with recent studies reporting this in 24–68 % of cases [57]. Of note, predictors of AIP relapse include failure of serum IgG4 levels to fall during steroid therapy and extrapancreatic disease, in particular biliary disease (i.e., IgG4-SC). In our own series from London, 54 % of patients with AIP who also had IgG4-SC subsequently relapsed or failed to wean steroids, compared to no relapse among AIP patients with isolated pancreatic disease [4]. This finding is similar to that of the Mayo Clinic, which demonstrated relapse in 53 % of IgG4-SC patients after an initial course of steroids. Proximal biliary stricturing more strongly predicted relapse than distal bile duct stricturing (64 % vs. 32 %) [28]. In those developing jaundice/biliary obstruction as the clinical manifestation of relapse, repeat ERCP may be necessary, both to enhance biliary drainage and to exclude the development of a malignant stricture (mindful that malignancy has been occasionally associated with AIP [58–60]). Biliary brush cytology should be taken from all dominant strictures. Endoscopic therapy is similar to that at first presentation. The medical management of relapse of IgG4-SC/AIP is discussed elsewhere.

## EUS/IDUS

### Ultrasonographic Features of IgG4-SC on EUS/IDUS

EUS and IDUS provide detailed images of the bile duct wall. The features to observe in EUS/IDUS are the following [38, 61]: (1) origin (wall thickness, extrinsic compression), (2) symmetry (circular-symmetric, circular-asymmetric, semicircular), (3) outer margin (smooth, notched), (4) inner margin (smooth, prickled, rigid, or papillary), (5) internal echo (homogeneous, linear-high, or heterogeneous), and (6) the bile duct wall thickness. Although EUS is useful to evaluate bile duct abnormalities, IDUS more readily evaluates "symmetry."

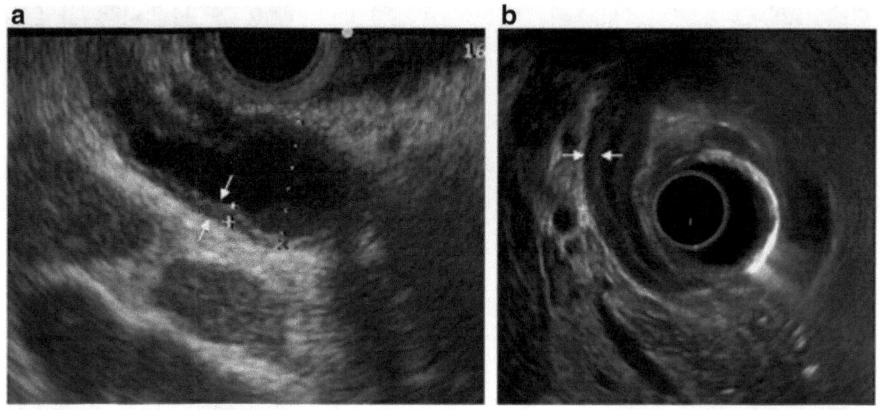

**Fig. 15.8** EUS findings in IgG4-SC. EUS demonstrates the diffuse thickening of the biliary wall (*between arrows*) of common bile duct with the following features (**a**, **b**): homogeneous and regular thickening which is characterized by an hypoechoic intermediate layer and hyperechoic outer and inner layers

The typical EUS feature of the bile duct in IgG4-SC/AIP is a homogeneous, regular thickening of the bile duct wall, which is characterized by an echopoor intermediate layer and hyperechoic outer and inner layers [62–64] (Fig. 15.8). Furthermore, characteristic bile duct wall thickening (diffuse and uniform thickening, circular-symmetric thickening) is generally recognizable on IDUS (Fig. 15.9). Naitoh et al. [38] reported that the origin of hilar strictures was wall thickening in all 9 of the patients (100 %) examined using IDUS. Moreover, the symmetry was circular-symmetric in 6 patients (67 %) and circular-asymmetric in 3 (33 %). In addition, a smooth outer margin and a smooth inner margin in the stricture are specific findings in EUS/IDUS. The internal echo in the thickening wall, whether it is homogeneous or heterogeneous, remains controversial.

The wall thickening can be visualized even if a cholangiogram on ERCP does not demonstrate a bile duct stricture. Slight sclerogenic changes of the extrapancreatic bile duct might not be clearly visible on ERCP. Naito et al. [38] evaluated the IDUS findings on proximal-middle CBD, where ERCP showed a normal appearance in 20 patients. The symmetry was circular-symmetric in 16 patients (80%) and circular-asymmetric in 4 (20 %). When they regarded wall thickness greater than 1 mm as indicating wall thickening, wall thickening was observed in 17 patients (85 %). From these data, it is considered that IDUS is superior to ERCP for evaluation of ductal change in IgG4-SC.

Contrast-enhanced EUS (CE-EUS) is increasingly performed. Hyodo et al. [65] evaluated CE-EUS findings of bile duct in five patients with AIP. They found that wall thickening is strongly enhanced by CE-EUS from 30 s after administration of contrast medium for ultrasound, peaking at 120 s in all patients. Moreover, in three patients, IDUS imaging showed concentric bile duct wall thickening with smooth configuration of the outermost layer, similar to that observed on EUS imaging. In addition, the thickened bile duct wall was markedly enhanced with contrast medium on IDUS.

## Role of EUS and IDUS in the Differential Diagnosis of IgG4-SC

EUS and IDUS enable visualization of the entire extrahepatic bile duct and may establish the diagnosis of a biliary stricture. As described above, ultrasound can reveal slight bile duct abnormalities, which are not normally detected by cholangiography. Hirano et al. reported [66] not only sclerogenic changes on ERCP but also wall thickening detected by IDUS or EUS as indicating biliary involvement in AIP. Furthermore, the frequency of biliary involvement in AIP was reported

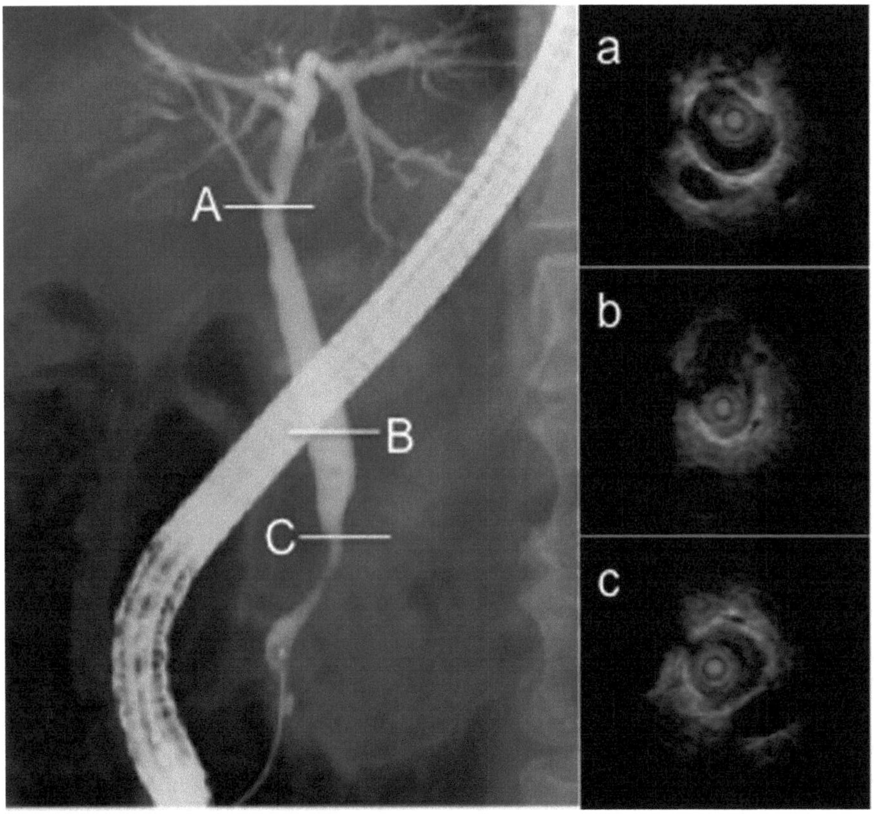


**Fig. 15.9** IDUS findings in IgG4-SC. Cholangiogram on ERCP shows intrahepatic and extrahepatic strictures. IDUS reveals the diffuse wall thickening of biliary duct in not only stricture but also normal appearance on cholangiogram. (**a**) IDUS shows circular-symmetric wall thickness in hilar stricture (line A). (**b**) IDUS shows slight wall thickness in middle extrahepatic bile duct in which cholangiogram is normal (line B). (**c**) IDUS shows wall thickness in the lower part of bile duct (line C); circular-symmetric thickening and smooth outer/inner margin with homogeneous internal echo

as 73.9 %, although it was 26.6 % if evaluation was made solely using ERCP. Therefore, ultrasound is an indispensable modality for the diagnosis of biliary abnormalities.

The most important role of EUS/IDUS in the differential diagnosis of IgG4-SC is the discrimination of IgG4-SC from PSC and/or cholangiocarcinoma. Biliary strictures can mimic both sclerosing cholangitis and biliary cancer. Fundamentally, EUS/IDUS findings showing circular-symmetric wall thickness, with inner and outer smooth margins, were typical for IgG4-SC.

Regarding discrimination from PSC, Kubota et al. [67] recently evaluated characteristic IDUS features that might discriminate eight patients with PSC from nine patients with IgG4-SC/AIP. The outcomes of IDUS (IgG4-SC/AIP vs. PSC) were as follows: symmetrical thickness, 89 % (8/9) vs. 25 % (2/8); wall thickness (mm), 3.0 +/−1.0 vs. 2.1+/−0.7; heterogeneous internal echo, 66.7 % (6/9) vs. 22.2 % (2/9); and lateral mucosal lesions continuous to the hilar, 55.6 % (5/9) vs. 11.1 % (1/9). Symmetrical thickness of the bile duct, a heterogeneous internal echo, and the presence of lateral mucosal lesions continuous to the hilar were significantly more detected in cases of IgG4-SC/AIP than in PSC ($p<.05$). Furthermore, the wall thickness tended to be more prominent in IgG4-SC/AIP than in the PSC.

Regarding discrimination of bile cancer, Naitoh et al. [38] evaluated IDUS findings in 23 patients with IgG4-SC. Their results show that circular-symmetry, wall thickness, smooth inner and outer margins, and a homogeneous intermediate layer within the stricture were significantly more common in AIP than in cholangiocarcinoma. The wall thickness in non-strictured regions of IgG4-SC was significantly greater than that in cholangiocarcinoma. Therefore, bile duct wall thickness exceeding 0.8 mm in regions of non-stricture on the cholangiogram was highly suggestive of IgG4-SC. In addition, Hyodo et al. [65] demonstrated that CE-EUS and IDUS showed an inflammatory pattern of the bile duct wall, with a long-lasting enhancement starting in the early phase instead of the poor enhancement found in bile duct cancer.

## EUS/IDUS and Response to Treatment

A change in the bile duct wall thickening after steroid therapy is regarded as an important feature for evaluating the therapeutic response. After initiation of steroid therapy, repeat EUS/IDUS shows attenuation of the bile duct thickening, whereas follow-up by CE-EUS reveals reduced enhancement of the bile duct wall, which reflects resolution of the inflammatory process with treatment [65]. However, Hoki et al. [64] reported that wall thickening persisted to some degree in almost all patients for an average of 5 months, even after steroid therapy. It remains unclear whether these changes are controllable using long-term therapy. Nevertheless, if the wall thickness does not improve at all after steroid therapy, then further assessment for malignancies is required.

## References


1. Cohen S, Bacon BR, Berlin JA, Fleischer D, Hecht GA, Loehrer Sr PJ, McNair Jr AE, Mulholland M, Norton NJ, Rabeneck L, Ransohoff DF, Sonnenberg A, Vannier MW. National Institutes of Health State-of-the-Science Conference Statement: ERCP for diagnosis and therapy, January 14–16, 2002. Gastrointest Endosc. 2002;56:803–9.
2. Ghazale A, Chari ST, Zhang L, Smyrk TC, Takahashi N, Levy MJ, Topazian MD, Clain JE, Pearson RK, Petersen BT, Vege SS, Lindor K, Farnell MB. Immunoglobulin G4-associated cholangitis: clinical profile and response to therapy. Gastroenterology. 2008;134(3):706–15.
3. Bjornsson E, Chari ST, Smyrk TC, Lindor K. Immunoglobulin G4 associated cholangitis: description of an emerging clinical entity based on review of the literature. Hepatology. 2007;45:1547–54.
4. Sandanayake NS, Church NI, Chapman MH, Johnson GJ, Dhar DK, Amin Z, Deheragoda MG, Novelli M, Winstanley A, Rodriguez-Justo M, Hatfield AR, Pereira SP, Webster GJ. Presentation and management of post-treatment relapse in autoimmune pancreatitis/immunoglobulin G4-associated cholangitis. Clin Gastroenterol Hepatol. 2009;7:1089–96.
5. Nakazawa T, Ohara H, Sano H, Ando T, Aoki S, Kobayashi S, Okamoto T, Nomura T, Joh T, Itoh M. Clinical differences between primary sclerosing cholangitis and sclerosing cholangitis with autoimmune pancreatitis. Pancreas. 2005;30:20–5.
6. Nishino T, Toki F, Oyama H, Oi I, Kobayashi M, Takasaki K, Shiratori K. Biliary tract involvement in autoimmune pancreatitis. Pancreas. 2005;30:76–82.
7. Nishino T, Oyama H, Toki F, Shiratori K. Differentiation between autoimmune pancreatitis and pancreatic carcinoma based on endoscopic retrograde cholangiopancreatography findings. J Gastroenterol. 2010;45:988–96.
8. Sugumar A, Levy MJ, Kamisawa T, Webster GJ, Kim MH, Enders F, Amin Z, Baron TH, Chapman MH, Church NI, Clain JE, Egawa N, Johnson GJ, Okazaki K, Pearson RK, Pereira SP, Petersen BT, Read S, Sah RP, Sandanayake NS, Takahashi N, Topazian MD, Uchida K, Vege SS, Chari ST. Endoscopic retrograde pancreatography criteria to diagnose autoimmune pancreatitis: an international multicentre study. Gut. 2011;60:666–70.
9. Cheng CL, Sherman S, Watkins JL, Barnett J, Freeman M, Geenen J, Ryan M, Parker H, Frakes JT, Fogel EL, Silverman WB, Dua KS, Aliperti G, Yakshe P, Uzer M, Jones W, Goff J, Lazzell-Pannell L, Rashdan A, Temkit M, Lehman GA. Risk factors for post-ERCP pancreatitis: a prospective multicenter study. Am J Gastroenterol. 2006;101:139–47.
10. Hamano H, Umemura T, Uehara T, Kawa S, Kiyosawa K. IgG4-related sclerosing cholangitis should be included as an exclusion criterion for the diagnosis of primary sclerosing cholangitis. Am J Gastroenterol. 2007;102:691–2.
11. Mendes FD, Jorgensen R, Keach J, Katzmann JA, Smyrk T, Donlinger J, Chari S, Lindor KD. Elevated serum IgG4 concentration in patients with primary sclerosing cholangitis. Am J Gastroenterol. 2006;101:2070–5.
12. Webster GJ, Pereira SP, Chapman RW. Autoimmune pancreatitis/IgG4-associated cholangitis and primary sclerosing cholangitis – overlapping or separate diseases? J Hepatol. 2009;51(2):398–402.

13. Hirano K, Kawabe T, Yamamoto N, Nakai Y, Sasahira N, Tsujino T, Toda N, Isayama H, Tada M, Omata M. Serum IgG4 concentrations in pancreatic and biliary diseases. Clin Chim Acta. 2006;367:181–4.
14. Epstein O, Chapman RW, Lake-Bakaar G, Foo AY, Rosalki SB, Sherlock S. The pancreas in primary biliary cirrhosis and primary sclerosing cholangitis. Gastroenterology. 1982;83:1177–82.
15. Zhang L, Lewis JT, Abraham SC, Leung S, Rosen C, Poterrucha J, Wu TT. IgG4+ plasma cell infiltrates in liver explants with primary sclerosing cholangitis. Mod Pathol. 2009;22:1480.
16. Buc E, Lesurtel M, Belghiti J. Is preoperative histological diagnosis necessary before referral to major surgery for cholangiocarcinoma? HPB (Oxford). 2008;10:98–105.
17. Cheung MT, Lo IL. IgG4-related sclerosing lymphoplasmacytic pancreatitis and cholangitis mimicking carcinoma of pancreas and Klatskin tumour. ANZ J Surg. 2008;78:252–6.
18. Chung DT, Tang CN, Lai EC, Yang GP, Li MK. Immunoglobulin G4-associated sclerosing cholangitis mimicking cholangiocarcinoma. Hong Kong Med J. 2010;16:149–52.
19. Hamano H, Kawa S, Uehara T, Ochi Y, Takayama M, Komatsu K, Muraki T, Umino J, Kiyosawa K, Miyagawa S. Immunoglobulin G4-related lymphoplasmacytic sclerosing cholangitis that mimics infiltrating hilar cholangiocarcinoma: part of a spectrum of autoimmune pancreatitis? Gastrointest Endosc. 2005;62:152–7.
20. Erdogan D, Kloek JJ, ten Kate FJ, Rauws EA, Busch OR, Gouma DJ, van Gulik TM. Immunoglobulin G4-related sclerosing cholangitis in patients resected for presumed malignant bile duct strictures. Br J Surg. 2008;95:727–34.
21. Oh HC, Kim MH, Lee KT, Lee JK, Moon SH, Song TJ, Eum J, Park do H, Lee SS, Seo DW, Lee SK. Clinical clues to suspicion of IgG4-associated sclerosing cholangitis disguised as primary sclerosing cholangitis or hilar cholangiocarcinoma. J Gastroenterol Hepatol. 2010;25:1831–7.
22. Kalaitzakis E, Levy M, Kamisawa T, Johnson GJ, Baron TH, Topazian MD, Takahashi N, Kanno A, Okazaki K, Egawa N, Uchida K, Sheikh K, Amin Z, Shimosegawa T, Sandanayake NS, Church NI, Chapman MH, Pereira SP, Chari S, Webster GJ. Endoscopic retrograde cholangiography does not reliably distinguish IgG4-associated cholangitis from primary sclerosing cholangitis or cholangiocarcinoma. Clin Gastroenterol Hepatol. 2011;9(9):800–803.e2.
23. Miglani RK, Murthy D, Bhat R, Kumar AK. Immunoglobulin G4-associated cholangitis mimicking cholangiocarcinoma in a young boy. J Postgrad Med. 2010;56:140–2.
24. Menias CO, Surabhi VR, Prasad SR, Wang HL, Narra VR, Chintapalli KN. Mimics of cholangiocarcinoma: spectrum of disease. Radiographics. 2008;28:1115–29.
25. Paik WH, Park YS, Hwang JH, Lee SH, Yoon CJ, Kang SG, Lee JK, Ryu JK, Kim YT, Yoon YB. Palliative treatment with self-expandable metallic stents in patients with advanced type III or IV hilar cholangiocarcinoma: a percutaneous versus endoscopic approach. Gastrointest Endosc. 2009;69:55–62.
26. Ayaru L, Kurzawinski TR, Shankar A, Webster GJ, Hatfield AR, Pereira SP. Complications and diagnostic difficulties arising from biliary self-expanding metal stent insertion before definitive histological diagnosis. J Gastroenterol Hepatol. 2008;23:315–20.
27. Webster G, Pereira S. Mesh-metal stents for hilar cholangiocarcinoma. Gastrointest Endosc. 2009;70:817–18.
28. Ghazale A, Chari ST, Zhang L, Smyrk TC, Takahashi N, Levy MJ, Topazian MD, Clain JE, Pearson RK, Petersen BT, Vege SS, Lindor K, Farnell MB. Immunoglobulin G4-associated cholangitis: clinical profile and response to therapy. Gastroenterology. 2008;134:706–15.
29. Kurzawinski TR, Deery A, Dooley JS, Dick R, Hobbs KE, Davidson BR. A prospective study of biliary cytology in 100 patients with bile duct strictures. Hepatology. 1993;18:1399–403.
30. Stewart CJ, Mills PR, Carter R, O'Donohue J, Fullarton G, Imrie CW, Murray WR. Brush cytology in the assessment of pancreatico-biliary strictures: a review of 406 cases. J Clin Pathol. 2001;54:449–55.
31. Temino Lopez-Jurado R, Cacho Acosta G, Arguelles Pintos M, Rodriguez Caravaca G, Lledo Navarro JL, Fernandez RC. Diagnostic yield of brush cytology for biliary stenosis during ERCP. Rev Esp Enferm Dig. 2009;101:385–9, 390–4.
32. Glasbrenner B, Ardan M, Boeck W, Preclik G, Moller P, Adler G. Prospective evaluation of brush cytology of biliary strictures during endoscopic retrograde cholangiopancreatography. Endoscopy. 1999;31: 712–17.
33. Boberg KM, Jebsen P, Clausen OP, Foss A, Aabakken L, Schrumpf E. Diagnostic benefit of biliary brush cytology in cholangiocarcinoma in primary sclerosing cholangitis. J Hepatol. 2006;45:568–74.
34. Levy MJ, Reddy RP, Wiersema MJ, Smyrk TC, Clain JE, Harewood GC, Pearson RK, Rajan E, Topazian MD, Yusuf TE, Chari ST, Petersen BT. EUS-guided trucut biopsy in establishing autoimmune pancreatitis as the cause of obstructive jaundice. Gastrointest Endosc. 2005;61:467–72.
35. Deshpande V, Mino-Kenudson M, Brugge WR, Pitman MB, Fernandez-del Castillo C, Warshaw AL, Lauwers GY. Endoscopic ultrasound guided fine needle aspiration biopsy of autoimmune pancreatitis: diagnostic criteria and pitfalls. Am J Surg Pathol. 2005;29:1464–71.
36. Deheragoda MG, Church NI, Rodriguez-Justo M, Munson P, Sandanayake N, Seward EW, Miller K, Novelli M, Hatfield AR, Pereira SP, Webster GJ. The use of immunoglobulin g4 immunostaining in

diagnosing pancreatic and extrapancreatic involvement in autoimmune pancreatitis. Clin Gastroenterol Hepatol. 2007;5:1229–34.
37. Alexander S, Bourke MJ, Williams SJ, Bailey A, Gill A, Kench JG. Diagnosis of autoimmune pancreatitis with intraductal biliary biopsy and treatment of stricture with serial placement of multiple biliary stents. Gastrointest Endosc. 2008;68(2):396–9.
38. Naitoh I, Nakazawa T, Ohara H, Ando T, Hayashi K, Tanaka H, Okumura F, Takahashi S, Joh T. Endoscopic transpapillary intraductal ultrasonography and biopsy in the diagnosis of IgG4-related sclerosing cholangitis. J Gastroenterol. 2009;44:1147–55.
39. Draganov PV, Lin T, Chauhan S, Wagh MS, Hou W, Forsmark CE. Prospective evaluation of the clinical utility of ERCP-guided cholangiopancreatoscopy with a new direct visualization system. Gastrointest Endosc. 2011;73:971–9.
40. Petersen BT. Cholangioscopy for special applications: primary sclerosing cholangitis, liver transplant, and selective duct access. Gastrointest Endosc Clin N Am. 2009;19:579–86.
41. Ramchandani M, Reddy DN, Gupta R, Lakhtakia S, Tandan M, Darisetty S, Sekaran A, Rao GV. Role of single-operator peroral cholangioscopy in the diagnosis of indeterminate biliary lesions: a single-center, prospective study. Gastrointest Endosc. 2011;74(3):511–9.
42. Itoi T, Osanai M, Igarashi Y, Tanaka K, Kida M, Maguchi H, Yasuda K, Okano N, Imaizumi H, Yokoyama T, Itokawa F. Diagnostic peroral video cholangioscopy is an accurate diagnostic tool for patients with bile duct lesions. Clin Gastroenterol Hepatol. 2010;8:934–8.
43. Webster GJ, Deheregoda MG, Church NI. Extrapancreatic manifestations in autoimmune pancreatitis. Minerva Gastroenterol Dietol. 2009;55:41–51.
44. Chang MC, Chang YT, Wei SC, Kuo CH, Liang PC, Wong JM. Autoimmune pancreatitis associated with high prevalence of gastric ulcer independent of *Helicobacter pylori* infection status. Pancreas. 2009;38(4):442–6.
45. Shinji A, Sano K, Hamano H, Unno H, Fukushima M, Nakamura N, Akamatsu T, Kawa S, Kiyosawa K. Autoimmune pancreatitis is closely associated with gastric ulcer presenting with abundant IgG4-bearing plasma cell infiltration. Gastrointest Endosc. 2004;59:506–11.
46. Kamisawa T, Tu Y, Nakajima H, Egawa N, Tsuruta K, Okamoto A. Usefulness of biopsying the major duodenal papilla to diagnose autoimmune pancreatitis: a prospective study using IgG4-immunostaining. World J Gastroenterol. 2006;12:2031–3.
47. Kamisawa T, Tu Y, Egawa N, Tsuruta K, Okamoto A. A new diagnostic endoscopic tool for autoimmune pancreatitis. Gastrointest Endosc. 2008;68:358–61.
48. Sepehr A, Mino-Kenudson M, Ogawa F, Brugge WR, Deshpande V, Lauwers GY. IgG4+ to IgG+ plasma cells ratio of ampulla can help differentiate autoimmune pancreatitis from other "mass forming" pancreatic lesions. Am J Surg Pathol. 2008;32(12):1770–9.
49. Sahin P, Pozsar J, Simon K, Illyes G, Laszlo F, Topa L. Autoimmune pancreatitis associated with immune-mediated inflammation of the papilla of Vater: report on two cases. Pancreas. 2004;29:162–6.
50. Chari ST. Current concepts in the treatment of autoimmune pancreatitis. JOP. 2007;8:1–3.
51. Alderlieste YA, van den Elzen BD, Rauws EA, Beuers U. Immunoglobulin G4-associated cholangitis: one variant of immunoglobulin G4-related systemic disease. Digestion. 2009;79:220–8.
52. Kamisawa T, Yoshiike M, Egawa N, Nakajima H, Tsuruta K, Okamoto A. Treating patients with autoimmune pancreatitis: results from a long-term follow-up study. Pancreatology. 2005;5:234–8; discussion 238–40.
53. Hamano H, Kawa S, Horiuchi A, Unno H, Furuya N, Akamatsu T, Fukushima M, Nikaido T, Nakayama K, Usuda N, Kiyosawa K. High serum IgG4 concentrations in patients with sclerosing pancreatitis. N Engl J Med. 2001;344:732–8.
54. Kaya M, Petersen BT, Angulo P, Baron TH, Andrews JC, Gostout CJ, Lindor KD. Balloon dilation compared to stenting of dominant strictures in primary sclerosing cholangitis. Am J Gastroenterol. 2001;96:1059–66.
55. Stiehl A, Rost D. Endoscopic treatment of dominant stenoses in patients with primary sclerosing cholangitis. Clin Rev Allergy Immunol. 2005;28:159–65.
56. Gotthardt DN, Rudolph G, Kloters-Plachky P, Kulaksiz H, Stiehl A. Endoscopic dilation of dominant stenoses in primary sclerosing cholangitis: outcome after long-term treatment. Gastrointest Endosc. 2010;71:527–34.
57. Kalaitzakis E, Webster GJ. Review article: autoimmune pancreatitis – management of an emerging disease. Aliment Pharmacol Ther. 2011;33(3):291–303.
58. Inoue H, Miyatani H, Sawada Y, Yoshida Y. A case of pancreas cancer with autoimmune pancreatitis. Pancreas. 2006;33:208–9.
59. Fukui T, Mitsuyama T, Takaoka M, Uchida K, Matsushita M, Okazaki K. Pancreatic cancer associated with autoimmune pancreatitis in remission. Intern Med. 2008;47:151–5.
60. Ghazale A, Chari S. Is autoimmune pancreatitis a risk factor for pancreatic cancer? Pancreas. 2007;35:376.
61. Tamada K, Kanai N, Wada S, Tomiyama T, Ohashi A, Satoh Y, et al. Utility and limitations of intraductal ultrasonography in distinguishing longitudinal cancer extension along the bile duct from inflammatory wall thickening. Abdom Imaging. 2001;26:623–31.
62. De Lisi S, Buscarini E, Arcidiacono PG, Petrone M, Menozzi F, Testoni PA, Zambelli A. Endoscopic ultrasonography findings in autoimmune pancreatitis: be aware of the ambiguous features and look for the pivotal ones. JOP. 2010;11:78–84.
63. Buscarini E, Frulloni L, De Lisi S, Falconi M, Testoni PA, Zambelli A. Autoimmune pancreatitis: a

challenging diagnostic puzzle for clinicians. Dig Liver Dis. 2010;42:92–8.
64. Hoki N, Mizuno N, Sawaki A, Tajika M, Takayama R, Shimizu Y, Bhatia V, Yamao K. Diagnosis of autoimmune pancreatitis using endoscopic ultrasonography. J Gastroenterol. 2009;44:154–9.
65. Hyodo N, Hyodo T. Ultrasonographic evaluation in patients with autoimmune-related pancreatitis. J Gastroenterol. 2003;38:1155–61.
66. Hamano H, Arakura N, Muraki T, et al. Prevalence and distribution of extrapancreatic lesions complicating autoimmune pancreatitis. J Gastroenterol. 2006;41:1197–205.
67. Kubota K, Kato S, Kobayashi N, Nakajima A. Intraductal ultrasonography can discriminate between sclerosing cholangitis associated with autoimmune pancreatitis and primary sclerosing cholangitis. Gastrointest Endosc. 2009;69:AB117.

# 16 Clinical Spectrum and Management

Einar S. Björnsson and Keith D. Lindor

## Abbreviations

| | |
|---|---|
| AIH | Autoimmune hepatitis |
| AIP | Autoimmune pancreatitis |
| ALP | Alkaline phosphatase |
| CCA | Cholangiocarcinoma |
| IBD | Inflammatory bowel disease |
| $IgG_4$-SC | $IgG_4$-related sclerosing cholangitis |
| ISD | IgG4 systemic disease |
| PSC | Primary sclerosing cholangitis |
| UC | Ulcerative colitis |

## Introduction

$IgG_4$-related disease ($IgG_4$-RD) is a relatively newly described entity. Although autoimmune pancreatitis (AIP) is its best characterized and most widely recognized manifestation, extrapancreatic lesions are common, such as cholangitis (sometimes sclerosing), sialadenitis, and retroperitoneal fibrosis. Thus, AIP has been considered to be the pancreatic manifestation of $IgG_4$-RD. Patients with biliary strictures similar to those that occur in primary sclerosing cholangitis (PSC), with concomitant pancreatic involvement, were reported in the early 1960s [1, 2]. Since the original reports, a wide variety of descriptive names appeared in the literature [3, 4]. "PSC mimicking chronic pancreatitis," "lymphoplasmacytic sclerosing pancreatitis with cholangitis" [5], "sclerosing pancreatocholangitis" [7–11], "lymphoplasmacytic sclerosing cholangitis without pancreatitis" [12], "immunoglobulin G4-related lymphoplasmacytic sclerosing cholangitis," and "autoimmune pancreatitis-associated sclerosing cholangitis," to name only a few. Patients with biliary strictures without pancreatic involvement, both intrahepatic and hilar, have been well documented [12–16]. In the first comprehensive review of the biliary manifestations of IgG4-associated systemic disease, we coined the term "$IgG_4$-associated cholangitis (IAC)" [3]. Subsequently the term "IgG4-related sclerosing cholangitis (IgG4-SC)" has been proposed for this entity even though biliary strictures diagnosed and treated with steroids early in the course can resolve and disappear after successful therapy. Since our original report [3], other reviews have been published that focus both on the clinical, pathological, and immunological and on the systemic nature of this condition [4, 17–23].

E.S. Björnsson, M.D., Ph.D.
Landspitali University Hospital, Hringbraut 101, Reykjavik, Iceland

Department of Internal Medicine, Division of Gastroenterology, The National University Hospital of Iceland, Reykjavik, Iceland
e-mail: einarsb@landspitali.is

K.D. Lindor, M.D. (✉)
Gastroenterology and Hepatology, Mayo Clinic, 200 1st ST., SW, Rochester, MN 55905, USA
e-mail: lindor.keith@mayo.edu

M.J. Levy and S.T. Chari (eds.), *Autoimmune (IgG4-related) Pancreatitis and Cholangitis*,
DOI 10.1007/978-1-4419-6430-4_16, © Springer Science+Business Media New York 2013

There is currently no published consensus that defines $IgG_4$-SC. Clinically it can best be described as "biliary strictures that respond to or improve with steroid therapy," and IgG4-SC is histologically characterized by infiltration of IgG4-bearing plasma cells [3, 4]. Most patients with $IgG_4$-SC have elevated serum levels of IgG4 [3, 4, 17–23]. However, strict criteria for $IgG_4$-SC are lacking. Although biliary strictures in $IgG_4$-SC typically respond to steroids, some strictures are refractory to steroid therapy. It is conceivable that long-standing $IgG_4$-SC may be dominated by fibrosis, which is one of the histological distinguishing features of $IgG_4$-SC but which may no longer resolve with steroids. The long-term effect of immunosuppressive therapy in these patients has not been reported, and the natural history after treatment that has been initiated is not well known. Because biliary strictures in $IgG_4$-SC and those in classic PSC seem to be indistinguishable by cholangiography alone, it is somewhat unclear and controversial if $IgG_4$-SC and PSC represent variations of the same disease spectrum or are separate entities [3, 4, 17–23]. Recent guidelines for PSC from the American Association for the Study of the Liver (AASLD) suggest measurement of serum IgG4 levels for all patients with possible PSC, to rule out IgG4-associated cholangiopathy [24]. Thus, the existence and the recognition of $IgG_4$-SC are not only of great academic interest but also of great therapeutic importance because these patients whether or not called PSC typically show steroid responsiveness which classic PSC does not.

## Epidemiology

Epidemiological data on IgG4-associated systemic disease, both AIP and $IgG_4$-SC, are largely lacking. No prospective studies on all patients in a population-based sample, including patients with both primary and secondary sclerosing cholangitides, exist in whom serum IgG4 measurements have been undertaken. Previous epidemiological studies, reporting prevalence figures among patients with biliary strictures, have mostly been on patients diagnosed with PSC. PSC is a rare disorder and the highest point prevalence reported to date was 16 cases per 100,000 in the total adult population [25]. A single-center study from Canada demonstrated that among PSC patients diagnosed and identified from 1972 to 2003, 5/72 (7 %) had associated pancreatic problems [26]. These pancreatic disorders included pancreatic insufficiency and acute pancreatitis, and three patients had a pancreatic mass. The patients presenting with a pancreatic mass were initially suspected on radiological and clinical grounds to have a pancreatic malignancy but were found to have a pancreatic pseudotumor associated with PSC [27] and therefore fulfilling at least some of the criteria for $IgG_4$-SC. From the same center, a recent analysis of 168 patients with radiological or biopsy-proven sclerosing cholangitis showed that classic large-duct PSC was present in 63 %, small-duct PSC in 8 %, overlap with autoimmune hepatitis (AIH) in 11 %, and secondary sclerosing cholangitis in 18 % [27]. Interestingly among the heterogeneous group of secondary etiologies, 14/30 (47 %) were diagnosed with $IgG_4$-SC [27]. Thus, 8 % of the total study population of sclerosing cholangitis had $IgG_4$-SC according to these results [27]. In a multicenter study of Japanese PSC patients diagnosed between 1975 and 2004, altogether 28/388 (7 %) patients were found to have PSC associated with AIP [28].

Serum IgG4 levels were measured in a large cohort of PSC attending the Mayo Clinic in Rochester, MN ($n = 128$), from stored samples [29]. Elevated levels were found in 9 % of the PSC patients whereas this was only found in one of 87 (1.1 %) PBC patients [29].

## Clinical Presentation

Since 1999, a prospective database on patients investigated for AIP has been maintained at the Mayo Clinic [16]. From this database, the largest cohort of $IgG_4$-SC patients was recently reported [16]. The mean age was 62 years, with 83 % older than 50 years of age and 85 % were of male gender. The most common clinical features on presentation were obstructive jaundice in approximately 80 % of patients, weight loss in 50 %, as well as steatorrhea in 15 % and less commonly diabetes mellitus and abdominal pain [16]. Similar results have been observed in other studies which have demonstrated that obstructive jaundice is the most common presentation [6, 7, 10, 11, 13, 28]. Many patients presenting with distal biliary strictures and a pancreatic mass and/or hilar strictures have been suspected to have a pancreatic malignancy or cholangiocarcinoma and have been operated on in the past. It was therefore only after major surgery such as pancreatoduodenectomy that their $IgG_4$-SC was detected [12, 13, 30].

In a more recent study, in which PSC patients were systematically screened with IgG4 measurements, approximately 50 % of patients with classic PSC who had elevated IgG4 levels presented with jaundice and 17 % had concomitant pancreatic disorders [15].

## $IgG_4$-SC and PSC

As previously stated, it is controversial and somewhat unclear if $IgG_4$-SC and PSC represent variation of the same disease spectrum or are separate conditions [3, 4, 17–23]. Demographics, clinical features, and associated conditions of $IgG_4$-SC seem to vary depending on whether patients are referred to a pancreatic clinic and investigated for AIP [16] or whether they found to have biliary strictures and considered to have PSC [15]. Intrahepatic strictures were observed in only 19/53 (36 %) in those investigated for AIP [16], but both intrahepatic and extrahepatic strictures were found in all PSC patients with elevated IgG4 serum levels [15], and only 4/24 (17 %) had an associated pancreatic disorder [15]. Only 6 % of the patients reported in the study by Ghazale et al. [16] had inflammatory bowel disease (IBD), whereas 75 % of PSC patients with elevated IgG4 levels had IBD [15], similar to other series of classic PSC patients [25]. This is in sharp contrast with $IgG_4$-SC patients in Japan who do not seem to have associated IBD [11, 19, 23, 31]. Recently, two HLA identical siblings exhibiting features of $IgG_4$-SC together with ulcerative colitis were reported from Belgium [32]. Thus, IBD-associated $IgG_4$-SC may in some cases be a part of $IgG_4$-RD highly responsive to steroid therapy [32].

Only a few studies have systematically assessed and reported the prevalence of elevated IgG4 serum levels in patients with PSC. In the first study of this kind, IgG4 levels were measured in stored sera from a large cohort of PSC patients ($n=128$) and elevated levels were found in 9 % of these patients [29]. A total of 33/285 (11.6 %) consecutive PSC patients seen and tested for IgG4 at the Mayo Clinic had elevated IgG4 levels (>140 mg/dL) during the period 2006–2008 [15]. In a recent population-based study of PSC patients from Sweden (published in abstract) [33], 7/111 (6.3 %) presented with IgG4 levels above the upper normal limit. Three out of these had signs of other organ involvement including autoimmune pancreatitis ($n=2$) and sialadenitis ($n=1$) suggesting IgG4-associated systemic disease. Patients with elevated serum IgG4 levels had a significantly greater frequency of combined involvement of both intra- and extrahepatic bile ducts on cholangiography (86 vs. 38 %; $p=0.02$) and jaundice at diagnosis (57 vs. 13 %, $p=0.01$). There was no significant difference in gender distribution, age at diagnosis (42 vs. 38 years), prevalence of IBD (57 vs. 73 %), or prevalence of other symptoms at diagnosis (i.e., cholangitis, pruritus, and abdominal pain) in IgG4-positive versus negative patients. The clinical picture at presentation of IgG4-positive and IgG4-negative patients was very similar in this and other series [15, 29], and analysis of IgG4 is therefore recommended in patients presenting with a suspicion of PSC. However, overall features of $IgG_4$-SC distinct from PSC suggest that $IgG_4$-SC affects older subjects more than PSC, obstructive jaundice is more common in $IgG_4$-SC, $IgG_4$-SC is more commonly associated with AIP but less with IBD, and last, but most importantly, $IgG_4$-SC is in most cases steroid responsive. Comparison between $IgG_4$-SC and PSC is shown in Table 16.1.

**Table 16.1** Comparison between clinical characteristics and biochemical findings in IAC and classic PSC

| | *$IgG_4$-SC* | Classic PSC |
|---|---|---|
| Older age | +++ | + |
| Jaundice at presentation | +++ | + |
| Pancreatic disorder | +++ | + |
| Other organ involvement | +++ | ++ |
| Association with IBD | + | +++ |
| Association with AIP | +++ | – |
| Association with CCA | – | +++ |
| Elevated IgG4 | +++ | + |
| Response to steroids | +++ | + |

IgG4-positive plasma cell infiltrates in liver explants from patients with PSC who had undergone liver transplantation for severe liver disease were recently analyzed [34]. Twenty-three (23 %) of liver explants showed periductal infiltration with IgG4-positive plasma cells and 18 cases (22 %) had elevated serum IgG4 levels, including eight false positives [34]. IgG4 positivity in the liver correlated strongly with moderate-marked periductal lymphoplasmacytic inflammation. None of the explants, however, showed histological features of $IgG_4$-SC. It is conceivable that end-stage $IgG_4$-SC could lose the characteristic features. Similarly, it can be very difficult to histologically distinguish end-stage PSC from other chronic biliary disorders [34]. It is possible that steroids might be helpful in early phases of PSC. Patients with PSC/AIH overlap can respond to steroids [35, 36], and PSC in children has unique features in children showing good response to immunosuppression [37].

## Diagnosis

No consensus exists for diagnostic criteria for $IgG_4$-SC. In clinical practice, the diagnosis of $IgG_4$-SC should be suspected in patient with obstructive jaundice due to a single or multiple biliary strictures in whom there is pancreatic disease or possible other organ involvement such as retroperitoneal fibrosis. The most important differential diagnoses are cholangiocarcinoma in a patient without a pancreatic manifestation and pancreatic malignancy when imaging shows pancreatic enlargement, pancreatic duct irregularities, or pancreatic tumor. Laboratory evaluation at baseline should include serum IgG4 and Ca 19-9. However, IgG4 levels may be elevated in other conditions including pancreatic cancer [38, 39]. Very high levels of CA 19-9 (>400 U/mL) suggest cholangiocarcinoma (CCA) but high CA 19-9 levels have also been reported in $IgG_4$-SC [10]. Once malignancy has been ruled out with appropriate diagnostic tests, PSC and $IgG_4$-SC are the most important differential diagnoses.

Clinicopathological features of patients with $IgG_4$-SC and PSC have been compared [11, 31]. Strictures of the lower common bile duct are more common in $IgG_4$-SC than in PSC [11]. Apart from the fact that patients with $IgG_4$-SC tend to be older and have higher IgG4 levels than those with PSC, the cholangiographic appearance may differ as well [31]. Segmental strictures and strictures in the distal third of the extrahepatic bile duct were common in the $IgG_4$-SC group, whereas band-like strictures with beaded and pruned-tree appearance of intrahepatic ducts were observed more commonly among PSC patients [31]. The sensitivity and specificity of the cholangiographic features of $IgG_4$-SC in comparison with PSC and CCA were recently assessed in a multicenter study [40]. Cholangiograms obtained during endoscopic retrograde cholangiography (ERC) of patients with a definitive diagnosis of $IgG_4$-SC, PSC, and CCA from centers in the USA, Japan, and the UK were compared by experienced endoscopists unaware of clinical diagnoses [40]. The specificity of ERC for detecting $IgG_4$-SC was high and did not differ significantly between centers. However, sensitivity was uniformly low in all centers. Neither reviewer specialty (endoscopist vs. radiologist) nor years of experience had any statistically significant effect on accuracy. Although intraobserver agreement was generally very good, the interobserver agreement was poor. It was concluded that the high specificity for diagnosing $IgG_4$-SC using ERC suggests that particular cholangiographic features support the diagnosis.

Poor sensitivity suggests that many patients with $IgG_4$-SC, who might benefit from steroid therapy, may be misdiagnosed with CCA or PSC. From these results, it seems that additional diagnostic strategies, including histology, are likely to be important in distinguishing these diseases. Diagnostic criteria have been proposed for AIP which require histology [38, 39]. Histology may be obtained via EUS TCB of the pancreas or from intraductal biopsy of the bile ducts. In a recent study of PSC patients with elevated serum IgG4 serum levels, 6/8 (75 %) of bile duct biopsies stained for IgG4 were positive [15]. These biopsies were mostly obtained in order to exclude CCA in a patient with a known PSC. If there is a clear indication for histology from the bile duct to exclude CCA, a positive staining for IgG4 in a patient without CCA supports the diagnosis of $IgG_4$-SC. However, moderate IgG4-positive bile duct plasma cell infiltrates were observed in 7 of 38 (18 %) of non-PSC-related cholangiocarcinoma specimens [34]. Liver histology has been proposed to be of value of distinguishing $IgG_4$-SC and PSC [31]. IgG4-positive cell infiltration was as expected more severe in $IgG_4$-SC than in PSC, and none of the $IgG_4$-SC patients had advanced liver fibrosis, corresponding to Ludwig's stages 3 and 4. Fibrous obliterative cholangitis was observed only in PSC [31]. Positive IgG4 immunostaining in liver biopsies from PSC was only found in a minority of patients with elevated serum IgG4 levels in previous studies [15, 29]. However, liver biopsies were not necessarily obtained at the same time as the serologic evaluation of IgG4 levels, which makes a firm conclusion regarding the value of liver histology in these patients unclear. Recently, liver histology was compared between $IgG_4$-SC and PSC patients in a Japanese study [41]. Small bile duct involvement of $IgG_4$-SC was defined histologically as damage small bile ducts associated with infiltration of ≥10 IgG4-positive plasma cells per high-power field (HPF). Clinicopathological characteristics were compared between $IgG_4$-SC patients with and without small bile duct involvement. Small bile duct involvement was observed in 5 (26 %) of the patients with $IgG_4$-SC. Patients with small bile duct involvement showed a higher incidence of intrahepatic biliary strictures on cholangiography (80 vs. 21 %, $p=0.038$). Conversely, 4 of 7 (57 %) patients with intrahepatic biliary strictures on cholangiography had histologically evident small duct involvement. The number of IgG4-positive plasma cells was significantly correlated with the site of the most proximal stricture on cholangiograms. The number of IgG4-positive plasma cells per HPF was significantly higher in $IgG_4$-SC patients with intrahepatic biliary strictures than in those with PSC (13.4 vs. 0.4 cells/HPF, $p<0.001$). According to these results, involvement of small bile ducts is more frequent in patients with intrahepatic biliary strictures on cholangiography, and liver biopsy could be of value in these patients.

In general the diagnosis of $IgG_4$-SC should be suspected with intrahepatic or proximal extrahepatic bile duct strictures or multifocal biliary strictures with a concomitant pancreatic disease. However, although pancreatic manifestations seem to be common in $IgG_4$-SC, these patients can have very similar biliary strictures as patients with CCA and PSC. In the study of patients with elevated IgG4 levels, the clinical and cholangiographic features were not different from other PSC patients with normal IgG4 levels [15]. Important aspects for the diagnosis and management of suspected $IgG_4$-SC are shown in Fig. 16.1.

## Treatment

Resolution of jaundice and improvement in liver tests associated with steroid treatment have been well documented in patients with $IgG_4$-SC [7, 11, 13–16, 31]. Improvement or resolution in biliary strictures has also been reported in these series. In the largest reported $IgG_4$-SC cohort, corticosteroid therapy was associated with normalization of liver tests in 61 % of patients and biliary stents could be removed in 17 of 18 patients [16]. Corticosteroid therapy was initiated in 30 patients as the first-line therapy, but surgical resection had been undertaken in 18 patients [16]. Relapses occurred in 53 % after corticosteroid withdrawal

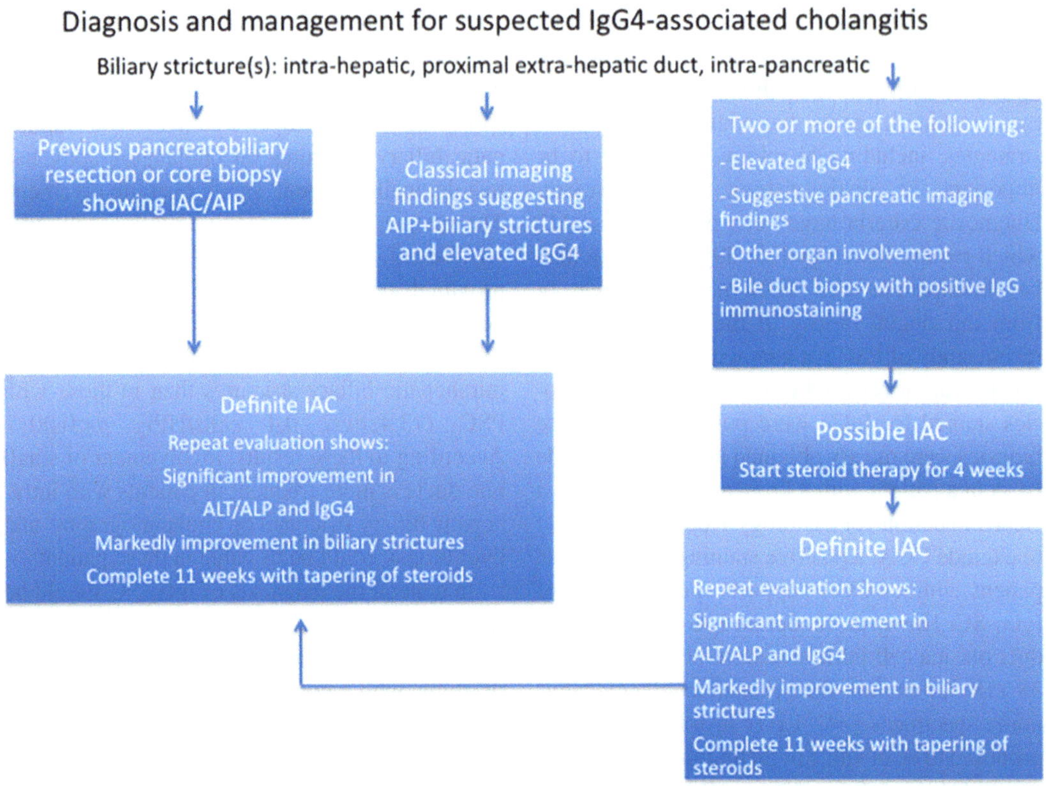


**Fig. 16.1** Algorithm for the diagnosis and management of $IgG_4$-SC (Adapted from [16])

and 44 % relapsed after surgery [16]. Subsequently, 15 patients required another course of steroids with each responding, whereas seven patients required further immunomodulatory treatment to achieve steroid-free remission [16]. Patients with intrahepatic or proximal extrahepatic strictures were more likely to relapse compared to those with isolated distal extrahepatic strictures (65 % vs. 23 %; $p=0.02$) [16]. It seems that some patients are in need of further immunosuppression. A recent report highlighted this, illustrating a patient refractory to conventional immunosuppressive therapy with steroids and 6-mercaptopurine who responded successfully with rituximab [42]. Treatment with immunosuppression of patients with PSC and elevated serum IgG4 levels was recently reported [15]. Overall 18 of 24 patients were treated with corticosteroids and 6 patients were managed conservatively. Ten of 11 (91 %) patients with jaundice had improvement and biliary stents could be removed in each [15]. It is conceivable that biliary stenting could be a contributor to the initial biochemical improvement, but medical therapy was required in all stented patients at follow-up and is unlikely that stenting is an important contributing factor for the long-term response [15]. In the treated group, 11/18 (61 %) decreased their alkaline phosphatase (ALP) values to less than two times the upper limit of normal (ULN) [15] compared to 19 % with budesonide treatment in PSC patients [43]. All existing studies reporting immunosuppressive therapy for $IgG_4$-SC have been retrospective and it remains to be determined if all IgG4-related strictures respond to steroids. It is conceivable that long-standing or "burnt-out" strictures may not respond, or incompletely respond, to steroid therapy. Although most patients with PSC and elevated IgG4 levels showed good biochemical response to steroids, relapse occurred in 50 % of patients [15]. In most cases, however, another course of steroids was

**Table 16.2** Treatment approach of an *$IgG_4$-SC* patient

| Initial treatment of *$IgG_4$-SC* | Treatment of relapse of *$IgG_4$-SC* |
|---|---|
| Prednisolone 40 mg daily for 4 weeks | No radiological or clinical but only biochemical relapse (AST, ALT, ALP, or IgG4), repeat imaging in 3 months. No medications |
| After 4 weeks: tapering of steroids 5 mg/week | Radiological, biochemical, and clinical relapse: initiate steroids (for 2–3 months) and azathioprine (2–2.5 mg/kg) for at least 2–3 years |
| No relapse: good clinical and biochemical response, discontinue steroids | Intolerance to azathioprine, mycophenolate mofetil can be tried |
| Suboptimal response: biliary stenting with ERCP, follow-up at 2 months | No or very limited response, rituximab can be tried |
| Improvement in strictures: stents removed | Difficult to treat patient: referral to a tertiary referral center |
| No improvement in strictures: consider surgical consultation | |

helpful. However, adverse effects were common, particularly in patients with cirrhosis [15]. Steroid-associated side effects were observed in 5/7 (71 %) of patients with cirrhosis, which might be due to increased systemic exposure to steroids due to decreased metabolism of steroids in the liver and shunting of steroids to the systemic circulation. The clinical significance of reduction of ALP and bilirubin in a short-term study of immunosuppression in PSC (and elevated IgG4 levels) is unclear. However, these patients seem to have a better response to steroids than has been observed in PSC before, and there seems to be a subset of PSC patients that not only have biochemical but also clinical and cholangiographic response to steroids [15]. A treatment approach for an $IgG_4$-SC patient is demonstrated in Table 16.2.

## Prognosis

The long-term prognosis and the natural history of patients with $IgG_4$-SC are not clear. Most case series have reported rather short follow-up, but as mentioned earlier, resolution of biliary strictures and jaundice has been well documented during short-term follow-up. In a Japanese study, the prognosis of $IgG_4$-SC patients was found to be better than of patients with classic PSC [28]. No patient with $IgG_4$-SC underwent liver transplantation, whereas transplantation was performed in a substantial proportion of patients with classic PSC [28].

In the first study measuring IgG4 levels in PSC, those patients with elevated IgG4 levels had higher bilirubin and ALP levels, higher Mayo risk score, and a shorter time to liver transplantation than the PSC patients with normal levels [29]. Thus, disease severity was more pronounced in this subset of PSC patients. These results seem to be confirmed by other studies [15, 16, 27, 34]. In a more recent study of PSC patients with elevated IgG4 serum levels, liver cirrhosis was observed in 50 % (12/24) of patients despite a median duration of PSC of only 4 years [15]. A subset of $IgG_4$-SC patients ($n=4$) in the study by Ghazale et al. [16] developed portal hypertension and liver cirrhosis presumably related to $IgG_4$-SC. Three out of four of these patients were untreated at the diagnosis of cirrhosis, whereas one was a nonresponder to immunosuppressive treatment [16]. The study of IgG4 positivity in explants from patients transplanted for PSC showed similar results [34]. PSC patients with positive IgG4 immunostaining had a more aggressive clinical course suggested by shorter time to liver transplantation and higher risk for recurrence post transplantation, although such findings were not based on the serum IgG4 data [16]. Recently, a study of unselected patients with secondary sclerosing cholangitis revealed that those with elevated IgG4 levels, apart from mainly being male and having a history of pancreatitis, also had higher ALP values and higher PSC Mayo risk score [27]. It is not yet completely clear whether treatment will halt or prevent progression of the hepatobiliary disease.

## Summary and Conclusions

$IgG_4$-SC is a fibroinflammatory hepatobiliary disorder which should be included in the differential diagnosis of all unexplained biliary strictures, particularly after the exclusion of malignancy. The biliary strictures have been found to resolve with a trial of steroids but relapse is common and the long-term outcome is unclear. Serum IgG4 levels should be measured as a part of the diagnostic work-up of all PSC patients. PSC patients with elevated IgG4 levels seem to have a worse prognosis than PSC patients with normal IgG4 levels.

## References

1. Bartholomew LG, Cain JC, Woolner LB, Utz DC, et al. Sclerosing cholangitis: its possible association with Riedel's struma and fibrous retroperitonitis. Report of two cases. N Engl J Med. 1963;269:8–12.
2. Wenger J, Gingrich GW, Mendeloff J. Sclerosing cholangitis – a manifestation of systemic disease. Increased serum gamma-globulin, follicular lymph node hyperplasia, and orbital pseudotumor. Arch Intern Med. 1965;116:509–14.
3. Bjornsson E, Chari ST, Smyrk TC, et al. Immunoglobulin G4 associated cholangitis: description of an emerging clinical entity based on review of the literature. Hepatology. 2007;45:1547–54.
4. Bjornsson E. Immunoglobulin G4-associated cholangitis. Curr Opin Gastroenterol. 2008;24:389–94.
5. Laszik GZ, Pap A, Farkas G. A case of primary sclerosing cholangitis mimicking chronic pancreatitis. Int J Pancreatol. 1988;3:503–8.
6. Kawaguchi K, Koike M, Tsuruta K, et al. Lymphoplasmacytic sclerosing pancreatitis with cholangitis: a variant of primary sclerosing cholangitis extensively involving pancreas. Hum Pathol. 1991; 22:387–95.
7. Erkelens GW, Vleggaar FP, Lesterhuis W, et al. Sclerosing pancreato-cholangitis responsive to steroid therapy. Lancet. 1999;354(9172):43–4.
8. Okazaki K, Uchida K, Ohana M, et al. Autoimmune-related pancreatitis is associated with autoantibodies and a Th1/Th2-type cellular immune response. Gastroenterology. 2000;118:573–81.
9. Horiuchi A, Kawa S, Hamano H, et al. Sclerosing pancreato-cholangitis responsive to corticosteroid therapy: report of 2 case reports and review. Gastrointest Endosc. 2001;53:518–22.
10. Hirano K, Shiratori Y, Komatsu Y, et al. Involvement of the biliary system in autoimmune pancreatitis: a follow-up study. Clin Gastroenterol Hepatol. 2003;1: 453–64.
11. Nakazawa T, Ohara H, Sano H, et al. Clinical differences between primary sclerosing cholangitis and sclerosing cholangitis with autoimmune pancreatitis. Pancreas. 2005;30:20–5.
12. Nakazawa T, Ohara H, Sano H, et al. Cholangiography can discriminate sclerosing cholangitis with autoimmune pancreatitis from primary sclerosing cholangitis. Gastrointest Endosc. 2004;60:937–44.
13. Zen Y, Harada K, Sasaki M, et al. IgG4-related sclerosing cholangitis with and without hepatic inflammatory pseudotumor, and sclerosing pancreatitis-associated sclerosing cholangitis: do they belong to a spectrum of sclerosing pancreatitis? Am J Surg Pathol. 2004;28:1193–203.
14. Hamano H, Kawa S, Uehara T, et al. Immunoglobulin G4-related lymphoplasmacytic sclerosing cholangitis that mimics infiltrating hilar cholangiocarcinoma: part of a spectrum of autoimmune pancreatitis? Gastrointest Endosc. 2005;62:152–7.
15. Bjornsson E, Chari S, Silveira M, et al. Primary sclerosing cholangitis associated with elevated immunoglobulinG4: clinical characteristics and response to therapy. Am J Ther. 2011;18(3):198–205.
16. Ghazale A, Chari ST, Zhang L, et al. Immunoglobulin G4-associated cholangitis: clinical profile and response to therapy. Gastroenterology. 2008;134: 706–15.
17. Nakanuma Y, Zen Y. Pathology and immunopathology immunoglobulin G4-related sclerosing cholangitis: the latest addition to the sclerosing cholangitis. Hepatol Res. 2007;37 Suppl 3:S478–86.
18. Kawa S, Hamano H, Umemura T, et al. Sclerosing cholangitis associated with autoimmune pancreatitis. Hepatol Res. 2007;37 Suppl 3:S487–95.
19. Kamisawa T, Okamuto A. IgG4-related sclerosing disease. World J Gastroenterol. 2008;14:3948–55.
20. Montana-Loza AJ, Lalor E, Mason AL. Recognizing immunoglobulin G4-related overlap in patients with pancreatic and hepatobiliary disease. Can J Gastroenterol. 2008;22:840–6.
21. Webster GJM, Pereira SP, Chapman RW. Autoimmune pancreatitis/IgG4-associated primary sclerosing cholangitis – overlapping or separate diseases? J Hepatol. 2009;51:398–402.
22. Alderlieste YA, van den Elzen BDJ, Rauws EAJ, Beuers U. Immunoglobulin G4-associated cholangitis: one variant of immunoglobulin G4-related systemic disease. Digestion. 2009;79:220–8.
23. Nishimori I, Otsuki M. Autoimmune pancreatitis and IgG4-associated sclerosing cholangitis. Best Pract Res Clin Gastroenterol. 2009;23:11–23.
24. Chapman R, Fevery J, Kalloo A, et al. Diagnosis and management of primary sclerosing cholangitis. Hepatology. 2010;51:660–78.
25. Lindkvist B, Benito de Valle M, Gullberg B, Björnsson E. Incidence and prevalence of primary sclerosing cholangitis in a defined adult population in Sweden. Hepatology. 2010;52:571–7.

26. Toosi MN, Heathcote J. Pancreatic pseudotumor with sclerosing pancreato-cholangitis: is this a systemic disease? Am J Gastroenterol. 2004;99:377–82.
27. Lee EY, May GR, Kortan PP, et al. IgG4-associated autoimmune cholangiopathy: a steroid responsive multi-systemic disease. Gastroenterology. 2010; 138(5):A-270.
28. Takikawa H, Takamori Y, Tanaka A, et al. Analysis of 388 cases of primary sclerosing cholangitis in Japan; presence of a subgroup without pancreatic involvement in older patients. Hepatol Res. 2004;29:153–9.
29. Mendes FD, Jorgensen R, Keach J, et al. Elevated serum IgG4 concentration in patients with primary sclerosing cholangitis. Am J Gastroenterol. 2006;101: 2070–5.
30. Stathopoulos G, Nourmand AD, Blackstone M, et al. Rapidly progressive sclerosing cholangitis following surgical treatment of pancreatic pseudotumor. J Clin Gastroenterol. 1995;21:143–8.
31. Nishino T, Oyama H, Hashimoto E, et al. Clinicopathological differentiation between sclerosing cholangitis with autoimmune pancreatitis and primary sclerosing cholangitis. J Gastroenterol. 2007;42: 550–9.
32. Dastis SN, Latinne D, Sempoux C, Geubel AP. Ulcerative colitis associated with IgG4 cholangitis: similar features in two HLA identical siblings. J Hepatol. 2009;51:601–5.
33. de Valle MB, Bjornsson E, Lindkvist B. Prevalence of elevated immunoglobulin G4 in a population based cohort of primary sclerosing cholangitis. Gastroenterology. 2010;138(5):S9–10.
34. Zhang L, Lewis JT, Abraham SC, et al. IgG4+ plasma cell infiltrates in liver explants with primary sclerosing cholangitis. Am J Surg Pathol. 2010;34:88–94.
35. Boberg KM, Egeland T, Schrumpf E. Long-term effect of corticosteroid treatment in primary sclerosing cholangitis. Scand J Gastroenterol. 2003;38:991–5.
36. Lindgren S, Glaumann H, Almer S, et al. High prevalence of small duct primary sclerosing cholangitis among patients with overlapping autoimmune hepatitis and primary sclerosing cholangitis. Eur J Intern Med. 2009;20:190–6.
37. Mieli-Vergani G, Vergani D. Unique features of primary sclerosing cholangitis in children. Curr Opin Gastroenterol. 2010;26(3):265–8.
38. Ghazale AH, Chari ST, Vege SS. Update on the diagnosis and treatment of autoimmune pancreatitis. Curr Gastroenterol Rep. 2008;10:115–21.
39. Ghazale A, Chari ST, Smyrk TC, et al. Value of serum IgG4 in the diagnosis of autoimmune pancreatitis and in distinguishing it from pancreatic cancer. Am J Gastroenterol. 2007;102:1646–53.
40. Kalaitzakis E, Johnson GJ, Levy M, et al. Utility of endoscopic retrograde cholangiography to diagnose IgG4-associated cholangitis: an international, double blind, randomized, multicenter study. Gastrointest Endosc. 2010;71(5):AB169.
41. Naitoh I, Zen Y, Nakazawa T, et al. Small bile duct involvement in IgG4-related sclerosing cholangitis: liver biopsy and cholangiography correlation. J Gastroenterol. 2011;46(2):269–76.
42. Topazian M, Witzig TE, Smyrk TC, et al. Rituximab therapy for refractory biliary strictures in immunoglobulin G-4 associated cholangitis. Clin Gastroenterol Hepatol. 2008;6:364–6.
43. Angulo P, Jorgensen RA, Keach JC, et al. Oral budesonide in the treatment of patients with primary biliary cirrhosis with a suboptimal response to ursodeoxycholic acid. Hepatology. 2000;31:318–23.

# Part III

# Other Organ Involvement

# Overview

# 17

Raghuwansh P. Sah and Suresh T. Chari

Establishment of autoimmune pancreatitis (AIP) as a distinct clinical entity and its increasing awareness have brought into recognition involvement of several extrapancreatic organs [1–6]. The affected organs demonstrate similar characteristic histopathologic pattern, IgG4-rich lymphoplasmacytic infiltrate, and a fibro-inflammatory process that is strikingly steroid responsive [7–11]. These observations led to the concept IgG4-related disease [12]. AIP (type 1) has been the most studied manifestation of IgG4-related disease [13]. Involvements of the biliary tract, lungs, kidneys, salivary glands, thyroid, retroperitoneum, and lymphoid system have been well characterized so far. Numerous other affected organs continue to be identified [12, 14]. Most of the affected organs were first recognized in patients with AIP. However, IgG4-related organ pathology is increasingly being recognized even in the absence of AIP. Thus, AIP seems to be only a part of the spectrum of IgG4-related disease. The population prevalence of a specific organ involvement or of IgG4-related disease itself is not known currently, though the recognition is increasing with awareness and experience [14].

R.P. Sah, M.B.B.S. (✉)
Internal Medicine, Mayo Clinic Rochester,
200 1st ST., SW, Rochester, MN 55905, USA
e-mail: sah.raghuwansh@mayo.edu

S.T. Chari, M.D.
Division of Gastroenterology and Hepatology,
Internal Medicine, Mayo Clinic College of Medicine,
200 First Street SW, Rochester, MN 55905, USA
e-mail: chari.suresh@mayo.edu

## Nomenclature

With several reports coming out from multiple centers around the world, there is a wide variety of published nomenclature related to IgG4-related disease. A unified nomenclature has recently been proposed by a panel of worldwide experts [15]. This panel recommended use of generic IgG4-related "organ" disease instead of the previously used specific terms, for example, IgG4-related sialadenitis instead of Mikulicz's disease for salivary gland involvement, IgG4-related pulmonary disease for lung involvement, and IgG4-related kidney disease for renal involvement. These have been described in the text.

## Significance of Recognizing Other Affected Organs in IgG4-Related Disease

A dramatic response to steroids is characteristic of IgG4-related disease [12]. A correct diagnosis leads to significant clinical improvement once steroids are started. For example, pulmonary involvement can progress to respiratory failure if unrecognized, while treatment rapidly resolves the pathology [16].

Manifestations of IgG4-related disease often mimic other commonly recognized autoimmune conditions. For example, involvement of salivary glands may be confused with Sjögren syndrome [17]. Involvement of biliary tract may be confused

M.J. Levy and S.T. Chari (eds.), *Autoimmune (IgG4-related) Pancreatitis and Cholangitis*,
DOI 10.1007/978-1-4419-6430-4_17, © Springer Science+Business Media New York 2013

with primary sclerosing cholangitis [18]. IgG4-related disease consistently shows striking response to steroids compared to the mimicked counterpart due to which it is essential to diagnose IgG4-related pathology correctly. The distinction may be often difficult in the absence of pathological analysis. For example, it is often difficult to separate IgG4-related sclerosing cholangitis which responds much more dramatically to steroids from primary sclerosing cholangitis, and biopsy may be often required [19]. It also turns out that some cases previously diagnosed as another well-known condition may actually be manifestations of IgG4-related disease. For example, several cases so far diagnosed as primary sclerosing cholangitis turn out to be IgG4-related sclerosing cholangitis [20]. Similarly, a condition of multifocal fibrosis that had been reported in literature several decades before recognition of AIP appears to be IgG4-related disease [21–23].

Some of the affected organs in IgG4-related disease may be clinically silent. For example, retroperitoneal fibrosis may be an incidental imaging finding. However, recognizing these silent manifestations is crucial in diagnosing AIP and differentiating it from pancreatic cancer. The commonly used diagnostic criteria for AIP including the ICDC [24] and the revised HISORt criteria [25] advocate for clinical and radiological review for evidence of other organ involvement before considering invasive alternatives for diagnosis.

## Biliary System

IgG4-related sclerosing cholangitis is the second most common extrapancreatic lesion in AIP [3, 4]. Intrapancreatic as well as extrapancreatic segments of the biliary tract may be affected. Most experts consider intrapancreatic bile duct involvement as a continuum of pancreatic involvement. The extrapancreatic bile duct involvement is accepted as IgG4-related sclerosing cholangitis. However, depending on the definition, the prevalence in AIP varies between reports. In one report [3], IgG4-related sclerosing cholangitis was noted in 84 % of AIP patients but only 39 % of these had extrapancreatic sclerosing cholangitis. Ghazale et al. reported biliary strictures confined to intrapancreatic bile duct in 51 % and involvement of proximal extrahepatic/intrahepatic ducts in 49 % of AIP patients [26]. While frequently seen in association with AIP, isolated IgG4-related sclerosing cholangitis without AIP is increasing being recognized [19, 26]. These cases have to be distinguished from primary sclerosing cholangitis [18, 19]. IgG4-related sclerosing cholangitis has been discussed in the next chapter in detail.

## Lymphoid System

Mediastinal or hilar lymphadenopathy is the most common extrapancreatic lesion observed in AIP seen in about 80 % [3, 4] of patients. Lymphadenopathy is usually found on imaging at the time of diagnosis of AIP [3]. Some authors have suggested that presence of lymphadenopathy in AIP may help differentiate it from pancreatic cancer though its utility is unclear [3]. Though mostly asymptomatic, the lymphoid proliferation may be associated with increased risk of non-Hodgkin lymphomas [27]. There is also increasing recognition of IgG4-related multiorgan lymphoproliferative syndrome which mimics multicentric Castleman's syndrome [28]. In fact, salivary and lacrimal gland involvement seen in IgG4-related disease appears to be organ-specific lymphoproliferative disease [28]. Some cases of IgG4-related myelodysplastic syndrome and cutaneous plasmacytomas have also been reported [29, 30].

## Salivary and Lacrimal Glands

IgG4-related sialadenitis is common, seen in 23–39 % of AIP patients [3, 4]. The salivary gland involvement may precede AIP in many patients [3, 31]. At least one study suggested that AIP patients with IgG4-related sialadenitis may have increased disease activity compared to AIP patients without IgG4-related sialadenitis [31].

In one series of IgG4-related sialadenitis, 83 % of cases did not have concomitant AIP [28]. Involvement of lacrimal gland known as IgG4-related dacryoadenitis has also been well described. The involvement of salivary and lacrimal glands had been previously known as Mikulicz's disease which was considered a spectrum of Sjögren syndrome [17]. However, despite clinical similarities, these patients lack anti-SSA and anti-SSB antibodies typically seen in primary Sjögren syndrome [17]. Characteristic histopathology with IgG4-rich infiltration, elevated serum IgG4 levels, and dramatic steroid response distinguish these from primary Sjögren syndrome [17].

## Kidneys

Kidney involvement is referred to as IgG4-related kidney disease which primarily constitutes tubulointerstitial nephritis with or without membranous nephropathy [32]. Tubulointerstitial nephritis was seen in 35 % of patients with AIP in one report [33]. These renal lesions deteriorated without therapy and regressed after steroid therapy [33]. Other forms of IgG4-associated kidney lesions have been described, including nodular lesions mimicking metastatic tumors [34] and inflammatory pseudotumors [35]. The association between membranous nephropathy in the absence of tubulointerstitial nephritis and IgG4-related kidney disease remains controversial with description of both isolated IgG4-related as well as the classical idiopathic form of membranous nephropathy [15, 36]. Kidney involvement has been discussed in detail in another chapter in this book.

## Lungs

IgG4-related pulmonary disease was recognized after initial observations of IgG4-rich infiltrates in a subgroup of patients with interstitial pneumonia [37, 38]. Further, interstitial pneumonia with IgG4-rich infiltrate was described in a few AIP patients with prevalence ranging from 3 % to 13 % [16, 39]. In one report, 2/4 patients with pulmonary involvement [16] developed respiratory failure. This report also noted that though pulmonary involvement shows good response to steroids, a higher dose was necessary to maintain remission than required in biliary involvement [16]. A detailed discussion of lung involvement is presented in a separate chapter.

## Retroperitoneum and Aorta

Retroperitoneal fibrosis (RPF) has been reported in 8–16 % of AIP patients [3, 4, 6]. A thick retroperitoneal fibrotic mass covers abdominal aorta and compresses ureters [40, 41]. Ureteral obstruction can lead to development of hydronephrosis and renal failure [42], while some patients may develop lower extremity edema [3]. In most cases, however, RPF is asymptomatic and may be discovered incidentally on imaging studies [41]. RPF was observed before AIP in only 20 % of patients while in 80 %, RPF developed during the course of AIP [3]. Steroid therapy leads to consistent histologic and radiologic improvement of RPF [6]. Meditational fibrosis is seen in some AIP patients though less commonly than RPF. Idiopathic RPF without evidence of IgG4-related mechanism has been described [43]. Additionally, a true aortitis with involvement of the media has been recognized [44]. The existence of true IgG4-related vasculitis remains to be explored.

## Thyroid

Fibrosis of thyroid gland (previously recognized as Riedel's thyroiditis) has been recently recognized as a manifestation of IgG4-related disease after demonstration of IgG4-rich lymphoplasmacytic infiltration and characteristic histological features [23]. Clinical hypothyroidism is more common in AIP patients than established Riedel's thyroiditis [45]. It is unclear if there is another mechanism of hypothyroidism in AIP in addition to Riedel's thyroiditis. There have been case reports of pituitary fibrosis related to IgG4 [46].

## Eyes

Lacrimal glands, extraocular muscles, and other parts of the orbit may be affected in IgG4-related disease. Lacrimal gland involvement has been discussed above. Orbital inflammation and pseudolymphoma have been discussed in detail later in a separate chapter.

## Liver

Pathological changes suggestive of an IgG4-associated process including IgG4-rich infiltrate were seen in liver biopsies from AIP patients and these were shown to be steroid responsive [47]. This led to recognition of IgG4-related hepatopathy. Another group [48] reported positive IgG4 staining in 9 of 24 liver biopsies of autoimmune hepatitis (AIH) patients and observed that IgG4-positive AIH responded markedly to prednisone compared to IgG4-negative AIH, thus suggesting that some of the previously recognized autoimmune hepatitis patients may have IgG4-related pathology.

## Other Extrapancreatic Lesions

Numerous other associations continue to be recognized: various inflammatory pseudotumors which may be IgG4-related organ-specific lymphoproliferation, prostatitis [49], pericarditis [50], gastric ulcer [51], gastric and colon polyps associated with IgG4 [52, 53], as well as cholecystitis [54]. These frequent case reports suggest that IgG4-related disease is a truly systemic disease and its spectrum of affected organs will continue to grow with our experience.

## References

1. Pearson RK, Longnecker DS, Chari ST, et al. Controversies in clinical pancreatology: autoimmune pancreatitis: does it exist? Pancreas. 2003;27(1):1–13.
2. Chari ST, Smyrk TC, Levy MJ, et al. Diagnosis of autoimmune pancreatitis: the Mayo Clinic experience. Clin Gastroenterol Hepatol. 2006;4(8):1010–16; quiz 934.
3. Naitoh I, Nakazawa T, Ohara H, et al. Clinical significance of extrapancreatic lesions in autoimmune pancreatitis. Pancreas. 2010;39(1):e1–5.
4. Hamano H, Arakura N, Muraki T, et al. Prevalence and distribution of extrapancreatic lesions complicating autoimmune pancreatitis. J Gastroenterol. 2006;41(12):1197–205.
5. Kamisawa T, Nakajima H, Egawa N, et al. IgG4-related sclerosing disease incorporating sclerosing pancreatitis, cholangitis, sialadenitis and retroperitoneal fibrosis with lymphadenopathy. Pancreatology. 2006;6(1–2):132–7.
6. Kamisawa T, Okamoto A. IgG4-related sclerosing disease. World J Gastroenterol. 2008;14(25):3948–55.
7. Kamisawa T. IgG4-positive plasma cells specifically infiltrate various organs in autoimmune pancreatitis. Pancreas. 2004;29(2):167–8.
8. Deshpande V, Chicano S, Finkelberg D, et al. Autoimmune pancreatitis: a systemic immune complex mediated disease. Am J Surg Pathol. 2006;30(12):1537–45.
9. Vlachou PA, Khalili K, Jang HJ, et al. IgG4-related sclerosing disease: autoimmune pancreatitis and extrapancreatic manifestations. Radiographics. 2011;31(5):1379–402.
10. Zhang L, Notohara K, Levy MJ, et al. IgG4-positive plasma cell infiltration in the diagnosis of autoimmune pancreatitis. Mod Pathol. 2007;20(1):23–8.
11. Zamboni G, Luttges J, Capelli P, et al. Histopathological features of diagnostic and clinical relevance in autoimmune pancreatitis: a study on 53 resection specimens and 9 biopsy specimens. Virchows Arch. 2004;445(6):552–63.
12. Stone JH, Zen Y, Deshpande V. IgG4-related disease. N Engl J Med. 2012;366(6):539–51.
13. Chari ST, Kloeppel G, Zhang L, et al. Histopathologic and clinical subtypes of autoimmune pancreatitis: the Honolulu consensus document. Pancreatology. 2010;10(6):664–72.
14. Carruthers MN, Stone JH, Khosroshahi A. The latest on IgG4-RD: a rapidly emerging disease. Curr Opin Rheumatol. 2012;24(1):60–9.
15. Stone JH, Khosroshahi A, Deshpande V, et al. IgG4-related disease: recommendations for the nomenclature of this condition and its individual organ system manifestations. Arthritis Rheum. 2012;64(10):3061–7.
16. Hirano K, Kawabe T, Komatsu Y, et al. High-rate pulmonary involvement in autoimmune pancreatitis. Intern Med J. 2006;36(1):58–61.
17. Yamamoto M, Harada S, Ohara M, et al. Clinical and pathological differences between Mikulicz's disease and Sjogren's syndrome. Rheumatology (Oxford). 2005;44(2):227–34.
18. Nakazawa T, Ohara H, Sano H, et al. Clinical differences between primary sclerosing cholangitis and sclerosing cholangitis with autoimmune pancreatitis. Pancreas. 2005;30(1):20–5.

19. Deshpande V, Sainani NI, Chung RT, et al. IgG4-associated cholangitis: a comparative histological and immunophenotypic study with primary sclerosing cholangitis on liver biopsy material. Mod Pathol. 2009;22(10):1287–95.
20. Koyabu M, Uchida K, Fukata N, et al. Primary sclerosing cholangitis with elevated serum IgG4 levels and/or infiltration of abundant IgG4-positive plasma cells. J Gastroenterol. 2010;45(1):122–9.
21. Comings DE, Skubi KB, Van Eyes J, et al. Familial multifocal fibrosclerosis. Findings suggesting that retroperitoneal fibrosis, mediastinal fibrosis, sclerosing cholangitis, Riedel's thyroiditis, and pseudotumor of the orbit may be different manifestations of a single disease. Ann Intern Med. 1967;66(5):884–92.
22. Bartholomew LG, Cain JC, Woolner LB, et al. Sclerosing cholangitis: its possible association with Riedel's struma and fibrous retroperitonitis. Report of two cases. N Engl J Med. 1963;269:8–12.
23. Dahlgren M, Khosroshahi A, Nielsen GP, et al. Riedel's thyroiditis and multifocal fibrosclerosis are part of the IgG4-related systemic disease spectrum. Arthritis Care Res (Hoboken). 2010;62(9):1312–18.
24. Shimosegawa T, Chari ST, Frulloni L, et al. International consensus diagnostic criteria for autoimmune pancreatitis: guidelines of the International Association of Pancreatology. Pancreas. 2011;40(3):352–8.
25. Chari ST, Takahashi N, Levy MJ, et al. A diagnostic strategy to distinguish autoimmune pancreatitis from pancreatic cancer. Clin Gastroenterol Hepatol. 2009;7(10):1097–103.
26. Ghazale A, Chari ST, Zhang L, et al. Immunoglobulin G4-associated cholangitis: clinical profile and response to therapy. Gastroenterology. 2008;134(3):706–15.
27. Takahashi N, Ghazale AH, Smyrk TC, et al. Possible association between IgG4-associated systemic disease with or without autoimmune pancreatitis and non-Hodgkin lymphoma. Pancreas. 2009;38(5):523–6.
28. Masaki Y, Dong L, Kurose N, et al. Proposal for a new clinical entity, IgG4-positive multiorgan lymphoproliferative syndrome: analysis of 64 cases of IgG4-related disorders. Ann Rheum Dis. 2009;68(8):1310–15.
29. Tabata R, Tabata C, Okamoto T, et al. Autoimmune pancreatitis associated with myelodysplastic syndrome. Int Arch Allergy Immunol. 2009;151(2):168–72.
30. Miyagawa-Hayashino A, Matsumura Y, Kawakami F, et al. High ratio of IgG4-positive plasma cell infiltration in cutaneous plasmacytosis – is this a cutaneous manifestation of IgG4-related disease? Hum Pathol. 2009;40(9):1269–77.
31. Kubota K, Wada T, Kato S, et al. Highly active state of autoimmune pancreatitis with mikulicz disease. Pancreas. 2010;39(1):e6–10.
32. Raissian Y, Nasr SH, Larsen CP, et al. Diagnosis of IgG4-related tubulointerstitial nephritis. J Am Soc Nephrol. 2011;22(7):1343–52.
33. Takahashi N, Kawashima A, Fletcher JG, et al. Renal involvement in patients with autoimmune pancreatitis: CT and MR imaging findings. Radiology. 2007;242(3):791–801.
34. Rudmik L, Trpkov K, Nash C, et al. Autoimmune pancreatitis associated with renal lesions mimicking metastatic tumours. CMAJ. 2006;175(4):367–9.
35. Cornell LD, Chicano SL, Deshpande V, et al. Pseudotumors due to IgG4 immune-complex tubulointerstitial nephritis associated with autoimmune pancreatocentric disease. Am J Surg Pathol. 2007;31(10):1586–97.
36. Watson SJ, Jenkins DA, Bellamy CO. Nephropathy in IgG4-related systemic disease. Am J Surg Pathol. 2006;30(11):1472–7.
37. Takato H, Yasui M, Ichikawa Y, et al. Nonspecific interstitial pneumonia with abundant IgG4-positive cells infiltration, which was thought as pulmonary involvement of IgG4-related autoimmune disease. Intern Med. 2008;47(4):291–4.
38. Kobayashi H, Shimokawaji T, Kanoh S, et al. IgG4-positive pulmonary disease. J Thorac Imaging. 2007;22(4):360–2.
39. Taniguchi T, Ko M, Seko S, et al. Interstitial pneumonia associated with autoimmune pancreatitis. Gut. 2004;53(5):770; author reply -1.
40. Kamisawa T, Matsukawa M, Ohkawa M. Autoimmune pancreatitis associated with retroperitoneal fibrosis. JOP. 2005;6(3):260–3.
41. Kamiya K, Yoshizu A, Nakazato T, et al. High serum immunoglobulin G4-related retrosternal fibrosclerosis. J Thorac Imaging. 2012;27:W190–2.
42. Hamano H, Kawa S, Ochi Y, et al. Hydronephrosis associated with retroperitoneal fibrosis and sclerosing pancreatitis. Lancet. 2002;359(9315):1403–4.
43. Swartz RD. Idiopathic retroperitoneal fibrosis: a review of the pathogenesis and approaches to treatment. Am J Kidney Dis. 2009;54(3):546–53.
44. Kasashima S, Zen Y, Kawashima A, et al. A clinicopathologic study of immunoglobulin G4-related sclerosing disease of the thoracic aorta. J Vasc Surg. 2010;52(6):1587–95.
45. Sah RP, Chari ST. Clinical hypothyroidism in autoimmune pancreatitis. Pancreas. 2010;39(7):1114–16.
46. Leporati P, Landek-Salgado MA, Lupi I, et al. IgG4-related hypophysitis: a new addition to the hypophysitis spectrum. J Clin Endocrinol Metab. 2011;96(7):1971–80.
47. Umemura T, Zen Y, Hamano H, et al. Immunoglobin G4-hepatopathy: association of immunoglobin G4-bearing plasma cells in liver with autoimmune pancreatitis. Hepatology. 2007;46(2):463–71.
48. Chung H, Watanabe T, Kudo M, et al. Identification and characterization of IgG4-associated autoimmune hepatitis. Liver Int. 2010;30(2):222–31.
49. Uehara T, Hamano H, Kawakami M, et al. Autoimmune pancreatitis-associated prostatitis: distinct clinicopathological entity. Pathol Int. 2008;58(2):118–25.
50. Nayar M, Charnley R, Scott J, et al. Autoimmune pancreatitis with multiorgan involvement. A case of pericardial involvement. JOP. 2009;10(5):539–42.

51. Shinji A, Sano K, Hamano H, et al. Autoimmune pancreatitis is closely associated with gastric ulcer presenting with abundant IgG4-bearing plasma cell infiltration. Gastrointest Endosc. 2004;59(4):506–11.
52. Kaji R, Okabe Y, Ishida Y, et al. Autoimmune pancreatitis presenting with IgG4-positive multiple gastric polyps. Gastrointest Endosc. 2009;71(2):420–2.
53. Matsui H, Watanabe T, Ueno K, et al. Colonic polyposis associated with autoimmune pancreatitis. Pancreas. 2009;38(7):840–2.
54. Leise MD, Smyrk TC, Takahashi N, et al. IgG4-associated cholecystitis: another clue in the diagnosis of autoimmune pancreatitis. Dig Dis Sci. 2011;56(5):1290–4.

# Tubulointerstitial Nephritis and Other Renal Involvement by IgG4-Related Disease

18

Lynn D. Cornell and Naoki Takahashi

It has been recognized only recently that pancreatitis due to autoimmune etiology, recognized first by Sarles et al. in 1961 [1], is part of a multi-organ disease called IgG4-related disease [2]. Now, manifestations of IgG4-related disease (IgG4-RD) have been described in nearly every organ system, including the liver, gallbladder, other gastrointestinal sites, kidney, salivary and lacrimal glands, orbit, breast, lung, retroperitoneum, aorta, lymph nodes, skin, pituitary gland, and prostate [3–9]. Involvement often consists of inflammatory masses in these organs.

IgG4-RD in the kidney may also present as an inflammatory mass, biopsy of which shows tubulointerstitial nephritis [10]. Takahashi et al. found radiographic evidence of renal parenchymal involvement in 30 % of patients with established autoimmune pancreatitis (AIP) [11], the renal radiographic lesions likely representing inflammatory masses due to the distinctive appearance of the lesions. Renal involvement by IgG4-RD more commonly presents as acute or progressive chronic renal failure; many of these cases also show radiographic abnormalities. Other presenting features are proteinuria due to associated glomerular disease or obstruction related to retroperitoneal fibrosis. The term used to refer to any form of renal involvement by IgG4-RD is "IgG4-related kidney disease" (IgG4-RKD) [12].

## Tubulointerstitial Nephritis

The most common pattern of renal IgG4-RKD is tubulointerstitial nephritis (TIN). This histologic pattern refers to interstitial inflammation accompanied by tubulitis, or inflammatory cells within the tubules intermingling with tubular epithelial cells. TIN is classified according to its cause. In general, TIN/nephropathy can be divided into broad categories of drug related, autoimmune, hereditary/toxic/metabolic, infection (direct or reactive to a distant infection), and idiopathic/other. Some overlap exists between the different categories; for example, some cases of BK polyomavirus tubulointerstitial nephritis (a direct infection) show tubular basement membrane immune complex deposits, which may indicate an additional autoimmune reaction.

The cause of TIN in a particular case can be determined by biopsy features by light microscopy, immunofluorescence (IF), and electron microscopy (EM) in conjunction with clinical history and clinical laboratory results and correlation with radiographic studies in some entities. By light microscopy, the renal pathologist

L.D. Cornell, M.D. (✉)
Laboratory Medicine and Pathology, Mayo Clinic, Hilton 10 200 1st ST., SW, Rochester, MN 55905, USA
e-mail: cornell.lynn@mayo.edu

N. Takahashi, M.D.
Department of Radiology, Mayo Clinic, 200 First Street SW, Rochester, MN 55905, USA
e-mail: takahashi.naoki@mayo.edu

M.J. Levy and S.T. Chari (eds.), *Autoimmune (IgG4-related) Pancreatitis and Cholangitis*, DOI 10.1007/978-1-4419-6430-4_18, © Springer Science+Business Media New York 2013

recognizes the pattern of inflammation and types of cells in infiltrate; by IF, the presence or absence of immune deposits and anatomic and immunophenotypic pattern of deposition; and by EM, the absence or presence of immune deposits, pattern of deposition, and presence of any substructure to the deposits.

TIN that occurs as part of IgG4-RD (IgG4-related TIN) is a specific type of immune-mediated TIN [13]. IgG4-RD can be recognized as the etiology by clinicopathologic features. Saeki et al. and Raissian et al. have collected data on the two largest biopsy series of IgG4-related TIN, at 23 and 35 cases, respectively [14, 15]. Both of these series showed many clinical and histologic features in the kidney that have also been encountered in the pancreas: presence of radiographic abnormalities, plasma cell-rich inflammatory infiltrates with increased IgG4+ plasma cells, elevated total IgG or IgG4 levels in the serum, presence of other organ involvement, and rapid response to steroid therapy. Features specific to the kidney are detailed below.

## Clinical Features of IgG4-Related TIN

Similar to AIP, most patients with IgG4-related TIN are men (~85 %), with a mean age of 65 years. Most patients (57 % and 76 %, respectively, in the Saeki and Raissian series) have acute or progressive chronic renal failure at the time of renal biopsy, while the primary indication for biopsy or nephrectomy in other patients usually is a renal radiographic lesion. In a radiographic series, in which renal lesions were incidentally found during evaluation for AIP, patients did not have renal-specific symptoms [11]. Renal function was normal or mildly diminished, with a serum creatinine range of 0.9–1.6, which was not different from those with AIP without radiographic evidence of renal involvement.

Eighty-five to ninety-six percentage of patients have other organ involvement, either prior to or concurrent with the renal involvement. The most common extrarenal sites affected are the pancreas and liver; other involved organs described include the salivary or lacrimal glands, lung, gallbladder, aorta (inflammatory abdominal aortic aneurysm), heart (pericarditis), skin (leukocytoclastic vasculitis or pseudolymphomatous infiltrate) [16, 17], retroperitoneum and/or ureter (retroperitoneal fibrosis), sinuses, lymph nodes, joints (inflammatory arthritis), prostate (prostatitis), pituitary, thyroid, and colon (inflammatory bowel disease) and pseudotumors in the orbit, paraspinal soft tissue, and testis. Most patients with extrarenal involvement have multiorgan involvement.

## Laboratory Features of IgG4-TIN

Elevated serum total IgG and IgG4 subclass levels have been observed in ~70–80 % of AIP patients [18] and can be a useful indicator of IgG4-RD in patients who have a positive serologic finding in the appropriate clinical setting. Similarly, in IgG4-related TIN, Raissian et al. found that almost 80 % of patients with measurements available in a series of IgG4-TIN had elevated serum total IgG or IgG4 levels, and 92 % had an elevated serum IgG4 level; some additional patients without IgG or IgG4 levels available had hypergammaglobulinemia [15]. (The patients with IgG4-TIN included in the Saeki series were in part defined by elevated serum IgG and IgG4 levels, and so this series may have excluded some cases of IgG4-TIN without this serologic feature.)

Other common laboratory features are hypocomplementemia (decreased serum C3 and/or C4 levels), seen in 56–78 % of IgG4-TIN patients, and peripheral blood eosinophilia, seen in 33–48 % of IgG4-TIN patients [14, 15]. Approximately 30 % of patients have a positive ANA, mostly low titer [15].

## Radiographic Features of IgG4-Related TIN

Renal involvement in patients with AIP is not uncommon and has been reported in 14–39 % of patients based on CT or MR findings [11, 19–21].

Renal lesions are commonly bilateral and multiple, predominantly involving renal cortex. Renal parenchymal lesions can be classified as small peripheral cortical nodules, round or wedge-shaped lesions, or diffuse patchy involvement [11]. Renal lesions may manifest as a large solitary mass that mimics a neoplasm. Another manifestation is bilateral diffuse marked enlargement of the kidneys [15]. On CT, the lesions are iso-attenuating on unenhanced CT images, hypo-attenuating on nephrographic phase images, and become iso-attenuating on delayed phase images. On MR, the lesions are often iso-intense on T1-weighted images and low intensity on T2-weighted images. After administration of gadolinium contrast material, the lesions are low intensity on parenchymal phase images. On ultrasound, the renal lesions usually appear as ill-defined, non-mass-like areas of decreased echogenicity or round mass-like area of decreased echogenicity [22], or kidneys are diffusely enlarged. The differential diagnosis of renal parenchymal lesions, when they are multiple, includes lymphoma, metastases, pyelonephritis, and vasculitis. A solitary round renal lesion of IgG4-related disease may be indistinguishable from a primary renal neoplasm. Diffuse involvement may mimic pyelonephritis or diffuse infiltrating neoplasms such as lymphoma or transitional cell carcinoma. Renal radiographic features are illustrated in Fig. 18.1.

In a histopathologic study of patients with IgG4-related TIN on a tissue specimen, 78 % with available radiographic data showed radiographic lesions. Overall, 77 % of these patients had renal insufficiency, which was usually the reason for renal biopsy. As would be expected, the mean serum creatinine was lower in patients with renal tissue specimens obtained primarily for mass lesions compared to those biopsied for renal failure (1.4 vs. 4.2 mg/dl, respectively) [15].

Extraparenchymal renal involvement is rare and includes a diffuse rim of soft tissue around the kidney, an irregular nodule in the renal sinus, and diffuse wall thickening of the renal pelvis on CT or MR [11]. The differential diagnosis of extraparenchymal renal involvement includes lymphoma and other hematologic malignancy, Erdheim-Chester disease, Rosai-Dorfman disease, extramedullary hematopoiesis, and retroperitoneal fibrosis. Retroperitoneal fibrosis, of course, may also be part of IgG4-related systemic disease.

## Histologic, Immunofluorescent, and Ultrastructural Features of IgG4-Related TIN

By light microscopy, IgG4-related TIN shows a plasma cell-rich interstitial inflammatory infiltrate. There is a range of histologic appearances, from an acute tubulointerstitial nephritis with minimal fibrosis (pattern "A"), to an intermediate pattern with some interstitial fibrosis but still a brisk inflammatory infiltrate (pattern "B"), to a densely fibrotic, pauci-cellular pattern (pattern "C") with extensive tubular destruction and atrophy (see Figs. 18.2, 18.3, and 18.4). Cases with fibrosis show an expansile fibrosis that pushes apart the tubules. All cases by definition show a diffuse or multifocal TIN with increased plasma cells, as well as mononuclear cells. Some cases show numerous eosinophils. Focal mild mononuclear cell tubulitis is seen in most cases, and plasma cell tubulitis is seen rarely. In cases with patterns "B" or "C," focal tubular basement membranes (TBMs) may be markedly thickened, and a trichrome stain can reveal reddish granular deposits within the TBMs and interstitium occasional cases with extensive immune complex deposits. In some cases, tubules are destroyed and only fragments of TBMs can be seen on PAS or silver-stained sections.

Glomeruli generally appear normal or show mild mesangial matrix expansion or hypercellularity. If there is a concurrent membranous glomerulonephritis (MGN), then glomeruli may show thickened glomerular capillary loops, glomerular basement membrane "spikes" on silver or PAS stains, or subepithelial immune deposits on a trichrome stain. Arteries show no specific features in IgG4-TIN.

By immunofluorescence, >80 % of cases show TBM immune complex deposits, which stain for IgG and kappa and lambda light chains

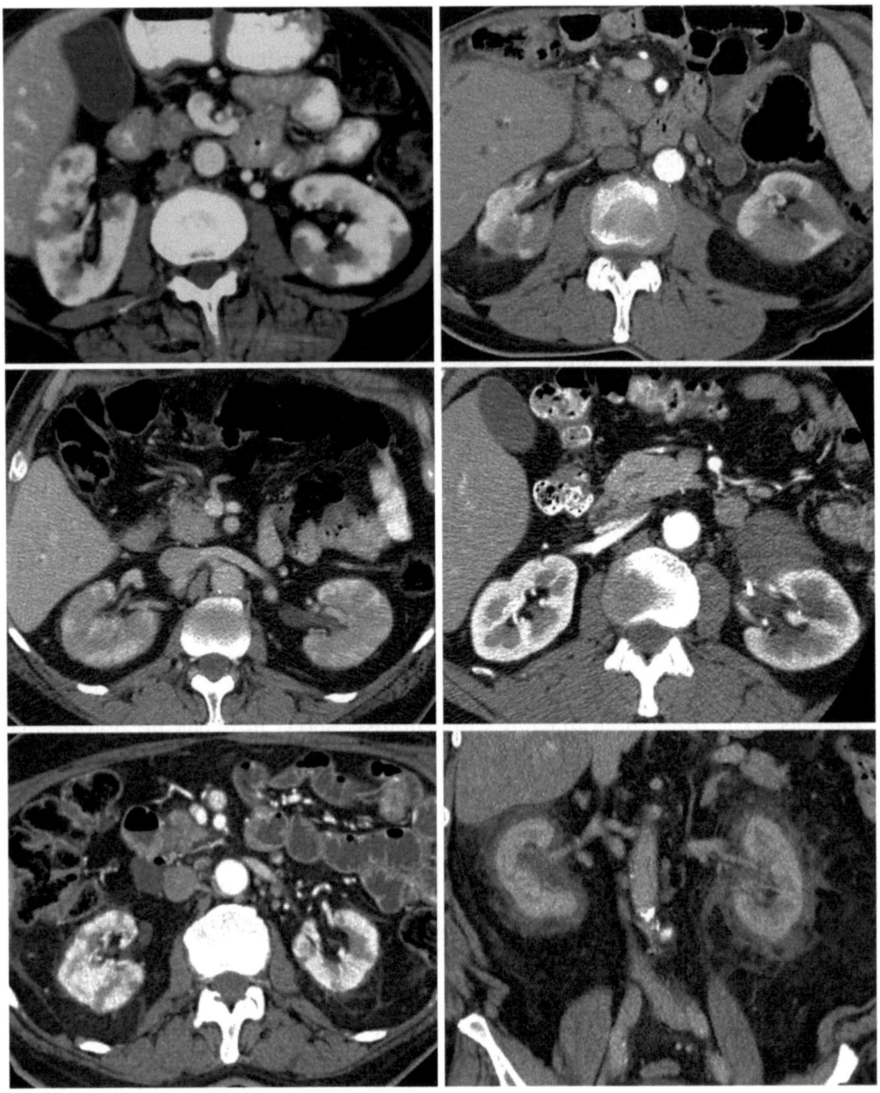

**Fig. 18.1** Renal radiographic features of IgG4-related systemic disease. (*Upper left*) Transverse contrast-enhanced CT image obtained during corticomedullary phase shows multiple well-defined round and wedge-shaped low-attenuation lesions in both kidneys. Open renal biopsy revealed tubulointerstitial nephritis with increased IgG4+ plasma cells. Images are from a 59-year-old woman with AIP. (*Upper right*) Transverse contrast-enhanced CT image obtained during corticomedullary phase shows two well-defined wedge-shaped low-attenuation lesions in the left kidney. Multiple scars are noted in the right kidney, which are fibrotic stage of renal involvement. The pancreas was atrophic likely due to fibrotic phase of the disease. The patient is a 76-year-old man with IgG4-related cholangitis. (*Middle left*) Transverse contrast-enhanced CT image shows diffuse heterogeneous enhancement of both kidneys. There were multiple low-attenuation masses in the pancreas (not shown). These images are from a 68-year-old man with AIP. The serum IgG4 level was markedly elevated. (*Middle right*) Transverse contrast-enhanced CT image obtained during corticomedullary phase shows a well-defined low-attenuation exophytic mass in left kidney. The pancreas appeared normal radiographically (not shown). The patient is a 62-year-old man who underwent partial nephrectomy. (*Lower left*) Transverse contrast-enhanced CT image shows multiple small low-attenuation nodules in both kidneys. The pancreas was diffusely enlarged (not shown). These images are from a 77-year-old man with AIP and normal serum IgG4 levels. (*Lower right*) Coronal reformat image of contrast-enhanced CT from a 71-year-old man shows diffuse soft tissue surrounding both kidneys. The pancreas was normal radiographically (not shown). This patient underwent biopsy of the perirenal soft tissue, which showed fibrosis and inflammation with increased IgG4+ plasma cells. The serum IgG4 level was normal

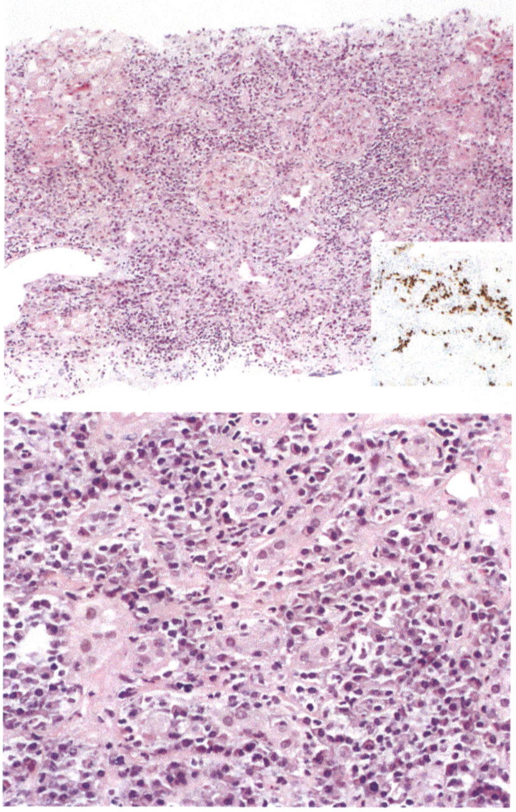

**Fig. 18.2** Acute interstitial nephritis (pattern "A") in IgG4-related TIN shows dense interstitial inflammation with minimal interstitial fibrosis (*upper panel*). An immunohistochemical stain for IgG4 shows markedly increased IgG4+ plasma cells (*insert*). (*Lower panel*) The infiltrate is composed of numerous plasma cells and mononuclear cells; eosinophils were also present. Mononuclear cell and plasma cell tubulitis are also seen (hematoxylin and eosin; *insert*, IgG4 immunoperoxidase). This case did not show tubular basement membrane immune complex deposits by immunofluorescence; tubular basement membrane deposits are often absent in pattern "A" cases

and usually stain for C3 and occasionally for C1q [15]. Most cases show diffuse TBM granular staining, but some cases can show focal staining. Several cases stained by immunofluorescence for IgG subclasses show IgG4-dominant staining of TBMs, although other IgG subclasses are also variably present (LD Cornell, unpublished data). TBM deposits are found more frequently in cases with patterns B or C (patterns with fibrosis) than in cases with pattern A (acute interstitial nephritis pattern) [15]. Glomeruli are usually negative by immunofluorescence unless there is a concurrent membranous glomerulonephritis, in which case glomeruli show granular subepithelial glomerular basement membrane staining for IgG, C3, and kappa and lambda light chains. Rare cases show mesangial immune deposits without a more specific glomerular disease assigned [10, 14].

Cases with deposits seen by immunofluorescence also show deposits by electron microscopy. TBM deposits are present in areas with inflammation and/or fibrosis and are not present in the unaffected areas of the kidney. The deposits may be small and scattered within thickened TBMs, or they may be massive and surround the TBMs and extend into the interstitium. The deposits appear finely granular and do not show substructure. Occasional interstitial deposits may also be seen within areas of fibrosis. Glomeruli typically are free of deposits, unless there is a concurrent membranous glomerulonephritis, in which case there are numerous subepithelial electron-dense deposits. Formalin-fixed, paraffin-embedded tissue from biopsy or nephrectomy samples done for a mass lesion may be deparaffinized for electron microscopy in order to visualize immune complex deposits.

## Value of IgG4 Staining

Zhang et al. and others have found that IgG4 staining in pancreas for increased IgG4+ plasma cells is useful to distinguish AIP from other forms of pancreatic inflammation, including chronic alcoholic pancreatitis and inflammatory infiltrates surrounding pancreatic cancers [23]. In the kidney, more types and causes of inflammatory infiltrates are recognized that give a pattern of TIN. Raissian et al. examined the concentration of IgG4+ plasma cells in IgG4-related TIN and in a variety of other forms of TIN that could mimic IgG4-TIN clinically and histologically [15]. We found a sensitivity of 100 % (95 % confidence interval (CI), 0.9–1) and specificity of 92 % (CI 0.86–0.95) using a cutoff of focal moderate (11–30 IgG4+ cells/40x field) to marked (>30 IgG4+ cells/40x field) increase in IgG4+ plasma cells for distinguishing

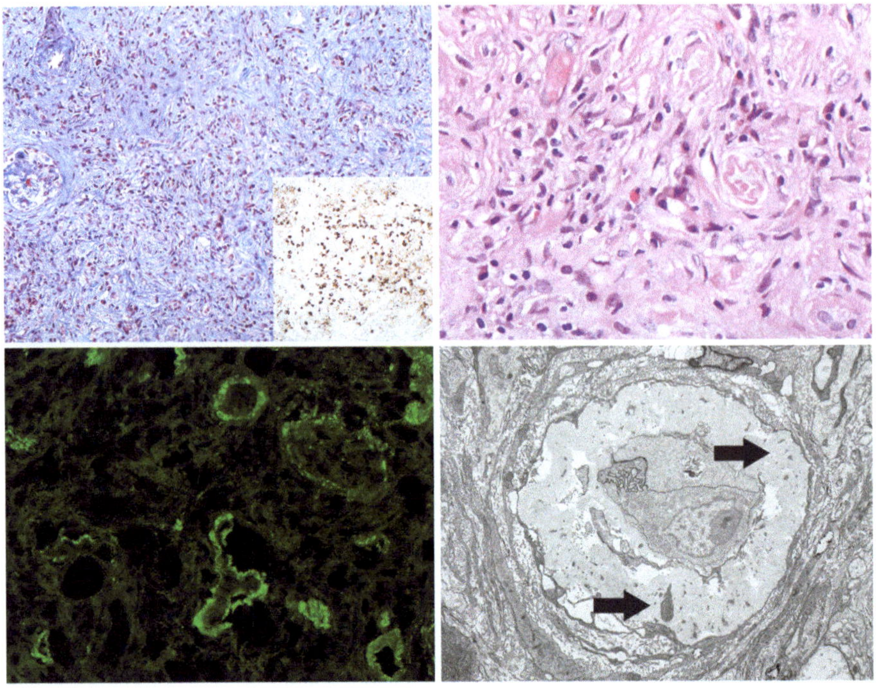

**Fig. 18.3** IgG4-related tubulointerstitial nephritis (pattern "B") shows an expansile interstitial fibrosis with marked interstitial inflammation and markedly increased IgG4+ plasma cells (*upper left*, Masson trichrome; *insert* IgG4 immunoperoxidase). (*Upper right*) On higher magnification, the infiltrate is composed of plasma cells, mononuclear cells, and eosinophils (hematoxylin and eosin). (*Lower left*) Immunofluorescence for IgG shows granular tubular basement membrane staining. (*Lower right*) Electron microscopy shows amorphous tubular basement membrane immune complex deposits (*arrow*)

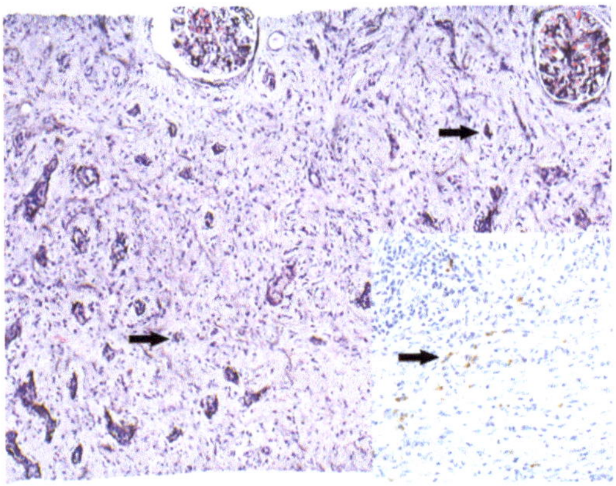

**Fig. 18.4** IgG4-related advanced sclerosing tubulointerstitial nephritis (pattern "C") shows a marked expansile interstitial fibrosis with lesser interstitial inflammation. Residua of destroyed tubular basement membranes can be seen on this silver stain (*arrows*) (Jones methenamine silver). Immunoperoxidase staining for IgG4 (*inset*) shows focally increased IgG4+ plasma cells (*arrow*), although fewer cells are present in this less inflammatory lesion than in cases with a denser inflammatory infiltrate. This case also showed tubular basement membrane immune complex deposits

IgG4-related TIN from other forms of TIN, with the exception of inflammatory infiltrates in pauci-immune necrotizing and crescentic glomerulonephritis. In pauci-immune glomerulonephritis, >30 % of cases showed a moderate to marked increase in IgG4+ plasma cells. Increased IgG4+ plasma cells have also been observed in granulomatosis with polyangiitis (Wegener's) affecting other organs [24]. The absence of a serum ANCA (or myeloperoxidase or proteinase 3 antibodies) and a necrotizing or crescentic glomerulonephritis on the tissue specimen helps to exclude pauci-immune glomerulonephritis as a cause of the interstitial inflammation in these cases. A few other causes of interstitial inflammation could also give focally increased IgG4+ plasma cells, including chronic pyelonephritis; these other causes usually can be distinguished by other clinical and histopathologic features. Notably, nearly all cases of Sjögren

**Table 18.1** Proposed diagnostic criteria for IgG4-related TIN [15]

| | |
|---|---|
| *Histology* | Plasma cell-rich tubulointerstitial nephritis with >10 IgG4+ plasma cells/hpf field in the most concentrated field[a] |
| | Tubular basement membrane immune complex deposits by immunofluorescence, immunohistochemistry, and/or electron microscopy[b] |
| *Imaging* | Small peripheral low-attenuation cortical nodules, round or wedge-shaped lesions, or diffuse patchy involvement |
| | Diffuse marked enlargement of kidneys |
| *Serology* | Elevated serum IgG4 or total IgG level |
| *Other organ involvement* | Includes autoimmune pancreatitis, sclerosing cholangitis, inflammatory masses in any organ, sialadenitis, inflammatory aortic aneurysm, lung involvement, retroperitoneal fibrosis |

Diagnosis of IgG4-TIN requires the histologic feature of plasma cell-rich TIN with increased IgG4+ plasma cells and at least one other feature from the imaging, serology, or other organ involvement categories

[a]Mandatory criterion

[b]Supportive criterion, present in >80 % of cases

syndrome-related TIN did not show increased IgG4+ plasma cells (Table 18.1).

## Response to Therapy

Similar to AIP, IgG4-related TIN also usually shows a rapid response to steroid therapy. In both the Saeki and Raissian series, 90 % of patients with elevated serum creatinine at presentation who were treated with steroids showed decreased creatinine at follow-up, from 1 to 36 months, including 90 % at 1-month follow-up in the Saeki series. While TIN of different causes may respond to steroid therapy, IgG4-related TIN tends to show a more brisk response, even in cases with severe interstitial fibrosis on the biopsy sample.

On imaging, renal lesions improve or resolve after steroid treatment. Focal cortical parenchymal loss (scars) may be present after treatment. Relapse of renal lesions may occur after cessation of steroid treatment. Without steroid treatment, renal lesions may progress to a diffuse pattern of involvement.

## Other Renal Involvement

### Glomerular Disease

Glomerular diseases have also been seen in patients with IgG4-RD. Membranous glomerulonephritis (MGN) is most commonly observed, present in approximately 7 % (4/58) of IgG4-RD patients in two biopsy series of renal parenchymal involvement by TIN, and has been noted in case reports [14, 15, 25, 26]. Of interest, MGN is also an IgG4-dominant disease in its primary (idiopathic) form [27]. This glomerular disease may also occur in patients without TIN but with other features of IgG4-RD. Currently, there is one published series of IgG4-related MGN, with or without concurrent IgG4-TIN, that included nine patients [28]. These patients all presented with proteinuria, typically nephrotic-range proteinuria. IgG4-MGN thus should be suspected in IgG4-RD patients with proteinuria, and conversely, patients with MGN on renal biopsy and an appropriate clinical history should be evaluated for IgG4-RD.

Other glomerular diseases have been variably reported in IgG4-RD, including IgA nephropathy and membranoproliferative glomerulonephritis [14, 29]. Although common in patients without AIP, diabetes mellitus may be a manifestation of AIP due to pancreatic endocrine insufficiency, and this may also affect the glomeruli as diabetic glomerulosclerosis. No specific radiographic features are present in patients with glomerular disease unless they have concurrent IgG4-related TIN.

### Obstruction Related to Retroperitoneal Fibrosis

The extrarenal manifestation of retroperitoneal fibrosis or ureteral inflammatory mass(es) may give rise to hydronephrosis, with or without accompanying renal parenchymal involvement. Histologic sections reveal storiform fibrosis with scattered areas of plasma cell-rich inflammation, similar to what is described in other organ systems. Radiographically, during the acute phase of urinary tract obstruction, nephrogram and excretion of contrast material from the kidney are delayed. The affected kidney is enlarged, and perinephric space strandings are present. The renal collecting system may or may not be dilated during the acute phase. During the subacute phase, the renal collecting system becomes dilated, while kidney enlargement and perinephric space strandings become less prominent. Renal parenchymal atrophy occurs in the chronic phase.

## Pathogenesis of IgG4-RD

IgG4 is an unusual immunoglobulin molecule, with some unusual physical characteristics. Compared to IgG1, IgG4 has weaker interchain bonds, resulting in a high rate of dissociation of immunoglobulin half-molecules. In this way, the IgG4 molecule cannot fix complement and cannot form large immune complexes. IgG4 may thus block antigen from the more pathogenic IgG1 or IgE.

Despite being thought of as an "anti-inflammatory" immunoglobulin, IgG4 nevertheless is often found in high levels in IgG4-related autoimmune disease, in both the serum and in the tissue as infiltrating plasma cells. This disease shows evidence of a T-helper 2-dominant immune response, both in examination of peripheral blood mononuclear cells and in affected tissue in this disease [30–34]. IgG4 class switching depends on IL-4 and/or IL-13, mainly secreted by T-helper 2 cells. IL-10 has an effect on IgG4 versus IgE class switching and may be required for IgG4 class-switched B cells to differentiate into IgG4-secreting plasma cells [34]. In IgG4-related systemic disease, one may speculate that an initial insult and process involving production of anti-inflammatory cytokines, including IL-10 and tumor necrosis factor-alpha, along with fibrogenic IL-13, drives increased fibrosis, induction of IgG4 class-switched B cells, and production and massive expansion of IgG4-secreting plasma cells. Details of a specific mechanism of this disease and its relationship to IgG4 and unusual histopathologic and radiographic features, however, remain to be elucidated.

## References


1. Sarles H, Sarles JC, Muratore R, et al. Chronic inflammatory sclerosis of the pancreas – an autonomous pancreatic disease? Am J Dig Dis. 1961;6:688–98.
2. Deshpande V, Mino-Kenudson M, Brugge W, et al. Autoimmune pancreatitis: more than just a pancreatic disease? A contemporary review of its pathology. Arch Pathol Lab Med. 2005;129:1148–54.
3. Cheuk W, Chan JK. IgG4-related sclerosing disease: a critical appraisal of an evolving clinicopathologic entity. Adv Anat Pathol. 2010;17:303–32.
4. Shrestha B, Sekiguchi H, Colby TV, et al. Distinctive pulmonary histopathology with increased IgG4-positive plasma cells in patients with autoimmune pancreatitis: report of 6 and 12 cases with similar histopathology. Am J Surg Pathol. 2009;33:1450–62.
5. Deshpande V, Chicano S, Finkelberg D, et al. Autoimmune pancreatitis: a systemic immune complex mediated disease. Am J Surg Pathol. 2006;30:1537–45.
6. Zen Y, Kasahara Y, Horita K, et al. Inflammatory pseudotumor of the breast in a patient with a high serum IgG4 level: histologic similarity to sclerosing pancreatitis. Am J Surg Pathol. 2005;29:275–8.
7. Uehara T, Hamano H, Kawa S, et al. Distinct clinicopathological entity 'autoimmune pancreatitis-associated sclerosing cholangitis'. Pathol Int. 2005;55:405–11.
8. Kitagawa S, Zen Y, Harada K, et al. Abundant IgG4-positive plasma cell infiltration characterizes chronic sclerosing sialadenitis (Kuttner's tumor). Am J Surg Pathol. 2005;29:783–91.
9. Kamisawa T, Funata N, Hayashi Y, et al. A new clinicopathological entity of IgG4-related autoimmune disease. J Gastroenterol. 2003;38:982–4.
10. Cornell LD, Chicano SL, Deshpande V, et al. Pseudotumors due to IgG4 immune-complex tubulointerstitial nephritis associated with autoimmune pancreatocentric disease. Am J Surg Pathol. 2007;31:1586–97.
11. Takahashi N, Kawashima A, Fletcher JG, et al. Renal involvement in patients with autoimmune pancreatitis: CT and MR imaging findings. Radiology. 2007;242:791–801.
12. Stone JH, Khosroshahi A, Deshpande V, et al. IgG4-related disease: recommendations for the nomenclature of this condition and its individual organ system manifestations. Arthritis Rheum. 2012;64(10):3061–7.

13. Cornell LD. IgG4-related tubulointerstitial nephritis. Kidney Int. 2010;78:951–3.
14. Saeki T, Nishi S, Imai N, et al. Clinicopathological characteristics of patients with IgG4-related tubulointerstitial nephritis. Kidney Int. 2010;78:1016–23.
15. Raissian Y, Nasr SH, Larsen CP, et al. Diagnosis of IgG4-related tubulointerstitial nephritis. J Am Soc Nephrol. 2011;22(7):1343–52.
16. Cheuk W, Lee KC, Chong LY, et al. IgG4-related sclerosing disease: a potential new etiology of cutaneous pseudolymphoma. Am J Surg Pathol. 2009;33:1713–19.
17. Garg M, Mackay S, Hill PA, et al. Leucocytoclastic and renal vasculitis in a patient with autoimmune pancreatitis: new associations. Intern Med J. 2010;40:376–80.
18. Sah RP, Chari ST. Serologic issues in IgG4-related systemic disease and autoimmune pancreatitis. Curr Opin Rheumatol. 2012;23:108–13.
19. Fujinaga Y, Kadoya M, Kawa S, et al. Characteristic findings in images of extra-pancreatic lesions associated with autoimmune pancreatitis. Eur J Radiol. 2010;76(2):228–38.
20. Khalili K, Doyle DJ, Chawla TP, et al. Renal cortical lesions in patients with autoimmune pancreatitis: a clue to differentiation from pancreatic malignancy. Eur J Radiol. 2008;67:329–35.
21. Triantopoulou C, Malachias G, Maniatis P, et al. Renal lesions associated with autoimmune pancreatitis: CT findings. Acta Radiol. 2010;51:702–7.
22. Sasiwimonphan K, Gorman B, Kawashima A, et al. Renal involvement in patients with autoimmune pancreatitis: ultrasound findings. Eur J Radiol. 2012;81:807–10.
23. Zhang L, Notohara K, Levy MJ, et al. IgG4-positive plasma cell infiltration in the diagnosis of autoimmune pancreatitis. Mod Pathol. 2007;20:23–8.
24. Chang SY, Keogh K, Lewis JE, et al. Increased IgG4-positive plasma cells in granulomatosis with polyangiitis: a diagnostic pitfall of IgG4-related disease. Int J Rheumatol. 2012;2012:121702.
25. Watson SJ, Jenkins DA, Bellamy CO. Nephropathy in IgG4-related systemic disease. Am J Surg Pathol. 2006;30:1472–7.
26. Merino JL, Fernandez Lucas M, Teruel JL, et al. Membranous nephropathy associated to autoimmune thyroiditis, chronic pancreatitis and suprarrenal insufficiency. Nefrologia. 2004;24:376–9.
27. Beck Jr LH, Bonegio RG, Lambeau G, et al. M-type phospholipase A2 receptor as target antigen in idiopathic membranous nephropathy. N Engl J Med. 2009;361:11–21.
28. Alexander MP, Larsen CP, Gibson IW, Nasr SH, Sethi S, Fidler ME, Raissian Y, Takahashi N, Chari S, Smyrk TC, Cornell LD. Membranous glomerulonephritis is a manifestation of IgG4-related disease. Kidney Int. 2013;83(3):455–62. doi:10.1038/ki.2012.382. Epub 2012 Dec 19. PubMed PMID: 23254897.
29. Morimoto J, Hasegawa Y, Fukushima H, et al. Membranoproliferative glomerulonephritis-like glomerular disease and concurrent tubulointerstitial nephritis complicating IgG4-related autoimmune pancreatitis. Intern Med. 2009;48:157–62.
30. Kanari H, Kagami S, Kashiwakuma D, et al. Role of Th2 cells in IgG4-related lacrimal gland enlargement. Int Arch Allergy Immunol. 2012;152 Suppl 1:47–53.
31. Kudo-Tanaka E, Nakatsuka S, Hirano T, et al. A case of Mikulicz's disease with Th2-biased cytokine profile: possible feature discriminable from Sjogren's syndrome. Mod Rheumatol. 2009;19:691–5.
32. Nirula A, Glaser SM, Kalled SL, et al. What is IgG4? A review of the biology of a unique immunoglobulin subtype. Curr Opin Rheumatol. 2012;23:119–24.
33. Zen Y, Nakanuma Y. Pathogenesis of IgG4-related disease. Curr Opin Rheumatol. 2012;23:114–18.
34. Zen Y, Fujii T, Harada K, et al. Th2 and regulatory immune reactions are increased in immunoglobin G4-related sclerosing pancreatitis and cholangitis. Hepatology. 2007;45:1538–46.

# 19 IgG4-Related Lung Disease

Jay H. Ryu, Hiroshi Sekiguchi, and Eunhee S. Yi

## Introduction

Over the past decade, it has become clear that the intrathoracic manifestations of IgG4-related disease (IgG4-RD) are varied and can result from involvement of not only the lung parenchyma but also the intrathoracic lymph nodes, mediastinum, and pleura. In a cross-sectional study, 16 of 114 patients (14 %) with IgG4-RD were found to have lung or pleural involvement [1]. However, intrathoracic lymphadenopathy may be detected in the majority of patients with IgG4-RD [2]. This intrathoracic involvement can occur in the presence or absence of extrapulmonary manifestations such as autoimmune pancreatitis (AIP) [1, 3–6].

## Epidemiology

The mean age of those with intrathoracic manifestations of IgG4-RD is 60–65 years and they are more commonly men (70–80 %) [1, 3, 4, 6]. With the possible exception of those patients with predominantly head and neck involvement in whom the male to female ratio is nearly equal [1], the epidemiologic features appear to be similar regardless of the organ involved. The role of tobacco smoking or other inhalational exposures in the development of pulmonary disease in patients with IgG4-RD has not been investigated.

J.H. Ryu, M.D. (✉)
Division of Pulmonary and Critical Care Medicine, Mayo Clinic College of Medicine, Gonda 18 South, Mayo Clinic 200 1st ST., SW, Rochester, MN 55905, USA
e-mail: ryu.jay@mayo.edu

H. Sekiguchi, M.D.
Division of Pulmonary and Critical Care Medicine, Mayo Clinic Rochester, Rochester, MN, USA

E.S. Yi, M.D.
Department of Laboratory Medicine and Pathology, Mayo Clinic, Rochester, MN, USA

## Clinical Features

Approximately one-half of patients with pulmonary IgG4-related disease have respiratory symptoms, while the remaining patients are noted to have intrathoracic findings by imaging studies in the absence of respiratory symptoms [4, 6]. Most common respiratory symptom is cough followed by dyspnea on exertion and chest pain [4, 6]. Constitutional symptoms such as fever and weight loss are uncommon [4, 6, 7]. Thus, the clinical presentation associated with IgG4-related lung disease is rather nonspecific.

## Intrathoracic Manifestations

Studies published over the past several years suggest that intrathoracic involvement in IgG4-RD can be seen in the lung parenchyma, airways, pleura, or mediastinum. Based on currently available data, intrathoracic manifestations can be categorized as shown in Table 19.1.

M.J. Levy and S.T. Chari (eds.), *Autoimmune (IgG4-related) Pancreatitis and Cholangitis*,
DOI 10.1007/978-1-4419-6430-4_19, © Springer Science+Business Media New York 2013

**Table 19.1** Intrathoracic involvement in IgG4-related sclerosing disease

| |
|---|
| Parenchymal |
| Nodules/masses |
| Interstitial lung disease |
| Airways |
| Tracheobronchial stenosis |
| Pleural |
| Pleural nodules |
| Pleural effusion |
| Mediastinal |
| Lymphadenopathy |
| Fibrosing mediastinitis |

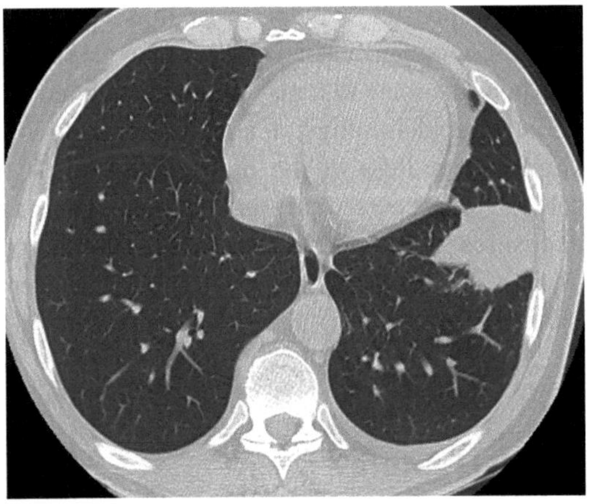

**Fig. 19.1** CT scan of the chest on a 60-year-old man revealing a 5 cm lung mass. Surgical lung biopsy showed an inflammatory pseudotumor with an increased number of IgG4-positive cells. He had transient submandibular lymphadenopathy several months before but no other manifestations

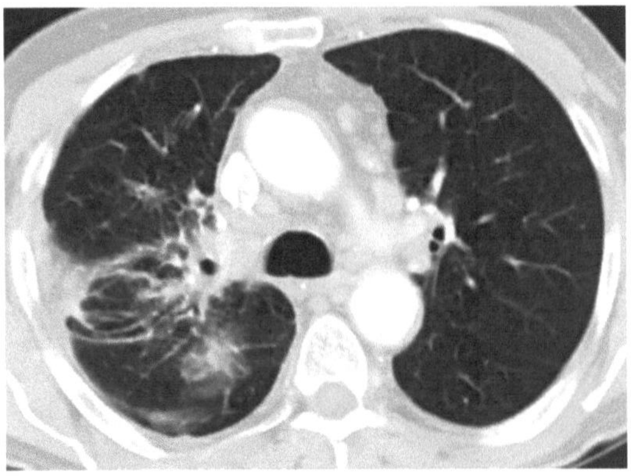

**Fig. 19.2** CT scan of the chest on a 74-year-old man demonstrating patchy consolidative infiltrate in the right lung. Surgical lung biopsy showed lymphoplasmacytic infiltrate with an increased number of IgG4-positive cells. He had undergone a radical pancreaticoduodenectomy the year before for a pancreatic mass which proved to be autoimmune pancreatitis

Multiple intrathoracic manifestations are commonly identified in an individual patient. For example, a lung nodule may be seen in combination with interstitial infiltrates and mediastinal lymphadenopathy.

## Parenchymal Disease

Lung parenchymal involvement in IgG4-RD consists mainly of rounded opacities (nodules [≤3 cm in diameter] and masses [>3 cm in diameter]) and interstitial lung disease. Rounded opacities (Fig. 19.1) may appear solid or of ground-glass attenuation (hazy increase in attenuation that does not obscure the underlying vascular structures) and range in size from less than 1 cm to greater than 5 cm in diameter [2, 4, 6, 8, 9]. Single or multiple rounded opacities may be revealed on chest radiography or CT and display no particular distribution characteristics [2, 4, 6, 8]. These rounded opacities commonly raise suspicion of malignancy, particularly when associated with spiculated margins [2, 6, 8]. Nodules of ground-glass attenuation may resemble bronchoalveolar carcinoma [6]. Thus, patients with these types of lung lesions have undergone wedge resection or lobectomy for suspected lung cancer.

Lung parenchymal involvement in IgG4-RD may also present as interstitial lung disease. Radiologic manifestations associated with this type of presentation are varied and are best defined on high-resolution CT of the chest rather than plain chest radiography (Fig. 19.2). Earlier reports described bilateral interstitial lung infiltrates consisting of ground-glass attenuation in the mid and lower lung zones associated with honeycombing [10]. Subsequent reports have described a wide array of parenchymal presentations including patchy ground-glass opacities or consolidation, reticular opacities (irregular lines), honeycombing, and thickening of the bronchovascular bundles and interlobular septa [2, 4, 6, 8, 11–15]. These CT findings resemble those found in other interstitial lung diseases such as idiopathic pulmonary fibrosis (usual interstitial pneumonia), nonspecific interstitial pneumonia, organizing pneumonia, and sarcoidosis.

## Airway Disease

Airway disease appears to be an uncommon manifestation of IgG4-RD. Ito and colleagues [16] described a 63-year-old woman with AIP who presented with cough and was noted to have irregular tracheobronchial stenosis on bronchoscopic examination. Bronchoscopy revealed edematous and hypervascular bronchial mucosa resembling findings seen in sarcoidosis. CT scanning showed intrathoracic lymphadenopathy along with thickening of the bronchovascular bundle.

Other airway manifestations seen in IgG4-related lung disease are extrinsic compression of the central airways due to fibrosing mediastinitis (see below) and bronchiectasis [4, 6, 17]. Bronchiectasis seen in this context appears to be that associated with parenchymal fibrosis in the peripheral zones of the lung, i.e., traction bronchiectasis, rather than of the proximal large airways [4, 6].

## Pleural Disease

Pleural involvement can be seen in patients with IgG4-related lung disease. For example, Zen and colleagues [4] reported 21 patients with intrathoracic manifestations of IgG4-RD of whom five had predominantly pleural disease. Pleural disease in this study consisted of nodular lesions involving the visceral or parietal pleura. Pleural effusion is an uncommon feature in patients with IgG4-related lung disease but has been described as the mode of presentation in one patient [8]. Histologically, pleuritis with fibrinous exudates and reactive changes are commonly seen in patients who undergo a surgical lung biopsy [3].

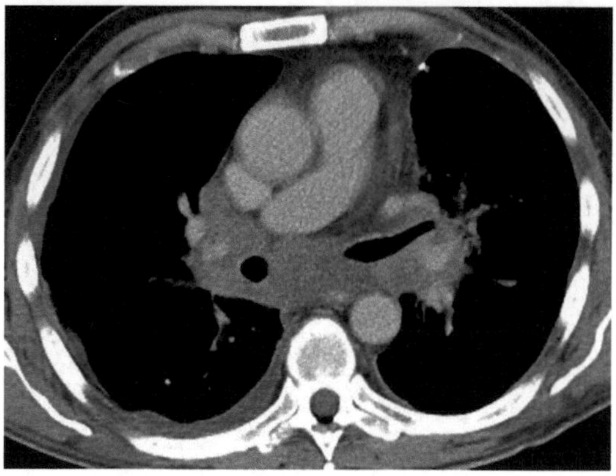

**Fig. 19.3** CT scan of the chest on a 59-year-old man showing mediastinal and bilateral hilar lymphadenopathy associated with mediastinal soft tissue thickening and a small right pleural effusion. Lymph node biopsy obtained by mediastinoscopy revealed findings consistent with IgG4-related lymphadenopathy

## Mediastinal Disease

The most common mediastinal manifestation is mediastinal and/or hilar lymphadenopathy seen in 40–90 % of patients with IgG4-RD (Fig. 19.3) [2, 4, 18–20]. For example, Hamano and colleagues [20] reported hilar lymphadenopathy detected by CT scanning and gallium-67 scintigraphy to be the most frequent extrapancreatic lesion (seen in 80 % of patients) in a survey of 65 patients with AIP. Other studies have identified intrathoracic lymphadenopathy by 18-fluorodeoxyglucose positron emission tomography (FDG-PET) [21, 22].

An unusual mediastinal manifestation of IgG4-RD is fibrosing mediastinitis. One case of fibrosing mediastinitis has been reported [17]. This patient improved with corticosteroid therapy which is noteworthy since fibrosing mediastinitis is generally considered to be a condition refractory to pharmacologic therapy.

## Histopathology

Histopathologic features associated with intrathoracic involvement in IgG4-RD are similar to those seen in extrapancreatic lesions with some exceptions. Features shared with extrapulmonary

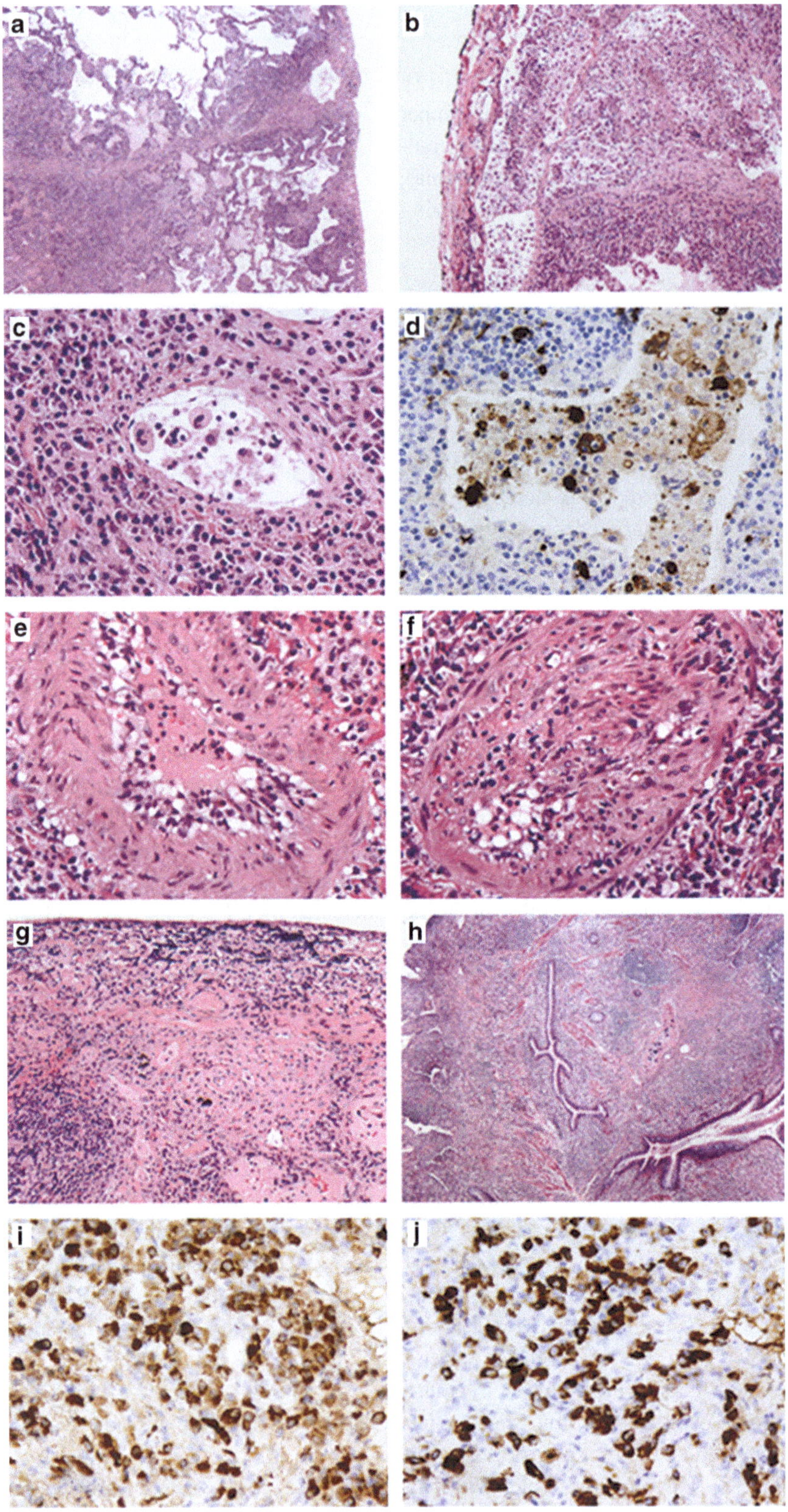

**Fig. 19.4** Pulmonary pathology in IgG4-related sclerosing disease. (**a**) Lower-power view of the lung biopsy showing a lymphangitic distribution of fibroinflammatory changes with focal consolidation shown in the lower field (HE, 40× original magnification). (**b**) Dilated lymphatic spaces filled with histiocytes seen in the visceral pleura, which shows mild fibrinous pleuritis (HE, 100×). (**c** and **d**) Emperipolesis in S100-positive histiocytes (HE and

IgG4-related lesions include lymphoplasmacytic inflammation, fibrosis, phlebitis, and increased numbers of IgG4-positive plasma cells (Fig. 19.4a–j) [1, 3, 6, 8, 23]. Plasma cells comprise the main cell type in the inflammatory infiltrate (usually greater than 50 %), followed by lymphocytes and histiocytes. Eosinophilic infiltration can be prominent, but granulomas are rarely present and are usually small and vague [1, 3]. These changes are better appreciated on surgical lung biopsies but can also be identified on bronchoscopic and needle biopsies [2, 3]. On surgical lung biopsies, prominent lymphangitic distribution involving the interlobular septa and visceral pleura is seen [3]. Dilated lymphatic spaces contain histiocytes showing emperipolesis of lymphocytes [3].

In contrast to histopathologic findings seen in the pancreas of AIP, characteristic storiform fibrosis seen in the pancreas is not as apparent in the lung biopsies [3]. In the lung, collagenized fibrosis and active fibroblastic proliferation are more prominent. In addition, both pulmonary arteries and veins are involved by intimal and mural inflammation in contrast to the findings in the involved pancreas which show obliterative phlebitis with sparing of the arteries [3]. Necrotizing vasculitis is not seen. Both the absolute number of IgG4-positive cells and the ratio of IgG4-/IgG-positive cells are increased, typically greater than 30 per high-power field and 30 %, respectively.

Increased number of IgG4-positive plasma cells is also seen in regional and non-regional lymph nodes in patients with IgG4-RD. However, other histopathologic features may be relatively nonspecific and have been broadly divided into three patterns: (1) Castleman disease-like, (2) follicular hyperplasia, and (3) interfollicular expansion [19].

As already discussed, intrathoracic manifestations of IgG4-RD may take several forms. IgG4-RD likely accounts for a subset of various idiopathic fibroinflammatory conditions involving the intrathoracic structures. For example, IgG4-RD involving the lung accounts for a portion of previously reported cases of pulmonary inflammatory pseudotumor (plasma cell granuloma) [9]. This is also true for cases of fibrosing mediastinitis [17]. IgG4-RD may also account for some cases of idiopathic interstitial pneumonias. For example, histopathologic features of organizing pneumonia and nonspecific interstitial pneumonia have been described in patients with IgG4-related lung disease [3, 12, 15, 24].

## Imaging

Chest imaging may reveal various patterns of abnormalities in patients with IgG4-related lung disease depending on the location, type, and extent of involvement. These findings are best characterized by CT (including high-resolution images of the lung parenchyma) rather than plain chest radiography. In the lung, main patterns of abnormalities include single or multiple rounded opacities or interstitial lung disease [2, 4, 6, 8, 11–15]. The rounded opacities may range in size from sub-centimeter to several centimeters in diameter. The density of these opacities may appear solid or of ground glass in attenuation, and the margin of the opacity may be smooth or irregular and spiculated.

The pattern of IgG4-related interstitial lung disease can take several forms. In some patients, patchy consolidation and ground-glass opacities may be seen suggestive of organizing pneumonia [3, 6, 11–13]. In others, reticular opacities and honeycombing may predominate similar to the

**Fig. 19.4** (continued) S100, 400×). (**e**) Endothelialitis characterized by subendothelial mixed inflammatory infiltrates with reactive endothelial cell changes (HE, 400×). (**f**) Intimal and mural inflammatory infiltrates accompanied by luminal occlusion owing to cellular myo-intimal proliferation (HE, 400×). (**g**) Fibroblastic proliferation in the center surrounded by mononuclear infiltrates at the periphery of field (HE, 100×). (**h**) Peribronchial inflammation without structural alteration of the involved airways (HE, 40×). (**i** and **j**) A marked increase in IgG and IgG4+ plasma cells among the inflammatory infiltrates showing a high IgG4/IgG ratio (IgG and IgG4, 400×). *HE* indicates hematoxylin and eosin (This figure is reproduced with permission from Shrestha et al. [3])

findings seen in nonspecific interstitial pneumonia or idiopathic pulmonary fibrosis [3, 6, 24]. Infiltrates along bronchovascular bundles and interlobular septa may be the predominant feature in some patients, raising the suspicion of sarcoidosis particularly when accompanied by intrathoracic lymphadenopathy [6].

Pleural involvement in IgG4-RD may manifest as pleural effusion or nodular lesions involving the pleura [4, 8]. Although pleural involvement is commonly seen histopathologically on lung biopsies, radiologically identifiable pleural involvement appears to be relatively uncommon.

Mediastinal involvement in IgG4-RD is most commonly seen in the form of mediastinal and/or hilar lymphadenopathy [1, 2, 18–20, 25]. Intrathoracic lymphadenopathy may be seen with or without parenchymal lung involvement. IgG4-related fibrosing mediastinitis radiologically manifests as a mediastinal mass or infiltrative process [17].

Aside from chest radiography and CT scanning, other imaging modalities may be helpful in the evaluation of patients suspected of intrathoracic involvement in IgG4-RD. On FDG-PET scanning, abnormal FDG uptake is observed in pancreatic and extrapancreatic lesions including the intrathoracic structures. This uptake in the thorax has been most commonly associated with intrathoracic lymphadenopathy [21, 22]. FDG uptake can also be seen in IgG4-related lung disease and fibrosing mediastinitis. Thus, FDG-PET will not distinguish lung cancer from an inflammatory lesion when evaluating a patient with a lung nodule or mass. Gallium-67 scintigraphy is rarely used in the evaluation of patients with pulmonary diseases but can also demonstrate uptake in involved intrathoracic structures including lung and lymph nodes [2, 25].

## Laboratory Tests

The serum IgG4 level is elevated in the majority of patients with IgG4-related lung disease [1–3, 6, 20]. The sensitivity and specificity of serum IgG4 level with respect to IgG4-related lung disease are not precisely known but are likely similar to those associated with IgG4-RD in general.

There are no blood tests that are specifically applicable to pulmonary involvement in IgG4-RD with the exception of serum Krebs von den Lungen-6 (KL-6) level. KL-6 is a circulating high molecular weight glycoprotein (MUC1 mucin) expressed by type II pneumocytes in the lung. Serum KL-6 level has been reported to be elevated in patients with various parenchymal lung diseases such as idiopathic pulmonary fibrosis. Circulating KL-6 level has been suggested to correlate with the extent of lung injury and has prognostic value but is not widely available outside of Japan [26–28]. Hirano and colleagues [12] identified pulmonary involvement in 4 of 30 patients with AIP, and the circulating level of KL-6 was noted to be elevated in all four patients.

Analysis of bronchoalveolar lavage (BAL) fluid obtained by bronchoscopy has been reported to show increased levels of IgG4 when compared to the specimens obtained from patients with sarcoidosis [2]. The BAL IgG4 level was observed to correlate with the serum IgG4 level. BAL cellular analysis typically reveals lymphocytosis as expected based on histopathologic findings [2, 16].

There are very few data regarding pulmonary function in patients with IgG4-related lung disease. Whether the pulmonary function results are normal or not, the pattern of abnormalities encountered is likely to be determined by the type of intrathoracic involvement and its severity. Patients with solitary lung nodule presentation will exhibit no impairment of their pulmonary function in the absence of preexisting cardiopulmonary disease such as emphysema. Those with interstitial lung disease associated with IgG4-RD are likely to manifest a reduced diffusing capacity and restrictive impairment (reduced lung volumes without airflow obstruction), particularly in the presence of extensive parenchymal infiltrates [12, 24]. On the other hand, an obstructive pattern will be encountered in rare patients with predominantly airway involvement [16].

## Diagnosis of IgG4-Related Lung Disease

IgG4-related lung disease can be encountered in the presence or absence of extrapulmonary disease including AIP. In patients who already have an established diagnosis of IgG4-RD, concern regarding IgG4-related lung disease will obviously arise when intrathoracic abnormalities are detected in such patients. Because intrathoracic manifestations of IgG4-RD are so varied, virtually any type of intrathoracic finding should raise suspicion including nodular or interstitial lung infiltrates, mediastinal or hilar lymphadenopathy, and pleural processes. In most cases, histopathologic examination of tissue biopsy from the intrathoracic lesion will be needed to distinguish intrathoracic manifestation related to IgG4-RD from a separate process such as lung cancer, lymphoma, sarcoidosis, or other distinct disease processes.

In patients without a known diagnosis of IgG4-RD, possibility of IgG4-related lung disease could easily be overlooked since various intrathoracic findings associated with this disorder are rather nonspecific and could be mistaken for pneumonia or some other more common disease processes. Here again, histopathologic examination of tissue biopsy of the intrathoracic lesion will be crucial in making the correct diagnosis. Bronchoscopic lung biopsy, whether transbronchial lung biopsy or transbronchial needle biopsy of mediastinal lymph nodes, may provide adequate amount of tissue to achieve the diagnosis of IgG4-related lung disease in the presence of appropriate clinical and radiologic context. If bronchoscopic biopsy does not yield sufficient amount of tissue for the diagnosis, surgical lung biopsy or mediastinoscopy will need to be considered depending on the predominant site of involvement.

It appears likely that the use of serum IgG4 level and immunostaining of lung biopsy specimens with anti-IgG4 antibody will increase in the evaluation of patients with various forms of pulmonary abnormalities. Although the presence of IgG4-positive lymphoplasmacytic infiltrate is characteristic of IgG4-RD, it is not specific for the diagnosis of IgG4-RD in the thorax or elsewhere [3, 23]. In addition, there is no single histopathologic parameter that distinguishes IgG4-related lung disease from other similar-appearing fibroinflammatory processes. Thus, it is crucial that histopathologic findings be correlated with the clinical and imaging findings to reach a correct diagnosis.

As in patients with AIP and other extrapulmonary lesions associated with IgG4-RD, the serum IgG4 level is elevated in the majority of patients with IgG4-related lung disease. However, an elevated serum IgG4 level is not seen in some of these patients, and the absence of such finding does not exclude the diagnosis of IgG4-related lung disease. Although BAL fluid analysis has been reported to show elevated IgG4 levels and lymphocytosis, the diagnostic utility of these measures has not been defined in the evaluation of patients with suspected IgG4-related lung disease.

Pulmonary involvement in IgG4-RD can be seen before, simultaneously, or after the diagnosis of AIP or other extrapulmonary IgG4-related lesion. The diagnosis of IgG4-related lung disease should be considered in the evaluation of any patient with fibroinflammatory disease of obscure etiology encountered in the thorax.

## Treatment

As with AIP and other extrapancreatic lesions of IgG4-RD, IgG4-related lung disease generally responds well to corticosteroid therapy [3, 4, 6, 8–10, 12, 13, 15, 16, 19–22]. This positive response to corticosteroid therapy is observed whether the predominant disease is in the lung parenchyma, airway, pleura, or mediastinum. The exact regimen of corticosteroids is not specified in many of the studies to date but generally consists of oral prednisone typically begun at a dose between 30 and 1 mg/kg/day for a duration of 1–2 weeks. Favorable response is usually observed by 2 weeks on treatment. The prednisone dose is then gradually tapered downward over the following several months with continued monitoring for possible recurrence or complete resolution.

The optimal dose and duration of corticosteroid therapy in the treatment of IgG4-related lung disease remain to be defined. A retrospective study on patients with AIP demonstrated the patients on low-dose maintenance dose of prednisone (10 mg/day or lower) to have a significantly lower relapse rate of AIP compared to those who had tapered off prednisone treatment [29]. These results have been extrapolated by some authors to patients with extrapancreatic IgG4-related disease manifestations. Thus, low-dose maintenance dose of prednisone has been used for some patient beyond several months of treatment to reduce the risk of recurrence. Spontaneous improvement in IgG4-related lung disease has not been described. Although corticosteroid is used widely in patients with IgG4-RD, it is probably not needed in the management of patients with IgG4-related lung disease who present with only a solitary pulmonary nodule or mass and undergo complete surgical resection of the lesion [4, 9].

There are few data on the treatment of IgG4-related lung disease with pharmacologic agents other than corticosteroids. The use of bortezomib, a proteasome inhibitor, and the addition of cyclosporine to corticosteroid therapy have been reported in two separate case reports describing patients with recurrent IgG4-related lung disease and appeared to provide benefit [11, 30]. In extrapulmonary IgG4-RD, azathioprine, mycophenolate, methotrexate, and cyclophosphamide have been used to prevent long-term relapse [31, 32]. Recently, rituximab therapy was reported to result in a rapid decline of serum IgG4 levels and prompt clinical improvement in four IgG4-RD patients with manifestations of AIP, sclerosing cholangitis, lymphoplasmacytic aortitis, salivary gland involvement, orbital pseudotumor, and lacrimal gland enlargement [32]. In this study, rituximab was used as a corticosteroid-sparing agent. Whether these nonsteroidal agents also have a role in IgG4-related lung disease remains to be determined.

## Prognosis

Although the response to corticosteroid therapy is favorable in most patients with IgG4-related lung disease, long-term follow-up data are currently not available. These patients may develop extrapulmonary lesions associated with IgG4-RD in the months and years following their initial diagnosis [1]. Some patients with IgG4-related lung disease may not experience complete resolution of their lung manifestations and have residual radiologic abnormalities. Zen and colleagues [4] described residual radiologic abnormalities in 3 of their 21 patients with IgG4-related lung disease and pleural disease after treatment.

Association with malignancies has been described in patients with IgG4-RD. These malignancies have included lymphoma, pancreatic cancer, as well as lung cancer [1, 4, 19, 33, 34]. It remains to be clarified whether there truly is an increased risk of malignancy in patients with IgG4-RD.

## Conclusions

Intrathoracic manifestations of IgG4-RD are varied and can involve any compartment of the respiratory system including the lung parenchyma, airway, pleura, as well as mediastinum. It appears likely that the spectrum of pulmonary involvement in IgG4-RD will continue to broaden with continuing investigations. In addition, the role of IgG4-related pathogenesis needs to be examined in various fibroinflammatory pulmonary diseases of unknown cause including various idiopathic interstitial pneumonias and fibrosing mediastinitis.

## Key Points

- Lung and pleural lesions are seen in approximately 10–20 % of patients with IgG4-RD, but intrathoracic lymphadenopathy can be detected in the majority of patients.
- Intrathoracic manifestations are varied and can involve the lung parenchyma, pleura, airways, and mediastinum.
- About one-half of patients with IgG4-related lung disease have no respiratory symptoms.
- Corticosteroid therapy is generally effective in the treatment of IgG4-related lung disease, but

some patients may be left with residual radiologic abnormalities.

- The role of IgG4-related pathogenesis needs to be evaluated in various fibroinflammatory pulmonary diseases of unknown cause including various idiopathic interstitial pneumonias and fibrosing mediastinitis.

## References


1. Zen Y, Nakanuma Y. IgG4-related disease: a cross-sectional study of 114 cases. Am J Surg Pathol. 2010;34(12):1812–19.
2. Tsushima K, Tanabe T, Yamamoto H, et al. Pulmonary involvement of autoimmune pancreatitis. Eur J Clin Invest. 2009;39(8):714–22.
3. Shrestha B, Sekiguchi H, Colby TV, et al. Distinctive pulmonary histopathology with increased IgG4-positive plasma cells in patients with autoimmune pancreatitis: report of 6 and 12 cases with similar histopathology. Am J Surg Pathol. 2009;33(10):1450–62.
4. Zen Y, Inoue D, Kitao A, et al. IgG4-related lung and pleural disease: a clinicopathologic study of 21 cases. Am J Surg Pathol. 2009;33(12):1886–93.
5. Shigemitsu H, Koss MN. IgG4-related interstitial lung disease: a new and evolving concept. Curr Opin Pulm Med. 2009;15(5):513–16.
6. Inoue D, Zen Y, Abo H, et al. Immunoglobulin G4-related lung disease: CT findings with pathologic correlations. Radiology. 2009;251(1):260–70.
7. Khosroshahi A, Stone JH. A clinical overview of IgG4-related systemic disease. Curr Opin Rheumatol. 2011;23(1):57–66.
8. Yamashita K, Haga H, Kobashi Y, Miyagawa-Hayashino A, Yoshizawa A, Manabe T. Lung involvement in IgG4-related lymphoplasmacytic vasculitis and interstitial fibrosis: report of 3 cases and review of the literature. Am J Surg Pathol. 2008;32(11):1620–6.
9. Zen Y, Kitagawa S, Minato H, et al. IgG4-positive plasma cells in inflammatory pseudotumor (plasma cell granuloma) of the lung. Hum Pathol. 2005;36(7):710–17.
10. Taniguchi T, Ko M, Seko S, et al. Interstitial pneumonia associated with autoimmune pancreatitis [comment]. Gut. 2004;53(5):770; author reply 770–1.
11. Kobayashi H, Shimokawaji T, Kanoh S, Motoyoshi K, Aida S. IgG4-positive pulmonary disease. J Thorac Imaging. 2007;22(4):360–2.
12. Hirano K, Kawabe T, Komatsu Y, et al. High-rate pulmonary involvement in autoimmune pancreatitis. Intern Med J. 2006;36(1):58–61.
13. Taniguchi T, Hamasaki A, Okamoto M. A case of suspected lymphocytic hypophysitis and organizing pneumonia during maintenance therapy for autoimmune pancreatitis associated with autoimmune thrombocytopenia. Endocr J. 2006;53(4):563–6.
14. Ohara H, Nakazawa T, Sano H, et al. Systemic extrapancreatic lesions associated with autoimmune pancreatitis. Pancreas. 2005;31(3):232–7.
15. Duvic C, Desrame J, et al. Retroperitoneal fibrosis, sclerosing pancreatitis and bronchiolitis obliterans with organizing pneumonia. Nephrol Dial Transplant. 2004;19(9):2397–9.
16. Ito M, Yasuo M, Yamamoto H, et al. Central airway stenosis in a patient with autoimmune pancreatitis. Eur Respir J. 2009;33(3):680–3.
17. Inoue M, Nose N, Nishikawa H, Takahashi M, Zen Y, Kawaguchi M. Successful treatment of sclerosing mediastinitis with a high serum IgG4 level. Gen Thorac Cardiovasc Surg. 2007;55(10):431–3.
18. Naitoh I, Nakazawa T, Ohara H, et al. Clinical significance of extrapancreatic lesions in autoimmune pancreatitis. Pancreas. 2010;39(1):e1–5.
19. Cheuk W, Yuen HKL, Chu SYY, Chiu EKW, Lam LK, Chan JKC. Lymphadenopathy of IgG4-related sclerosing disease. Am J Surg Pathol. 2008;32(5):671–81.
20. Hamano H, Arakura N, Muraki T, Ozaki Y, Kiyosawa K, Kawa S. Prevalence and distribution of extrapancreatic lesions complicating autoimmune pancreatitis. J Gastroenterol. 2006;41(12):1197–205.
21. Nakajo M, Jinnouchi S, Fukukura Y, Tanabe H, Tateno R, Nakajo M. The efficacy of whole-body FDG-PET or PET/CT for autoimmune pancreatitis and associated extrapancreatic autoimmune lesions. Eur J Nucl Med Mol Imaging. 2007;34(12):2088–95.
22. Hamed G, Tsushima K, Yasuo M, et al. Inflammatory lesions of the lung, submandibular gland, bile duct and prostate in a patient with IgG4-associated multifocal systemic fibrosclerosis. Respirology. 2007;12(3):455–7.
23. Smyrk TC. Pathological features of IgG4-related sclerosing disease. Curr Opin Rheumatol. 2011;23(1):74–9.
24. Takato H, Yasui M, Ichikawa Y, et al. Nonspecific interstitial pneumonia with abundant IgG4-positive cells infiltration, which was thought as pulmonary involvement of IgG4-related autoimmune disease. Intern Med. 2008;47(4):291–4.
25. Saegusa H, Momose M, Kawa S, et al. Hilar and pancreatic gallium-67 accumulation is characteristic feature of autoimmune pancreatitis. Pancreas. 2003;27(1):20–5.
26. Yokoyama A, Kondo K, Nakajima M, et al. Prognostic value of circulating KL-6 in idiopathic pulmonary fibrosis. Respirology. 2006;11(2):164–8.
27. Al-Salmi QA, Walter JN, Colasurdo GN, et al. Serum KL-6 and surfactant proteins A and D in pediatric interstitial lung disease. Chest. 2005;127(1):403–7.
28. Kinoshita F, Hamano H, Harada H, et al. Role of KL-6 in evaluating the disease severity of rheumatoid lung disease: comparison with HRCT. Respir Med. 2004;98(11):1131–7.

29. Kamisawa T, Shimosegawa T, Okazaki K, et al. Standard steroid treatment for autoimmune pancreatitis. Gut. 2009;58(11):1504–7.
30. Khan ML, Colby TV, Viggiano RW, Fonseca R. Treatment with bortezomib of a patient having hyper IgG4 disease. Clin Lymphoma Myeloma Leuk. 2010;10(3):217–19.
31. Ghazale A, Chari ST, Zhang L, et al. Immunoglobulin G4-associated cholangitis: clinical profile and response to therapy. Gastroenterology. 2008;134(3):706–15.
32. Khosroshahi A, Bloch DB, Deshpande V, Stone JH. Rituximab therapy leads to rapid decline of serum IgG4 levels and prompt clinical improvement in IgG4-related systemic disease. Arthritis Rheum. 2010;62(6):1755–62.
33. Takahashi N, Ghazale AH, Smyrk TC, Mandrekar JN, Chari ST. Possible association between IgG4-associated systemic disease with or without autoimmune pancreatitis and non-Hodgkin lymphoma. Pancreas. 2009;38(5):523–6.
34. Fukui T, Mitsuyama T, Takaoka M, Uchida K, Matsushita M, Okazaki K. Pancreatic cancer associated with autoimmune pancreatitis in remission. Intern Med. 2008;47(3):151–5.

# Part IV

# World-Wide Experience with AIP and IgG4-Related Sclerosing Cholangitis

# Italian Experience

# 20

Luca Frulloni and Giuseppe Zamboni

## Introduction

Autoimmune pancreatitis (AIP) is an inflammatory disease of the pancreas which is clinically and pathologically different from all other types of pancreatitis [1]. Many papers have been published after the introduction of the term "autoimmune pancreatitis" by Yoshida et al. in 1995 [2], based mainly on the dramatic and quick response to steroid therapy.

The knowledge of the disease was initially based on the Japanese experience that defined the AIP as a diffuse disease involving the entire pancreas and responsive to steroid therapy [3–5]. Later, the focal involvement (mass forming) of the pancreas by inflammation has been reported [6]. Consequently, the clinical approach changed, since in the presence of a hypodense mass, a diagnosis of pancreatic cancer should be excluded before the introduction of steroid therapy.

Recently, the disease has been classified in type 1 and type 2 AIPs [7]. These two forms are characterized by different clinical profiles; whereas type 1 AIP is associated with other organ involvement (biliary tract, salivary glands, gastrointestinal tract, kidney, retroperitoneum) and frequent relapses, type 2 AIP is associated with ulcerative colitis and does not relapse.

The diagnostic criteria for AIP vary largely around the world, though they all are based on four cardinal criteria: histology, imaging, association with other autoimmune diseases or other organ involvement, and response to steroids [8]. Serological profile, in particular the presence of high serum level of IgG4, has been also proposed as a diagnostic criteria, but sensitivity and specificity of all tests are not yet satisfactory [9, 10].

Based on the high prevalence of focal AIP form (60 %) in Italy, the most important clinical goal is to differentiate AIP from pancreatic cancer to safely use steroid therapy [11].

## Pathology

### Surgical Specimens

We report the pathological experience on 19 cases of AIP, resected with suspicion of pancreatic cancer (16 pancreaticoduodenectomies and 3 distal pancreatectomies).

Macroscopically, an ill-defined mass in the head of the pancreas was found in 16 cases.

A narrowed or mild dilated pancreatic duct was present in all cases, differently to that observed in pancreatic cancer. Pseudocysts and pancreatic calculi were not observed. The bile duct stenosis was present in 12 cases. Type 1 and type 2 AIPs were macroscopically indistinguishable.

L. Frulloni, M.D., Ph.D. (✉)
Department of Medicine, University of Verona, Policlinico G.B. Rossi P.le L.A. Scuro, 10, Verona 37134, Italy
e-mail: luca.frulloni@univr.it

G. Zamboni, M.D.
Servizio di Anatomia-Istologia Patologica, Università di Verona, Ospedale S.Cuore-Don Calabria, Negrar-Verona, Italy

M.J. Levy and S.T. Chari (eds.), *Autoimmune (IgG4-related) Pancreatitis and Cholangitis*,
DOI 10.1007/978-1-4419-6430-4_20, © Springer Science+Business Media New York 2013

Microscopically, 9 cases (47 %) were classified as type 1 AIP and 10 cases (53 %) as type 2 AIP (Tables 20.1 and 20.2).

Type 1 AIP was characterized by a dense lymphoplasmacytic infiltration centered on the pancreatic ducts, prominent storiform fibrosis, inflammatory cellular stroma, obliterative phlebitis, and acinar atrophy (Fig. 20.1a–c). Prominent lymphoid aggregates were also frequently present.

The density and distribution of the inflammatory infiltration changed from case to case and within the same case from mild, focal, and periductal infiltration with mild fibrosis to heavy periductal and acinar infiltration with severe periductal fibrosis, duct obstruction and duct destruction, and acinar atrophy. The venulitis was always prominent.

In most cases, the distribution of the lesions was patchy. In a few cases, the storiform fibrosis mimicked a fibroinflammatory pseudotumor [13–20]. The inflammatory process was usually well demarcated from the surrounding peripancreatic fatty tissue and only occasionally showed some small tonguelike extensions. The peripancreatic lymph nodes were enlarged and showed follicular hyperplasia. The distal common bile duct presented with marked fibroinflammatory thickening in six cases (67 %), whereas the gallbladder was involved in two cases (22 %).

Tissue IgG4-positive plasma cells were abundant (>50 per HPF) in all cases (Fig. 20.1d).

The pathognomic lesion in type 2 AIP was the "granulocytic epithelial" lesions (GELs) (Tab1) [12], characterized by the granulocytic invasion of the ductal structures, with detachment, disruption, and destruction of the duct epithelium (Fig. 20.2a, b). In almost all cases, the granulocytes extended from large-medium ducts to small ductules within the acinar parenchyma (Fig. 20.2c). Immunohistochemically, the IgG4-positive plasma cells were absent or very few in number (Fig. 20.2d).

The common feature of both AIP types was the presence of periductal lymphoplasmacytic infiltrate, whereas storiform fibrosis, inflammatory cellular stroma, obliterative phlebitis, and lymphoid aggregates were less prominent or inconspicuous in type 2 AIP.

## Fine-Needle Aspiration Cytology and Biopsy

A useful diagnostic tool in clinically and radiologically suspected AIP could be fine-needle aspiration cytology (FNAC) or fine-needle core biopsy (FNCB) [13–20].

The role of FNAC is to rule out a carcinoma and in some cases to suggest or to be in accordance with the diagnosis of AIP. The cytological features of AIP, more pleomorphic than cancers, are characterized by an underrepresentation of ductal cells, lack of significant nuclear atypia, and the presence of lymphocytes, plasma cells, and cellular stromal fragments (Fig. 20.3). The presence of stromal fragments infiltrated by granulocytes may only suggest a possible diagnosis of type 2 AIP (Fig. 20.4).

The (EUS) Tru-Cut biopsy, providing a core of tissue, enables the histologic evaluation as well as the immunohistochemical detection of IgG4 [17]. The diagnosis of AIP on biopsy relies on the recognition of the combination of lymphoplasmacellular infiltration, especially around ducts, cellular stroma, venulitis, and the presence of abundant IgG4-positive cells (Fig. 20.5) and the presence of GELs (Fig. 20.6). The presence of IgG4-positive plasma cells on the one hand and GELs on the other can be considered the hallmarks of the two subtypes of AIPs [17].

In our experience, the diagnosis of AIP in core biopsy is possible in half of cases, whereas in the presence of few morphological criteria, the diagnosis may be only suggestive or negative.

## Imaging of AIP

In our series of AIP patients, the imaging techniques of the pancreas showed a higher frequency of focal type (60 %). In clinical practice, computed tomography (CT) and magnetic resonance imaging (MRI) are the imaging techniques more frequently used.

In a recent paper, we reported the CT findings on 21 AIP patients showing pancreatic parenchyma enlargement, focal in 14 (67 %) cases and diffuse enlargement in the remaining 7 (33 %)

**Table 20.1** Clinical, pathological, and tissue IgG4 findings in 19 resected AIPs

| GEL | Sex | Age | Site | Jaundice | Periductal LPL infiltrate | Acinar PMN infiltrate | Inflammatory cellular stroma | Storiform fibrosis | Obliterative phlebitis | Lymphoid aggregates | Bile duct involvement | Papilla involvement | IgG4 tissue |
|---|---|---|---|---|---|---|---|---|---|---|---|---|---|
| | M | 66 | Head | 1 | 2 | 0 | 2 | 1 | 1 | 1 | 1 | 1 | 2 |
| | F | 54 | Tail | 0 | 2 | 0 | 2 | 2 | 2 | 1 | 0 | 0 | 2 |
| | M | 49 | Head | 1 | 2 | 0 | 2 | 2 | 2 | 2 | 1 | 1 | 2 |
| | F | 48 | Tail | 0 | 2 | 0 | 2 | 2 | 2 | 2 | 0 | 0 | 2 |
| | M | 78 | Head | 0 | 2 | 0 | 2 | 1 | 2 | 1 | 0 | 1 | 2 |
| | M | 49 | Head | 1 | 2 | 0 | 2 | 2 | 2 | 1 | 2 | 1 | 2 |
| | F | 68 | Head | 1 | 2 | 0 | 2 | 2 | 2 | 1 | 1 | 1 | 2 |
| | M | 48 | Head | 1 | 2 | 0 | 2 | 2 | 2 | 1 | 1 | 1 | 2 |
| | M | 73 | Head | 1 | 2 | 0 | 2 | 2 | 2 | 1 | 2 | 1 | 2 |
| GEL-pos | M | 36 | Head | 0 | 1 | 0 | 1 | 0 | 0 | 0 | 0 | 0 | 0 |
| GEL-pos | M | 56 | Head | 1 | 1 | 1 | 1 | 0 | 1 | 1 | 1 | 1 | 0 |
| GEL-pos | M | 52 | Tail | 0 | 1 | 1 | 1 | 0 | 1 | 1 | 0 | 0 | 0 |
| GEL-pos | F | 62 | Head | 1 | 1 | 2 | 2 | 1 | 1 | 1 | 1 | 1 | 1 |
| GEL-pos | M | 32 | Head | 1 | 1 | 2 | 1 | 1 | 1 | 1 | 1 | 1 | 0 |
| GEL-pos | M | 41 | Head | 0 | 1 | 2 | 1 | 1 | 1 | 1 | 0 | 0 | 0 |
| GEL-pos | F | 46 | Head | 1 | 1 | 1 | 1 | 0 | 1 | 0 | 1 | 1 | 0 |
| GEL-pos | M | 26 | Head | 1 | 1 | 2 | 1 | 0 | 1 | 0 | 1 | 1 | 0 |
| GEL-pos | M | 48 | Head | 0 | 1 | 2 | 1 | 2 | 1 | 2 | 0 | 0 | 0 |
| GEL-pos | F | 57 | Head | 1 | 2 | 2 | 2 | 1 | 1 | 2 | 2 | 1 | 0 |

IgG4 (counting three hot spots: 0, negative or <5HPF; 1>20<50HPF;2>50HPF

*LPL* lymphoplasmacytic, *GEL* granulocytic epithelial lesion, *PMN* polymorphonuclear cells, Grading: *0* absent, *1* present, *2* prominent

**Table 20.2** Clinicopathological features: type 1-GEL-neg AIP versus type 2-GEL-pos AIP

| | Type 1-GEL-neg ($n$=9) | Type 2-GEL-pos ($n$=10) |
|---|---|---|
| *Age* | 59.2 (range 48–78) | 45.6 (range 26–60) |
| *Gender* | | |
| Male | 6 (67 %) | 7 (70 %) |
| Female | 3 (33 %) | 3 (30 %) |
| *Site* | | |
| Head | 7 (78 %) | 9 (90 %) |
| Tail | 2 (22 %) | 1 (10 %) |
| *Jaundice* | 6 (67 %) | 6 (60 %) |
| *Autoimmune diseases* | 1 Sjogren, 1 asthma, 1 psoriasis | 3 ulcerative colitis, 1 Crohn |
| *Prominent tissue IgG4* | 9 (100 %) | 1 (10 %) |
| *Acinar PMN* | 0 (0 %) | 10 (100 %) |
| *Prominent storiform fibrosis* | 6 (67 %) | 1 (10 %) |
| *Prominent obliterative phlebitis* | 8 (89 %) | 0 (0 %) |
| *Prominent lymphoid follicles* | 6 (67 %) | 2 (20 %) |
| *Bile duct involvement* | 6 (67 %) | 6 (60 %) |
| *Papilla involvement* | 7 (78 %) | 6 (60 %) |

[21]. In both types, parenchyma affected by AIP appeared hypoattenuating in 19 (90 %) patients and isoattenuating in 2 (10 %). During the portal venous phase, pancreatic parenchyma showed delayed enhancement in 18 (86 %) patients and washout in 3 (14 %). The main pancreatic duct was never visible within the enlarged pancreatic parenchyma. In focal AIP, the upstream main pancreatic duct was dilated in 8 out of 14 patients. After steroid treatment, there was a reduction in the size of enlarged pancreatic parenchyma, with normal enhancement pattern in 15 (71 %) of the 21 patients, as well as a normal main pancreatic duct within the lesion was observed in all patients.

The findings of MR of 27 AIP patients showed a focal enlargement of the pancreatic parenchyma in 13 (48 %) and diffuse in 14 (53 %) [22]. The pancreatic parenchyma appeared hypointense on T1-weighted images in all 27 (100 %) patients, hyperintense on T2-weighted images in 25 (93 %), and isointense in 2 (7 %). After contrast-medium injection, enlarged pancreatic parenchyma appeared hypointense during arterial phases in 25 (93 %) patients and isointense in 2 (7 %). During the portal venous and delayed phases, the images of 19 (70 %) patients showed delayed enhancement. The main pancreatic duct was not visible within the enlarged pancreatic parenchyma in all 27 AIP patients (100 %), suggesting compression. In focal type, there is a stricture of the main pancreatic duct with mild dilation upstream. After steroid treatment, there was a normalization of the signal intensity on the T1-weighted images, whereas on the T2-weighted images, the involved pancreatic parenchyma appeared normally hypointense in 14 (52 %), isointense in 7 (26 %), and remained hyperintense in 6 (22 %) patients. After steroids, the dynamic study after contrast-medium injection in arterial, parenchymal, and venous phase is similar to that observed at CT scan, and the main pancreatic duct became normal in 23 (85 %) and remained narrowed in 4 (15 %) patients.

CT imaging can be used in the differential diagnosis between the diffuse form of AIP and nonnecrotizing acute pancreatitis (NNAP) [23]. The main parameters used for this purpose are the "relative enhancement rate" (RER) and the presence of peripancreatic stranding and retroperitoneal fluid film. The RER is the rate of relative variation in enhancement from the previous phase, and it is calculated from dynamic pancreatic density data of the quadriphasic MDCT study by qualitative changes of pancreatic density. Compared to the spleen, the pancreas appears hypodense in diffuse AIP, with progressive retention of contrast media in the involved pancreas, whereas in edematous acute pancreatitis, the pancreas appears isodense in nearly all patients, with progressive washout of the contrast medium. The RER in the delayed phase (RER3) has 100 % sensitivity and 100 % specificity for differentiating between AIP and NNAP. Peripancreatic stranding and retroperitoneal fluid is observed in NNAP.

In our experience, contrast-enhanced ultrasonography (CEUS) proved useful to differentiate focal AIP from pancreatic cancer. CEUS may differentiate inflammation from cancer on the basis of enhancement of the mass in an early phase after contrast-medium injection with high

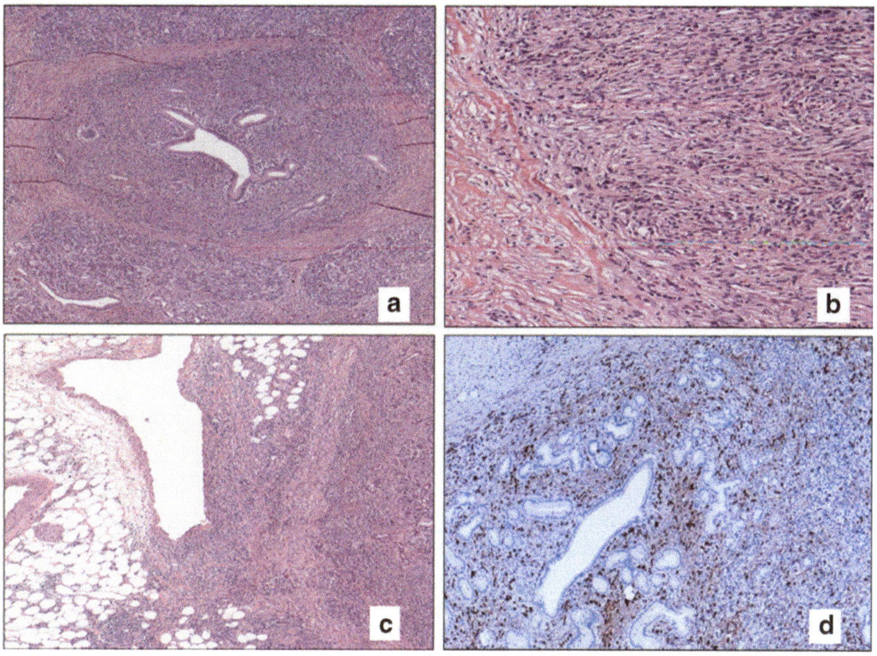


**Fig. 20.1** (**a**–**d**) Type 1 AIP features: periductal fibrosis and inflammatory cell infiltration, characterized by lymphocytes, plasma cells, and macrophages (**a**); inflammatory cellular stroma with prominent storiform fibrosis (**b**); phlebitis (**c**); heavy periductal infiltration of IgG4-positive plasma cells (**d**)

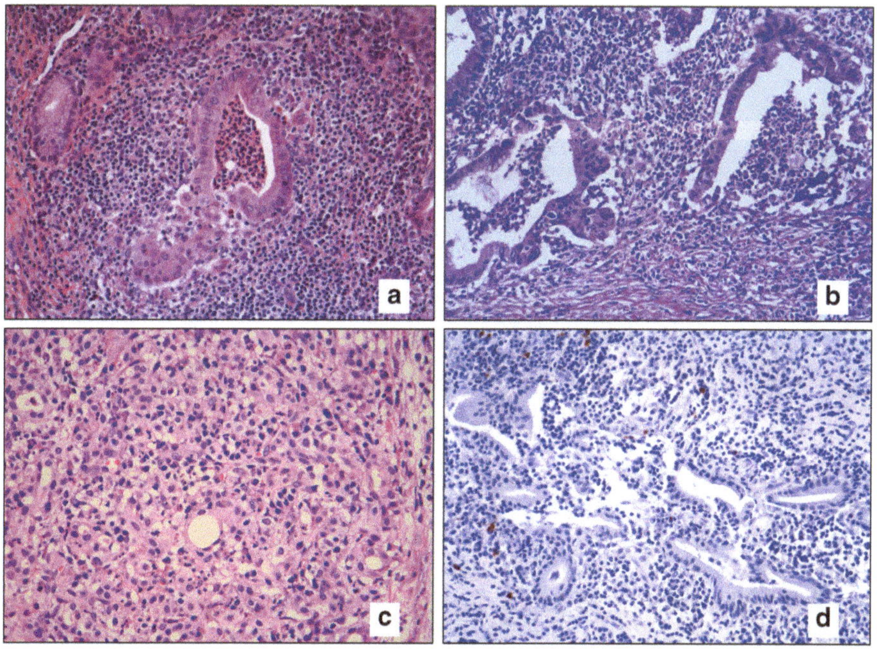


**Fig. 20.2** (**a**–**d**) Granulocytic epithelial lesion (*GEL*), characterized by the invasion of the ductal structures by neutrophilic granulocytes, with detachment, disruption, and destruction of the duct epithelium (**a**, **b**); acinar-type GELs with granulocytes extension into the intra-acinar small ducts (**c**); GEL with very few IgG4-positive plasma cells (**d**)

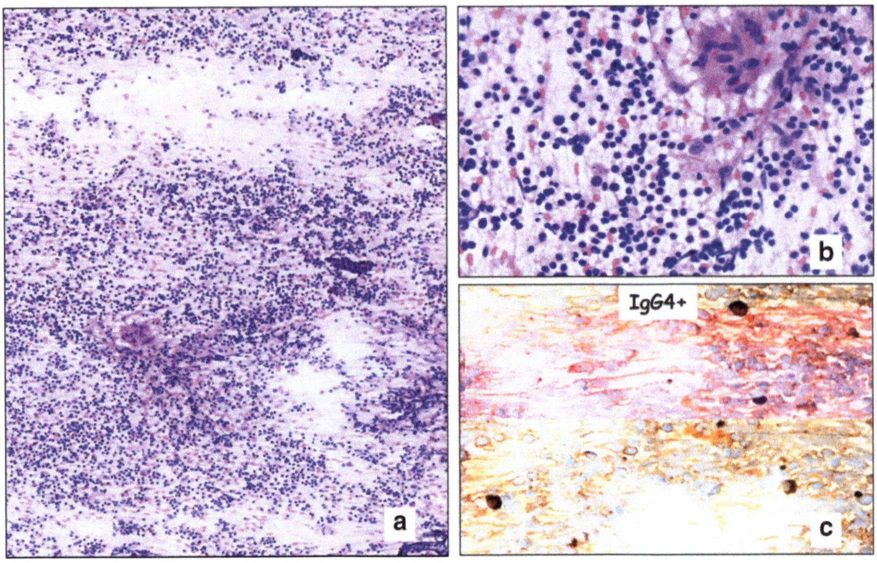


**Fig. 20.3** (**a**–**c**) The cytological smear is characterized by an underrepresentation of ductal cells, lack of significant nuclear atypia, and the presence of lymphocytes, plasma cells, and cellular stromal fragments (**a**, **b**); few IgG4-positive plasma cells (**c**)

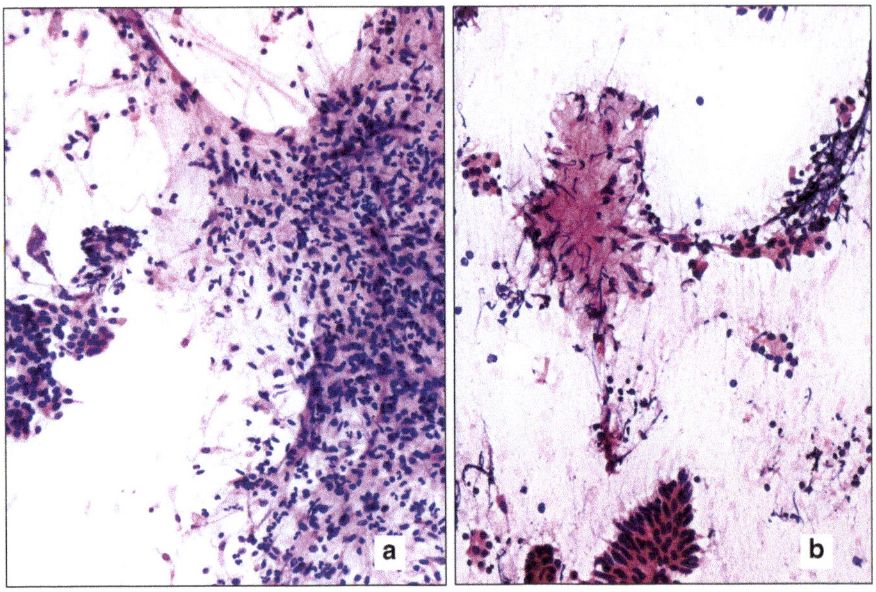


**Fig. 20.4** (**a**–**b**) The presence of stromal fragments infiltrated by granulocytes suggesting a possible diagnosis of type 2 AIP (**a**, **b**)

sensitivity (88.6 %), specificity (97.8 %), and overall accuracy of 96 % [24].

In Italy, the endoscopic retrograde pancreatography (ERP) findings are no longer included as criteria for the diagnosis of AIP [25, 26], since ERP was replaced by secretin-enhanced MR cholangiopancreatography (MRCP). ERP has a higher spatial resolution than MRCP, but it is an invasive and operator-dependent procedure.

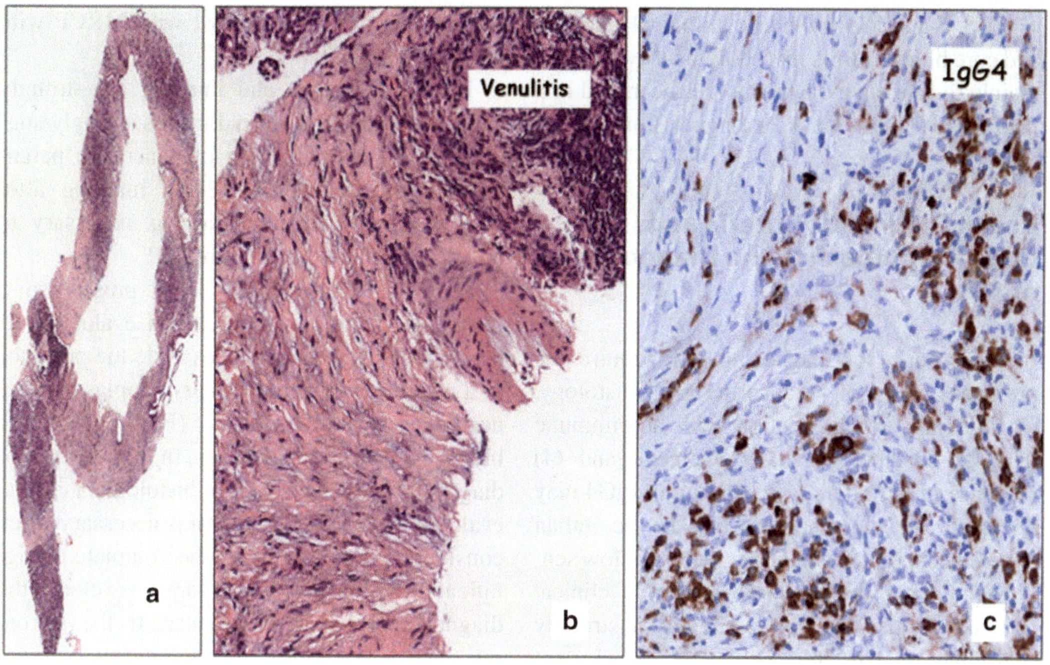


**Fig. 20.5** (**a**–**c**) Tru-Cut biopsy: extensive fibroinflammatory infiltration with focally spared parenchyma (**a**); venulitis (**b**); IgG4-positive plasma cells (**c**)

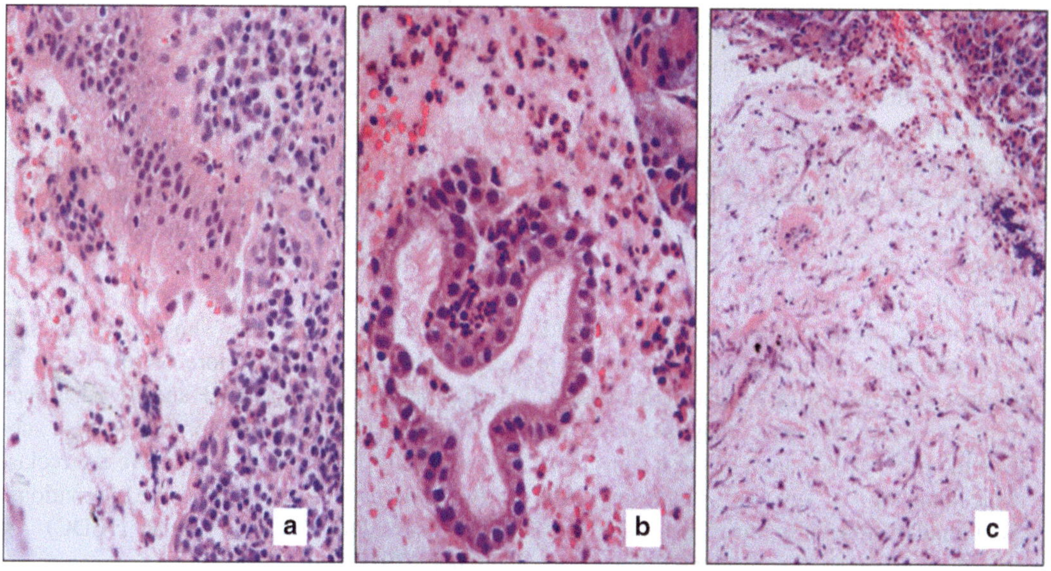


**Fig. 20.6** (**a**–**c**) Tru-Cut biopsy: a granulocytic-rich inflammation with GELs formation (**a**, **b**); myxoid stroma with plump myofibroblasts (**c**)

EUS is used to provide cytological material and core biopsies for a morphological evaluation, mainly to rule out a diagnosis of cancer, and in a minority of cases to make a diagnosis of AIP.

## Italian Diagnostic Criteria and Clinical Approach to the Diagnosis of AIP

Italian criteria for diagnosing AIP require the presence of 3 out of 4 main criteria: (1) histology, (2) imaging, (3) association with autoimmune diseases or other organ involvement, and (4) response to steroid therapy [6]. Serum IgG4 may be useful for the diagnosis but, in the Italian experience, provides high specificity but low sensitivity [27]. Carrying this evidence in clinical practice, high serum levels of IgG4 are strongly indicative of AIP, but normal levels do not exclude AIP. Furthermore, IgG4 may be mildly elevated in patients with pancreatic cancer [9].

Since response to steroids is by definition an "a posteriori" diagnostic criterion, the main clinical problem is when and how to safely administer a steroid trial. The approach to a patient with a suspicion of AIP is different in diffuse and focal forms of the disease [11].

In the diffuse form, a suspicion of AIP is based on the clinical profile and imaging. The clinical profile of AIP patients is peculiar and different from "classic" acute pancreatitis. A history of autoimmune diseases may be present, etiologic factors of acute pancreatitis (biliary lithiasis, alcohol abuse) are absent, pain is generally mild, not infrequently jaundice is present secondary to bile duct stenosis, and a persistent increase of serum amylase and lipase may be observed. Given the nonspecific nature of these signs, pancreatic imaging is key for diagnosing AIP. Abdominal imaging also investigates the presence of other organ involvement (biliary tree, kidney) that strongly supports the diagnosis of AIP. In diffuse-type AIP, cytology and core biopsy are not mandatory for diagnosing AIP and not employed in our practice due to the potential risk of fistula in the presence of acute pancreatitis. We also discourage ERCP, since similar information may be obtained with MRCP with secretin stimulation.

If clinical profile and imaging are strongly suggestive of AIP, a steroid trial is strongly suggested. The normalization of pancreatic parenchymal and ductal changes at imaging after 3–4 weeks of steroid therapy is necessary to make a definitive diagnosis of AIP.

In focal AIP, particularly in the presence of a low-density mass, a more careful evaluation of the patients is necessary to exclude the presence of a pancreatic or periampullary neoplasm. Fine-needle aspiration cytology (FNAC) or core biopsy is therefore mandatory. In the presence of diagnostic or suggestive AIP histology, a careful evaluation of the other criteria is necessary when considering a steroid trial. The complete or significant response to steroids largely excludes the diagnosis of pancreatic cancer. If the steroid response is absent or not significant, surgery should be performed as soon as possible.

## Clinical Profile of the Italian Patients Suffering from AIP

In September 2010, 114 patients (75 males, 39 females, mean age at clinical onset 46.8 ± 15.9 years) with a definitive diagnosis of AIP based on Italian criteria were included in our database from 1995. The main characteristics of AIP patients, divided in focal and diffuse forms, are reported in Table 20.3.

Histology to classify AIP as type 1 or 2 was available only in patients who underwent surgery. We estimated that more or less 60 % of Italian patients had type 1 AIP and 40 % had type 2 AIP. However, the clinical profile of these subtypes of AIP is not yet available. We are reclassifying AIP patients according to the International Consensus Diagnostic Criteria (ICDC) of Fukuoka 2011 [28].

The clinical profile of AIP in Italy differs from other forms of pancreatitis. AIP patients are usually of male gender, have a negative history of smoking and drinking, more often manifest jaundice or atypical pancreatitis, frequently have other autoimmune diseases or other organ

**Table 20.3** Clinical and radiological differences between focal and diffuse type of AIP

| | All patients | Focal AIP | Diffuse AIP | *P* |
|---|---|---|---|---|
| N. | 114 | 68 | 46 | – |
| Males | 75 (66 %) | 51 (75 %) | 24 (52 %) | 0.016 |
| Age at clinical onset *(years)* | 43.4 ± 15.3 | 51 ± 15 | 40 ± 16 | <0.001 |
| Duration of follow-up *(years)* | 6±5 | 6±5 | 6±6 | Ns |
| Heavy drinkers *(>80 g alcohol/day)* | 2 (2 %) | 1 (1.5 %) | 1 (2 %) | Ns |
| Smokers | 39 (36 %) | 27 (43 %) | 12 (27 %) | Ns |
| Elevated serum IgG4 (>135 mg/L) | 35 (43 %) | 22 (45 %) | 13 (39 %) | Ns |
| Associated autoimmune diseases | 58 (50 %) | 29 (43 %) | 28 (61 %) | Ns |
| Associated ulcerative colitis | 32 (28 %) | 16 (23 %) | 16 (35 %) | Ns |
| Pancreatic surgery | 24 (21 %) | 24 (35 %) | 0 | <0.001 |
| Calcifications | 11 (10 %) | 9 (13 %) | 4 (9 %) | Ns |
| Diabetes | 29 (26 %) | 23 (34 %) | 6 (13 %) | 0.015 |
| Steatorrhea | 24 (21 %) | 17 (25 %) | 7 (15 %) | Ns |
| Steroid treatment | 81 (71 %) | 41 (60 %) | 40 (89 %) | <0.001 |
| Immunosuppressant | 30 (26 %) | 18 (27 %) | 12 (26) | Ns |
| Recurrences | 22 (25 %) | 18 (33 %) | 4 (12 %) | 0.043 |

involvement, and have significant weight loss at clinical onset secondary to a combination of pancreatic exocrine and endocrine insufficiency [29]. The main sign of focal AIP is jaundice, whereas acute pancreatitis is more commonly observed in the diffuse form. Acute pancreatitis is generally "atypical," since it is characterized by mild pain not requiring analgesics and it may be diagnosed only by imaging.

All of our patients respond quickly to steroid therapy [6]. One third of these patients experienced disease relapses with 30 patients receiving immunosuppressant treatment, 21 for the pancreatic disease and 9 for associated autoimmune diseases. Predictors of disease relapse in our series were elevated serum IgG4 at clinical onset and/or after steroid treatment and cigarette smoking [6].

## Conclusions

The differentiation between focal and diffuse forms of AIP is important for guiding patient evaluation and management. In focal forms, it is primarily necessary to exclude pancreatic cancer. Since the use of steroids is a diagnostic criterion, the diagnosis of AIP may be achieved after exclusion of a pancreatic cancer. Fine-needle aspiration cytology seems to be the best tools to exclude cancer. In diffuse forms, AIP should be differentiated from NNAP that may be best achieved with CT. The distinction of type 1 and 2 AIPs provides prognostic information that may impact patient follow-up and care. However, we do not have yet Italian data to confirm this hypothesis that can be obtained only after the reclassification in type 1 and 2 AIPs of Italian patients suffering from AIP.

## References

1. Finkelberg DL et al. Autoimmune pancreatitis. N Engl J Med. 2006;355(25):2670–6.
2. Yoshida K et al. Chronic pancreatitis caused by an autoimmune abnormality. Proposal of the concept of autoimmune pancreatitis. Dig Dis Sci. 1995;40(7):1561–8.
3. Ito T et al. Autoimmune pancreatitis as a new clinical entity. Three cases of autoimmune pancreatitis with effective steroid therapy. Dig Dis Sci. 1997;42(7):1458–68.
4. Furukawa N et al. Autoimmune pancreatitis: radiologic findings in three histologically proven cases. J Comput Assist Tomogr. 1998;22(6):880–3.
5. Okazaki K et al. Autoimmune-related pancreatitis is associated with autoantibodies and a Thl/Th2-type cellular immune response. Gastroenterology. 2000;118(3):573–81.
6. Frulloni L et al. Autoimmune pancreatitis: differences between the focal and diffuse forms in 87 patients. Am J Gastroenterol. 2009;104(9):2288–94.
7. Chari ST et al. Histopathologic and clinical subtypes of autoimmune pancreatitis: the Honolulu consensus document. Pancreas. 2010;39(5):549–54.

8. Chari ST. Diagnosis of autoimmune pancreatitis using its five cardinal features: introducing the Mayo Clinic's HISORt criteria. J Gastroenterol. 2007;42 Suppl 18:39–41.
9. Ghazale A et al. Value of serum IgG4 in the diagnosis of autoimmune pancreatitis and in distinguishing it from pancreatic cancer. Am J Gastroenterol. 2007;102(8):1646–53.
10. Morselli-Labate AM, Pezzilli R. Usefulness of serum IgG4 in the diagnosis and follow up of autoimmune pancreatitis: a systematic literature review and meta-analysis. J Gastroenterol Hepatol. 2009;24(1):15–36.
11. Frulloni L et al. A practical approach to the diagnosis of autoimmune pancreatitis. World J Gastroenterol. 2011;17(16):2076–9.
12. Zamboni G et al. Histopathological features of diagnostic and clinical relevance in autoimmune pancreatitis: a study on 53 resection specimens and 9 biopsy specimens. Virchows Arch. 2004;445(6):552–63.
13. Deshpande V et al. Endoscopic ultrasound guided fine needle aspiration biopsy of autoimmune pancreatitis: diagnostic criteria and pitfalls. Am J Surg Pathol. 2005;29(11):1464–71.
14. Levy MJ et al. EUS-guided Tru-Cut biopsy in establishing autoimmune pancreatitis as the cause of obstructive jaundice. Gastrointest Endosc. 2005;61(3):467–72.
15. Khalid A et al. Endoscopic ultrasound fine needle aspirate DNA analysis to differentiate malignant and benign pancreatic masses. Am J Gastroenterol. 2006;101(11):2493–500.
16. Levy MJ. Endoscopic ultrasound-guided Tru-Cut biopsy of the pancreas: prospects and problems. Pancreatology. 2007;7(2–3):163–6.
17. Detlefsen S et al. Diagnosis of autoimmune pancreatitis by core needle biopsy: application of six microscopic criteria. Virchows Arch. 2009;454(5):531–9.
18. Mizuno N et al. Histological diagnosis of autoimmune pancreatitis using EUS-guided Tru-Cut biopsy: a comparison study with EUS-FNA. J Gastroenterol. 2009;44(7):742–50.
19. Imai K et al. Endoscopic ultrasonography-guided fine needle aspiration biopsy using 22-gauge needle in diagnosis of autoimmune pancreatitis. Dig Liver Dis. 2011;43(11):869–74.
20. Iwashita T et al. Use of samples from endoscopic ultrasound-guided 19-gauge fine-needle aspiration in diagnosis of autoimmune pancreatitis. Clin Gastroenterol Hepatol. 2012;10(3):316–22.
21. Manfredi R et al. Autoimmune pancreatitis: CT patterns and their changes after steroid treatment. Radiology. 2008;247(2):435–43.
22. Manfredi R et al. Autoimmune pancreatitis: pancreatic and extrapancreatic MR imaging-MR cholangiopancreatography findings at diagnosis, after steroid therapy, and at recurrence. Radiology. 2011;260(2):428–36.
23. Graziani R et al. Autoimmune pancreatitis and non-necrotizing acute pancreatitis: computed tomography pattern. Dig Liver Dis. 2012;44(9):759–66.
24. D'Onofrio M et al. Mass-forming pancreatitis: value of contrast-enhanced ultrasonography. World J Gastroenterol. 2006;12(26):4181–4.
25. Okazaki K et al. Japanese clinical guidelines for autoimmune pancreatitis. Pancreas. 2009;38(8):849–66.
26. Otsuki M et al. Asian diagnostic criteria for autoimmune pancreatitis: consensus of the Japan-Korea symposium on autoimmune pancreatitis. J Gastroenterol. 2008;43(6):403–8.
27. Frulloni L, Lunardi C. Serum IgG4 in autoimmune pancreatitis: a marker of disease severity and recurrence? Dig Liver Dis. 2011;43(9):674–5.
28. Shimosegawa T et al. International consensus diagnostic criteria for autoimmune pancreatitis: guidelines of the International Association of Pancreatology. Pancreas. 2011;40(3):352–8.
29. Frulloni L et al. Exocrine and endocrine pancreatic function in 21 patients suffering from autoimmune pancreatitis before and after steroid treatment. Pancreatology. 2010;10(2–3):129–33.

# British Experience

# 21

Evangelos Kalaitzakis, Robert Sutton, and George Webster

## Abbreviations

| | |
|---|---|
| AIP | Autoimmune pancreatitis |
| IgG4-SC | IgG4-related sclerosing cholangitis |
| NHS | National Health Service |
| UCH | University College Hospital |

## Nomenclature

Autoimmune pancreatitis (AIP) and IgG4-related sclerosing cholangitis (IgG4-SC) are fibroinflammatory diseases of the pancreaticobiliary system, which may be seen as part of a multiorgan disorder involving a range of organs (IgG4-related diseases) [1–6]. Both conditions were initially described more than 40 years ago [7, 8] but have been better defined by Japanese groups since 1995 [9]. However, our understanding of this condition has been constrained for many years by a lack of consensus over nomenclature. AIP and IgG4-SC have had many descriptive names in the literature [6], such as "sclerosing pancreato-cholangitis," "sclerosing pancreatitis-associated sclerosing cholangitis," and "primary sclerosing pancreatitis and cholangitis."

In view of the marked increase in reports of AIP/IgG4-SC worldwide over the last few years, it is perhaps surprising that as recent as 2003 there was an ongoing debate as to whether AIP was of relevance in the West [10]. However, case series from the USA and Europe in the last 5 years have led to an acceptance that AIP is a global disease [11–14]. "AIP" is now the term commonly used to describe the pancreatic manifestations of IgG4-related diseases, whereas the term "IgG4-associated cholangitis" was introduced in 2007 [6].

## Diagnostic Criteria

Until the recent publication of international consensus criteria for AIP, there are no uniformly accepted diagnostic criteria for the disease, but several sets of criteria have been published, including the Asian diagnostic criteria (proposed jointly by researchers in Japan and Korea) [15], the Italian criteria [13], and the diagnostic criteria developed at the Mayo Clinic [11]. All systems utilize imaging and histopathological data as well as a response to steroids to diagnose AIP [11, 13, 15]. The HISORt criteria of the Mayo Clinic, in which five cardinal features of AIP and IgG4-SC

E. Kalaitzakis, M.D., Ph.D. (✉)
Department of Gastroenterology, Skåne University Hospital, Lund 221 85, Sweden
e-mail: evangelos.kalaitzakis@medicine.gu.se

R. Sutton, D.Phil., FRCS
NIHR Pancreas Biomedical Research Unit, Royal Liverpool University Hospital, Daulby Street, Liverpool L69 3GA, UK
e-mail: r.sutton@liverpool.ac.uk

G. Webster, B.Sc., M.D., FRCP
GI Services, University College London Hospitals, Ground Floor West 250 Euston Road, London NW1 2PG, United Kingdom
e-mail: george.webster@uclh.nhs.uk

M.J. Levy and S.T. Chari (eds.), *Autoimmune (IgG4-related) Pancreatitis and Cholangitis*, DOI 10.1007/978-1-4419-6430-4_21, © Springer Science+Business Media New York 2013

are taken into consideration (histology, imaging, serology, other organ involvement, and response to steroid therapy), are most commonly utilized in the UK for the diagnosis of this condition [11, 16]. Of 52 patients with AIP/IgG4-SC diagnosed at University College Hospital in London, from 2004 to 2010, 89 % fulfilled HISORt criteria, whether applied retrospectively (in those diagnosed prior to publication of HISORt criteria in 2006) or prospectively [17].

Both the Asian and the HISORt diagnostic criteria take account of pancreatic histological findings of lymphoplasmacytic infiltrate with IgG4-positive plasma cells [11, 15], but the HISORt criteria also take into consideration extrapancreatic disease showing histologically abundant IgG4-positive plasma cells [11]. The diagnostic use of IgG4 immunostaining of pancreatic and extrapancreatic tissues in AIP has been recently assessed in a study from the UK [18]. Seventeen biopsy specimens and three gallbladder resections were assessed from 11 consecutive patients with clinical and radiologic features of AIP. In both pancreatic and extrapancreatic tissues, high levels of IgG4 immunostaining (>10 IgG4-positive plasma cells/high power field) were found in 17/20 (85 %) specimens from AIP patients, compared with 1/175 (0.6 %) specimens from controls ($p<0.05$) (Fig. 21.1). Positive extrapancreatic IgG4 immunostaining was found in 8/11 (73 %) patients. Positive IgG4 immunostaining enabled a definitive diagnosis in 10/11 (91 %) AIP patients (Fig. 21.2) [18]. However, IgG4 immunopositivity is not mandatory for the diagnosis [16].

## Historical Perspective: Published UK Experience of AIP and IgG4-SC

The first two probable cases of AIP/IgG4-SC from the UK were published in the literature in 1975, consisting of two siblings with "chronic pancreatitis, sclerosing cholangitis, and sicca complex" [19]. It is uncertain whether a case series of three patients with apparently steroid-responsive primary sclerosing cholangitis in 1991 in fact represented an early UK report of therapy in IgG4-SC [20]. The first series of patients with well-defined AIP from the UK was published in 2007 [12]. A total of 11 consecutive patients with AIP presenting to University College Hospital (UCH) in London with jaundice were included. All showed pancreatic duct strictures and 8 had diffuse pancreatic enlargement. Following diagnosis, prednisolone 30 mg was commenced in all patients and gradually reduced over 2–3 months, tailored to the disease response. All patients showed a rapid symptomatic response within 4 weeks of commencing steroids, with the resolution of jaundice, improvement of pancreatic imaging (Fig. 21.3), and reduction in abdominal discomfort. Improvement in liver function tests mirrored the clinical response (Figs. 21.4 and 21.5). Steroid therapy allowed biliary stent removal without recurrence of jaundice [12].

In a subsequent study of 28 consecutive patients with AIP treated at UCH, the frequency and clinical management of relapse after steroid treatment were reported [21]. In addition to pancreatic changes, 23/28 (82 %) of patients had proximal, hilar, or intrahepatic biliary stricturing (i.e., IgG4-SC). Failure to wean steroids occurred in 5/28 (18 %) of patients treated with prednisolone and disease relapse in 8/28 (29 %) of patients achieving remission (Fig. 21.6) [21]. Interestingly, all patients who relapsed or failed weaning of steroids had IgG4-SC, and relapse occurred in the biliary tree or other extrapancreatic sites, but not in the pancreas. Steroids were restarted or increased in all 13 patients with a relapse or failure to wean steroids, while 10/13 also received azathioprine at a dose of 2 mg/kg with remission being achieved in 7/13 [21]. The finding that IgG4-SC predicts relapse is similar to the data from the Mayo Clinic, which demonstrated relapse in 53 % of IgG4-SC patients after an initial course of steroids and that proximal biliary stricturing more strongly predicted relapse than distal bile duct stricturing (64 % vs. 32 %) [16]. Furthermore, according to our experience surgery (pylorus-preserving pancreatoduodenectomy) itself may elicit IgG4-SC in a predisposed individual, with need for long-term prednisolone to control disease manifestations.

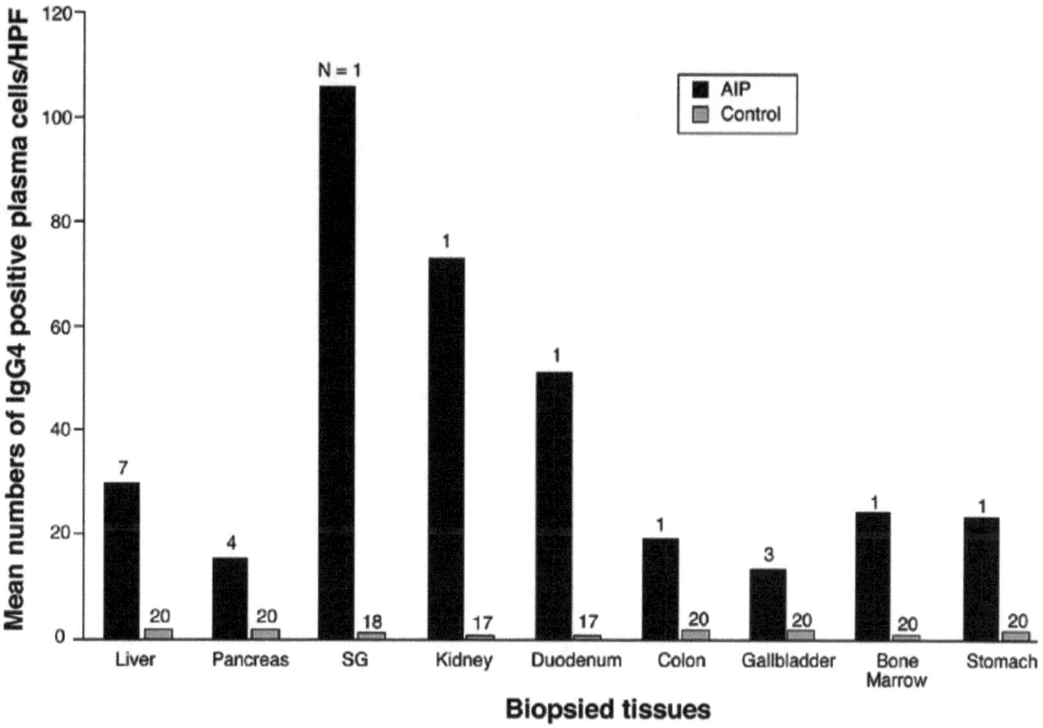


**Fig. 21.1** Mean numbers of IgG4-positive plasma cells in AIP patients versus normal and inflamed controls. *SG* salivary gland (From Clin Gastroenterol Hepatol 2007;5:1229–1234 with permission)

## Formalization of Pancreatic Cancer Care in the UK

The differentiation of AIP from pancreatic cancer and IgG4-SC from cholangiocarcinoma is central to the diagnostic workup of these conditions, as the clinical presentation and imaging may mimic pancreatic or biliary malignancy [22–25]. Of note, > 70 % of patients in the first UK series of AIP were referred with suspected pancreaticobiliary malignancy [12]. Prior to 2008, most patients had been told at their referring hospital/clinic that they had cancer and were being referred on for further management of malignancy.

The ability to diagnose AIP and IgG4-SC on cholangiopancreatographic criteria alone has been shown to be limited [26, 27]. Differentiating AIP/IgG4-SC from pancreaticobiliary malignancy can be very challenging, and it should be performed in the context of a structured strategy [24, 25], in which a multidisciplinary team of physicians, surgeons, radiologists, and pathologists familiar with the two diseases is involved [28]. In a series of 1287 patients from the USA who had undergone pancreaticoduodenectomies for presumed pancreatic malignancy, 3 % were subsequently found to have AIP [23]. In the same study, 8/29 patients (28 %) diagnosed with AIP following surgery developed relapse after a median of 11 months postoperatively [23]. Similarly, in a recent study from the Netherlands, 15/185 (8 %) of patients undergoing resection for suspected hilar cholangiocarcinoma were found to have histological features consistent with IgG4-SC [22]. These reports emphasize that a misdiagnosis of pancreatic cancer or cholangiocarcinoma in patients with AIP/IgG4-SC may lead to high-risk, unnecessary surgery and that this surgery may frequently not "cure" the disease while potentially delaying beneficial

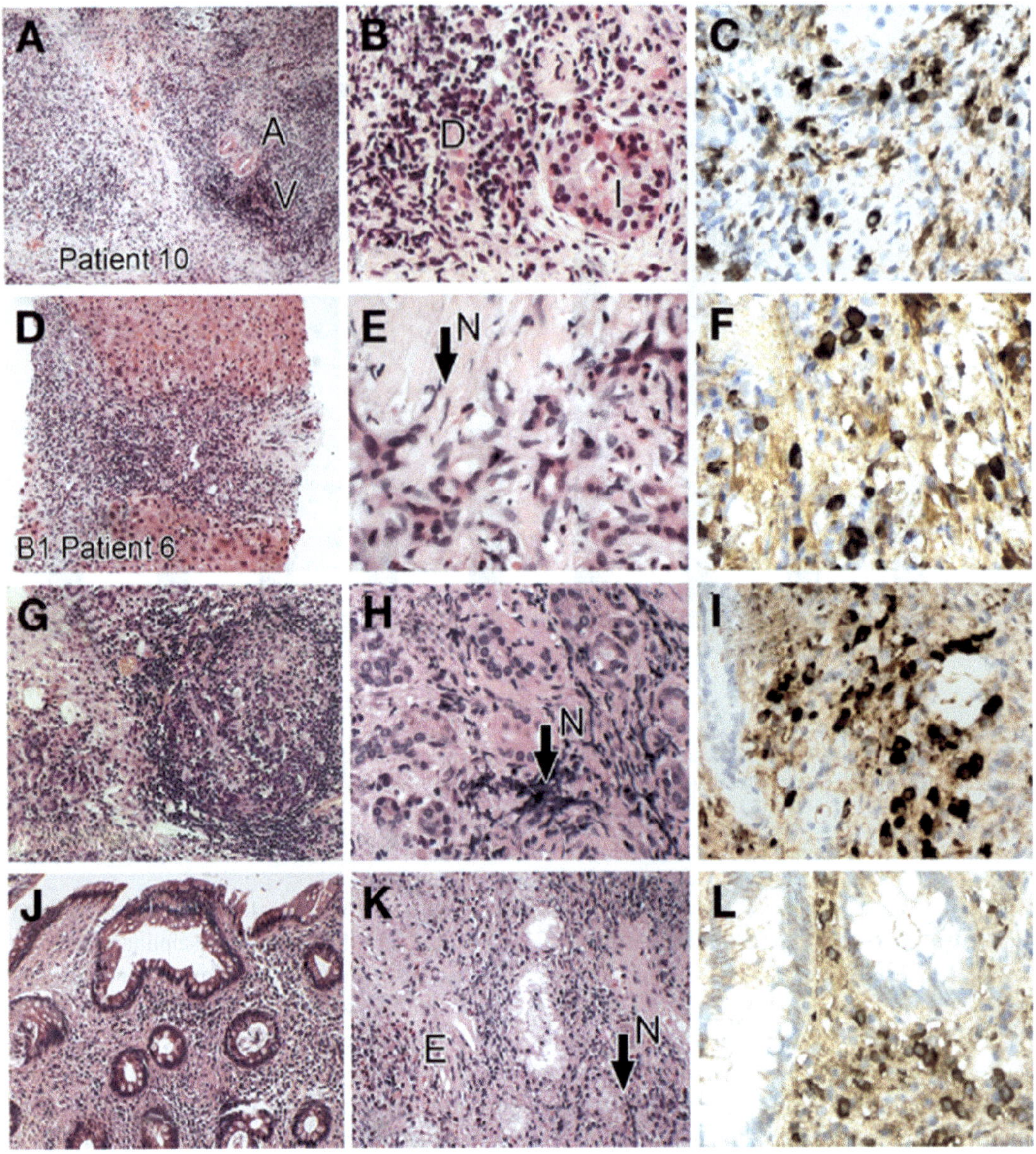


**Fig. 21.2** (**a**) H&E-stained section (magnification, 100) of a pancreatic biopsy specimen from a patient with AIP showing fibrosis, a lymphoplasmacytic infiltrate within pancreatic lobules, with nuclear streaming artifact surrounding a venule showing obliterative phlebitis (*V*). There is a relative preservation of arterioles (*A*). (**b**) H&E-stained section of the same pancreatic biopsy (magnification, 200) with a lymphoplasmacytic infiltrate surrounding pancreatic ducts (*D*). There is atrophy of exocrine pancreatic tissue with preservation of islets (*I*). (**c**) IgG4 immunostaining of plasma cells within the same pancreatic biopsy (magnification, 400). (**d**) H&E-stained section (magnification, 100) of a liver biopsy from a patient with AIP showing the lymphoplasmacytic infiltrate within portal tracts. (**e**) H&E-stained section of a portal tract from the same liver biopsy showing the features of large duct obstruction with a mild increase in eosinophils and nuclear streaming artifact (*N*) (magnification, 200). (**f**) IgG4 immunostaining of plasma cells within portal tracts from the same liver biopsy (magnification, 400). (**g**) H&E-stained section (magnification, 100) of salivary gland from another patient with AIP showing a lymphoplasmacytic infiltrate with lymphoid follicle formation. (**h**) H&E-stained section (magnification, 200) of salivary gland (from the same as in G) showing a lymphoplasmacytic infiltrate and nuclear streaming artifact (*N*) within lobules (magnification, 200). (**i**) IgG4 immunostaining of plasma cells within salivary gland from the same patient (magnification, 400). (**j**) H&E-stained section (magnification, 100) of duodenum from

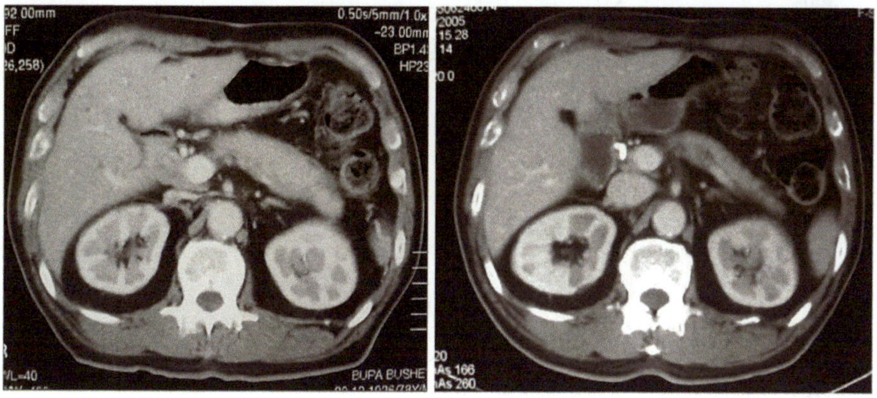

**Fig. 21.3** Abdominal computed tomography scan of the pancreas in a patient with AIP showing a diffusely enlarged "sausage" pancreas (**a**), with subsequent radiological remission after 2 months of steroid therapy (**b**) (From Am J Gastroenterol 2007; 102: 2417–2425 with permission)

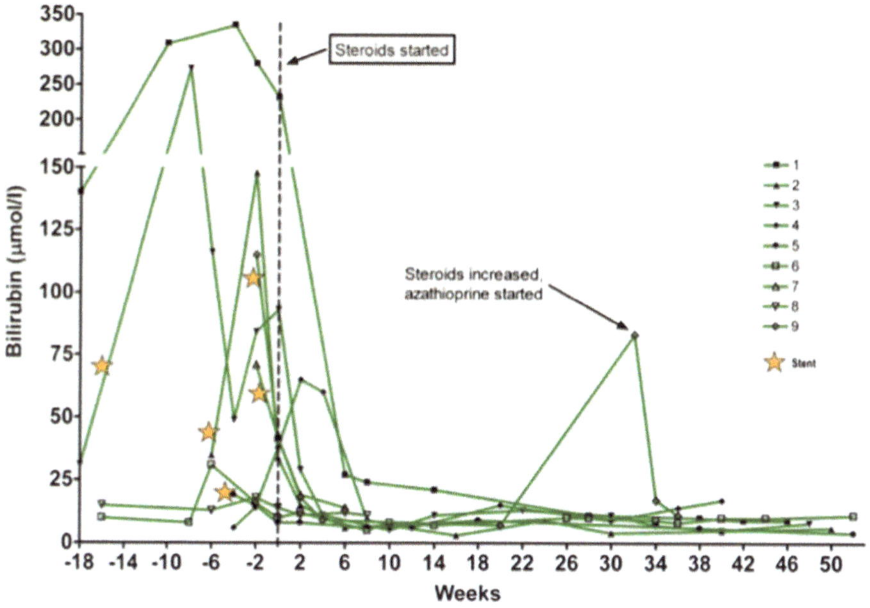


**Fig. 21.4** Response of serum bilirubin to steroid therapy in 11 patients with AIP (From Am J Gastroenterol 2007; 102: 2417–2425 with permission)

**Fig. 21.2** (continued) patient 3. (**k**) H&E-stained section of duodenal biopsy from the same patient (magnification, 200) of duodenum showing fibrosis with nuclear streaming artifact (*N*) and a lymphoplasmacytic infiltrate with a prominence of eosinophils (*E*). (**l**) IgG4 immunostaining of the same duodenal biopsy (magnification, 400). Plasma cells expressing IgG4 were identified on the basis of CD138 staining of adjacent tissue sections and characteristic plasma cell morphology (an eccentrically placed nucleus that has a clock face appearance and abundant cytoplasm) (From Clin Gastroenterol Hepatol 2007;5 : 1229–1234 with permission)

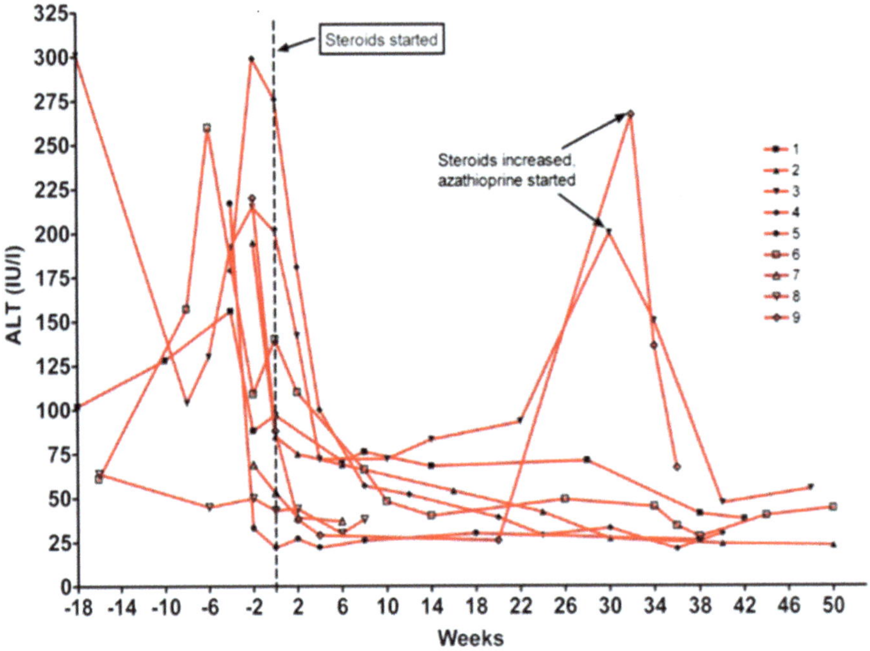


**Fig. 21.5** Response of serum ALT to steroid therapy in 11 patients with AIP (From Am J Gastroenterol 2007; 102: 2417–2425 with permission)

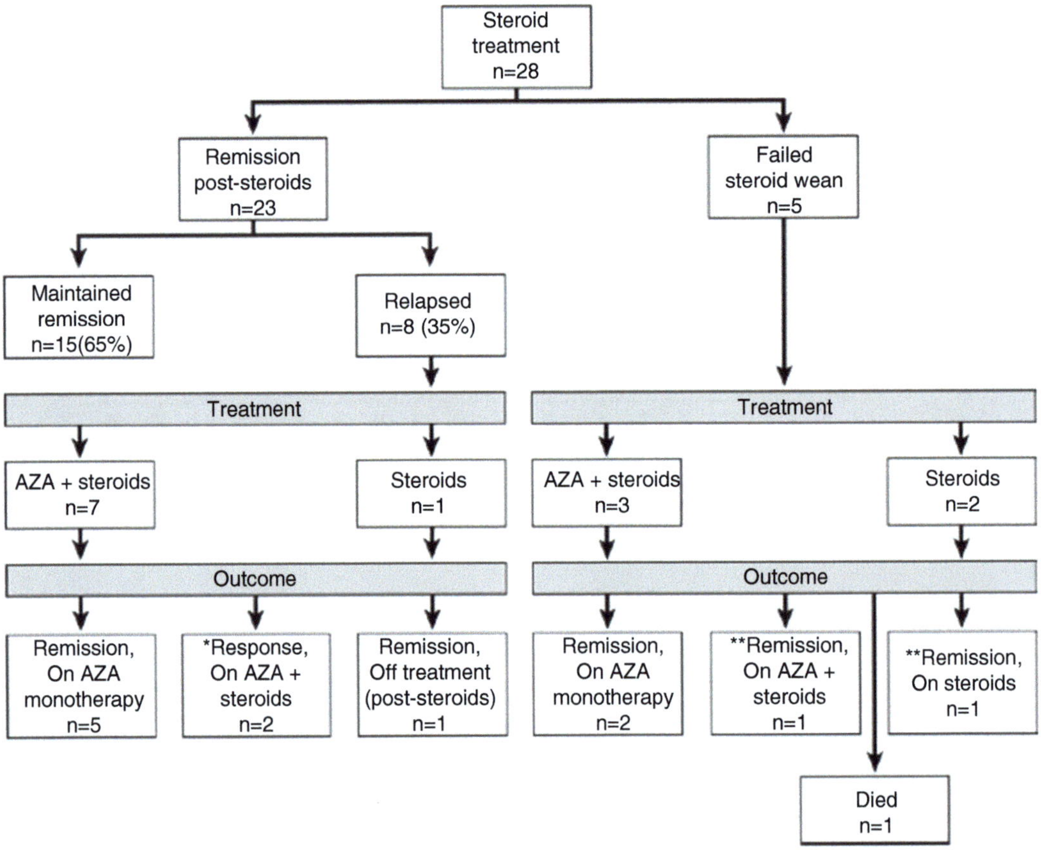


**Fig. 21.6** Response and outcome to treatment in 28 patients with AIP (From Clin Gastroenterol Hepatol 2009; 7: 1089–1096 with permission)

treatment (i.e., steroids). However, approximately 30 % of undiagnosed patients with AIP will not fit imaging, serologic, or other involvement criteria of the HISORt scheme, and thus, a core biopsy or surgery may be needed for diagnosis [25].

In the UK, publication of the National Cancer Plan within the National Health Service (NHS) led to the establishment since 2004 of approximately 30 regional cancer networks, in order to improve speed, quality, and equality of cancer services [29]. Each regional cancer network has developed a strategic service delivery plan in the region encompassing all levels of cancer-related care from prevention and screening to diagnosis and treatment and serves a resident population of 2–4 million [29]. Each network is served by a specialized pancreaticobiliary cancer center to which all cases of potential pancreaticobiliary cancer are referred for diagnosis and treatment. In this way, multidisciplinary teams familiar with pancreaticobiliary cancers and their differential diagnoses are linked to the diagnostic process earlier on with outcomes improved through centralized and higher-volume specialist services. Although to date the awareness, incidence, and diagnostic workup of potential AIP and IgG4-SC cases within each pancreaticobiliary center have not been audited, the focus of care within specialist teams is likely to lead to improved case identification and management. Anecdotally, our experience in the UK is that since 2008 a greater proportion of patients who are eventually diagnosed as having AIP have had the diagnosis considered prior to tertiary referral than was the case in the past.

## Clinical Profile of AIP in the UK

### Prevalence/Incidence

It is widely accepted that AIP/IgG4-SC is a global disease. Although the prevalence of AIP in Japan has been estimated to be 0.82/100,000 [30], the prevalence or incidence of AIP/IgG4-SC in the general UK population is unknown. In the pancreaticobiliary unit of UCH, London, 55 patients were diagnosed with AIP/IgG4-SC between 2004 and 2010, with a diagnostic rate of approximately 10 cases per year for the last 3 years [12, 21, 31]. With a referral catchment population of approximately three million, this suggests an estimated incidence of 0.3/100,000. It is not certain whether this incidence is reflected nationwide, but it seems very likely that the disease remains underdiagnosed. The incidence of pancreatic cancer in the UK is approximately 10/100,000. It is of interest that this relative incidence of AIP and pancreatic cancer exactly mirrors surgical data from the USA, in whom 3 % of patients undergoing pancreatoduodenectomy for presumed pancreatic cancer were found to have AIP (at a time when there was little diagnostic awareness of AIP) [23].

### Demographics

Although the majority (64 %) of patients who have been diagnosed with AIP in the UK are Caucasians, a range of racial groups is represented in the UK cohort including South Asian, Far Eastern, and Afro-Caribbean patients [12]. This is in line with published evidence that AIP is a global disease, and it also reflects the variety in the background composition of the general population in the country.

Both AIP and IgG4-SC have occurred predominantly in males (86 %) with a mean age at diagnosis of 61 years (range 27–81 years) [21], which is in keeping with data from Asia and the USA [11, 32, 33].

### Clinical Presentation

The initial presentation of UK patients with AIP is usually obstructive jaundice (82 %), whereas a minority (14 %) present with abdominal/back pain alone or with abnormal imaging findings, e.g., incidental pancreatic mass (4 %) [21]. Although acute pancreatitis [34] and isolated pancreatic exocrine insufficiency [11] have been previously described as initial presentations in AIP, these appear to be unusual presentations in

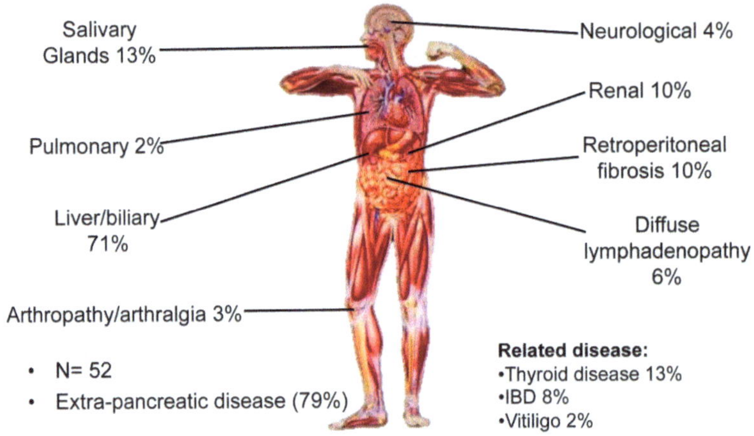


**Fig. 21.7** Extrapancreatic manifestations in patients with AIP diagnosed at University College Hospital, London, 2004–2010

UK experience [12, 21, 31], although it has to be noted that AIP is not usually searched for in such patients. Overall, 18 % of patients diagnosed with AIP have undergone surgery after initial presentation (before AIP diagnosis) in view of the suspicion of pancreatic cancer [31].

## Extrapancreatic Disease

Extrapancreatic disease is recognized to occur in 40–90 % of patients with AIP [11, 12, 35, 36]. Involvement of extrapancreatic organs is considered part of the spectrum of IgG4-related diseases as a similar lymphoplasmacytic infiltrate, containing IgG4 positive plasma cells, is seen within both pancreatic and extrapancreatic lesions (Fig. 21.1) [11, 18]. As outlined above, extrapancreatic disease and in particular positive extrapancreatic IgG4 immunostaining may aid in the diagnosis of AIP [11, 18].

Although IgG4-SC can occur in patients without AIP, the biliary tree proximal to the intrapancreatic portion of the common bile duct is the most common extrapancreatic site involved in AIP, and thus, the two conditions are frequently diagnosed in the same patient [11, 16, 21, 37]. In 52 patients with AIP at UCH in London, IgG4-SC has been found in 71 % of patients, renal abnormalities in 10 % (including infiltrates and scarring), sialadenitis in 13 %, retroperitoneal fibrosis in 10 %, extensive lymphadenopathy in 6 %, and neurological involvement in 4 % [17]. See Fig. 21.7. Twenty percent of AIP patients did not show any extra-pancreatic involvement.

Other autoimmune conditions (non-IgG4 related) occur frequently in patients with AIP/IgG4-SC and include several diseases, such as Sjögren's syndrome, vitiligo, and psoriasis [12]. Inflammatory bowel disease, either ulcerative colitis or Crohn's disease, is described in up to 30 % of patients in Western series [37] but is rare in Japan [38]. In our experience, 8 % of patients with AIP also have inflammatory bowel disease. Interestingly, although in the initial description of IgG4-SC inflammatory bowel disease was considered to argue against the diagnosis of IgG4-SC [6], 75 % of patients with AIP and inflammatory bowel disease in our series also had IgG4-SC [31].

## Serum IgG4 Levels

Raised serum IgG4 is considered to be an important diagnostic landmark of AIP/IgG4-SC and is thus included in both the Mayo Clinic [11] and Asian [15] diagnostic criteria. Interestingly, although both raised serum IgG4 and raised number of tissue IgG4-positive plasma cells are

**Table 21.1** Disease profile of non-histologically proven AIP worldwide

| Country | Japan ($n=127$) | Korea ($n=86$) | Taiwan ($n=33$) | India ($n=36$) | USA ($n=28$) | Germany ($n=36$) | Italy ($n=87$) | UK ($n=28$) |
|---|---|---|---|---|---|---|---|---|
| Mean age, years | 65 | 59 | 66 | N/A | 64 | 43 | 43 | 58 |
| % male | 83 | 71 | 90 | 69 | 79 | 42 | 62 | 82 |
| Presentation | | | | | | | | |
| Jaundice (%) | 61 | 50 | 70 | 56 | 79 | 14 | 44 | 64 |
| Abdominal pain (%) | 13 | 23 | 18 | 86 | 50 | 13 | 20 | 18 |
| Acute pancreatitis (%) | 2 | 13 | 18 | 22 | 25 | 64 | 32 | 0 |
| Other organ involvement (%) | 63 | 41 | 33 | 31 | 75 | 44 | 15 | 82 |
| IBD (%) | 3 | 3 | 0 | 6 | 11 | 8 | 30 | 14 |
| Elevated serum IgG4 (%) | 91 | 52 | 100 | 100 | 85 | 59 | 50 | 54 |
| Relapse poststeroids (%) | 15 | 26 | 18 | 25 | 64 | 15 | 37 | 54 |

important findings in AIP/IgG4-SC, increased tissue IgG4 may be found irrespective of serum IgG4 level [18].

Early data from Japan reported that raised IgG4 levels are highly specific and sensitive for differentiating AIP from pancreatic cancer [39]. However, in UK cohorts, a raised serum IgG4 has been found only in 68 % of AIP patients at presentation [21]. This is similar to 71 % of patients with raised IgG4 in a US series [11], while lower proportions have been reported in other Western series [13, 32]. As raised levels of serum IgG4 have also been found in patients with pancreatic cancer, they cannot be used for the exclusion of pancreaticobiliary malignancy. This distinction, as mentioned above, should be made in the context of a structured strategy [24, 25] that includes data from pancreatic imaging, serum IgG4 levels, determination of other organ involvement, and pancreatic histopathology [25]. In a recent paper from the UK, researchers from Oxford analyzed serum IgG in 196 patients, suffering from AIP and other diseases, to address the specific question as to whether the level could help differentiate AIP from cancer [40]. Patients with AIP possessed a mean serum IgG level that was significantly higher compared with all other groups (mean serum IgG level = 19.0 g/l+/−2.5, $p<0.001$) and specifically compared with cancer patients (mean IgG4 level = 3.7 g/l+/−0.5, $p<0.001$). They concluded that while serum IgG4 could help in the differentiation of AIP from cancer in the UK patient group, it should only be used to do so in conjunction with other imaging, histological, and clinical criteria [40].

Although a marked elevation in IgG4 levels has been used to define or predict relapse in Japanese series of AIP [33], it is currently unclear whether early disease relapse can be predicted solely based on a rise in serum IgG4, as also highlighted in the Japanese guidelines for AIP [39]. In a recent study from the UK, no statistically significant correlation was found between serum IgG4 levels and relapse [21]. Thus, in our practice, we do not define AIP relapse according to changes in serum IgG4 levels.

## Clinical Parameters: Comparison of UK with Worldwide Data

The Autoimmune Pancreatitis International Cooperative Study Group (APICS) met in Honolulu in 2010. Experience was pooled from groups from Asia, North America, and Europe, which included data on patients diagnosed with AIP but without histological confirmation (Table 21.1). Demographic and clinical features were similar between USA, Japanese, and UK groups, but different to patient groups from Germany and Italy. The explanation for this is unclear, but seems more likely to be due to differences in diagnostic criteria and nomenclature, rather than marked differences in disease phenotype across Europe.

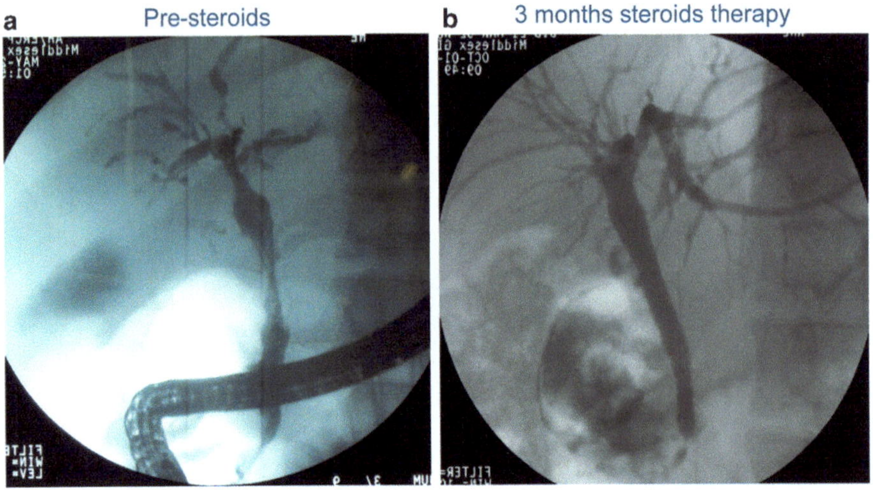


**Fig. 21.8** Cholangiography in a UK patient with IgG4-SC, before (**a**) and 3 months after steroid therapy (**b**)

## Treatment

Despite the fact that a response to steroids is a characteristic (and diagnostic) feature of AIP/IgG4-SC, there are no prospective randomized placebo-controlled data related to steroid use. This is true for all aspects of AIP/IgG4-SC management, which is based on nonrandomized data and expert opinion. In our practice, we treat patients with AIP and symptomatic disease, e.g., obstructive jaundice, abdominal pain, and/or the presence of symptomatic extrapancreatic disease, which is also in accordance with the Japanese guidelines for AIP [39].

### Initial Management

The majority of patients with AIP present with obstructive jaundice and, thus, should be considered for biliary drainage prior to steroid therapy. Also, ERCP may demonstrate the biliary features of IgG4-SC or characteristic pancreatic duct changes [26], and it allows biliary cytology to be taken (to help to exclude malignancy) and ampullary biopsies to identify an IgG4 positive lymphoplasmacytic infiltrate [41], thus contributing to the diagnostic workup of these patients. In the event of diagnostic uncertainty, we also perform endoscopic ultrasound-guided fine-needle aspiration in the context of a structured strategy to exclude pancreaticobiliary malignancy [25]. In published series, 14–64 % of AIP patients underwent transhepatic or endoscopic biliary drainage prior to steroid therapy [12, 32, 42–45]. Nevertheless, in our initial experience of AIP we found that bilirubin and liver enzymes fell most reliably in response to steroid therapy, not biliary stenting, even in the presence of a dominant extrahepatic biliary stricture (Figs. 21.4 and 21.5). In the minority of patients in whom there is no biliary obstruction and no diagnostic doubt about AIP, we do not perform an ERCP. In IgG4-SC, obstructive jaundice due to dominant hilar or extrahepatic biliary stricturing is usually managed initially with endoscopic polyethylene stent insertion. The presence of IgG4-SC within the differential diagnosis of complex hilar stricturing with an associated mass [22] emphasizes the importance of avoiding self-expanding uncovered mesh metal stent insertion for presumed malignancy without a cytological/histological diagnosis [46]. Although stenting at the diagnosis of IgG4-SC may be indicated, long-term stenting rarely appears necessary, since improvements with steroid therapy often allow subsequent management without stents (Fig. 21.8). Of 30 patients with IgG4-SC who received steroids in the Mayo Clinic series, nor-

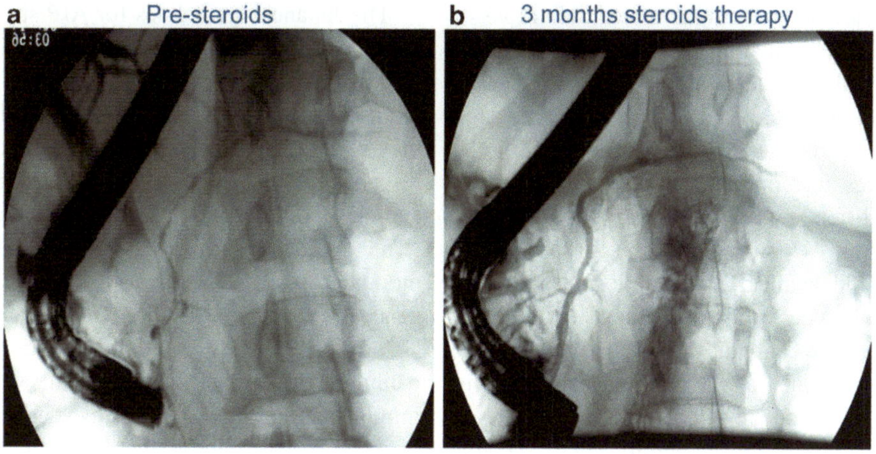


**Fig. 21.9** Pancreaticography in a patient with AIP, before (**a**) and after (**b**) steroid therapy

malization of liver function tests occurred in 61 %, and biliary stents could be removed in 17 of 18 patients [16], and this experience mirrors our own.

Diabetes mellitus is common in AIP and often requires treatment prior to steroids. In our experience, diabetes mellitus is present in 37 % of AIP patients [31], which is similar to the prevalence of diabetes of 31 % in a recent large retrospective study from Japan [33]. Although improvement in diabetic control following the introduction of steroids for AIP has been reported [43–45, 47–49], we have seen this infrequently in our practice. Furthermore, exocrine pancreatic dysfunction occurs in 56 % of British patients with AIP [31], but a prevalence of up to 88 % has been reported in some series [43, 44, 48]. Thus, we routinely measure pancreatic fecal elastase levels in these patients and prescribe pancreatic enzyme supplements generously, since fecal elastase levels are but a rough guide, and the consequences of long-term digestive insufficiency are significant. Pancreatic exocrine function may improve after steroid therapy in up to 2/3 of patients [43, 44, 48], although worsening has also been reported poststeroids [44]. In our AIP cohort, pre-steroid pancreatic insufficiency persisted in most patients despite steroids, overall clinical improvement [31], and even dramatic improvement in pancreatic duct stricturing (Fig. 21.9).

## Initial Steroid Treatment

Various starting prednisolone doses have been used for the treatment of AIP ranging from 5 to 60 mg od [33, 45, 47, 50], but most clinicians use 30–40 mg daily [11, 12, 21, 32, 33, 42, 43, 45, 47, 50]. Retrospective studies indicate that there is no correlation between the degree of morphological improvement on imaging or the time required to induce remission and the initial prednisolone dose (30 mg/day vs. 40 mg/day) [33, 45]. Thus, in UK clinical practice 30 mg of prednisolone is commonly used as a starting dose for induction of remission in AIP [12, 21].

Different patterns of tapering steroids have been proposed. In Japan, the dose of prednisolone is reduced after 2 weeks in 75 % of cases and after 3–4 weeks in the rest, followed by an extended tapering period [33]. Tapering by 5 mg/week after an initial period of 2–4 weeks has been generally reported from the USA and the UK [11, 12, 21, 32]. An attempt to withdraw steroids is usually made early on, although an extended tapering period or a few months' treatment with low-dose steroids may be necessary. In our practice, patients are followed closely, especially in the first months of treatment, undergoing radiological, serological, and biochemical evaluation as well as assessment of symptomatic relief, in line with published reports [11, 12, 21, 32, 33, 45].

There are no generally accepted definitions of response to treatment and remission, in terms of radiological, biochemical, or serological variables. Differences in the definition of remission and steroid regimens probably account for the differences in reported frequency of remission among different series, ranging from 22 % to 100 % [51]. We define disease response as symptomatic, biochemical, and radiological improvement following commencement of steroid therapy. In a recent study, we found that disease remission, defined as the maintenance of symptomatic, biochemical, and radiologic disease control after cessation of prednisolone and the removal of previously sited biliary stents, occurred in 82 % of patients after a median of 5 months of treatment (range 1.5–17 months) [21].

## Treatment of Relapse

Over recent years, disease relapse following steroid therapy has become increasingly recognized, with series reporting frequencies ranging from 0 % to 68 % [51]. This variability may reflect differences between clinical groups with respect to the definition of relapse, the length of clinical follow-up, and perhaps the use or not of very slow tapering regimens or maintenance therapy. In a recent study from the UK, relapse was defined as recurrence of disease activity after achievement of remission and cessation of steroids, and it was discriminated from failed weaning of steroids, the latter being defined by a flare of disease activity while tapering initial steroid course or an inability to wean steroids completely due to biochemical and/or radiological deterioration [21]. Failure to wean steroids occurred in 18 % and disease relapse in 35 % of patients (Fig. 21.6) [21]. We restart/increase oral prednisolone to 30 mg in all patients with a relapse or failure to wean steroids and also start azathioprine treatment, with a target dose of 2 mg/kg per day. Steroid therapy is tailored to clinical, biochemical, and radiological response. In our experience, the majority of patients are able to cease their steroid course within 3–9 months.

The Japanese guidelines for AIP suggest that maintenance therapy be instituted from the outset [39], as it has been reported to be related to lower relapse rates [33]. It is possible that AIP/IgG4-SC may be analogous to autoimmune hepatitis in this respect, as both conditions are steroid responsive and show high relapse rates necessitating long-term immunosuppressive treatment. Azathioprine monotherapy is effective as long-term maintenance treatment in autoimmune hepatitis [52]. However, disease relapse is almost universal in patients with autoimmune hepatitis who stop immunosuppression early [53], whereas relapse of AIP following steroid therapy is frequent [21, 51] but not universal. Further studies may help to define subgroups with a high risk of relapse, where long-term immunosuppression should be considered from diagnosis.

## Key Points

- First two UK cases of probable AIP and IgG4-SC in two siblings with "chronic pancreatitis, sclerosing cholangitis, and sicca complex" published in 1975.
- Widening recognition in UK literature of condition in the West in 2005.
- Following international adoption of nomenclature (AIP/IgG4-SC), a UK series of patients with AIP was published in 2007, providing further evidence of global disease.
- An estimated UK incidence of AIP/IgG4-SC of 0.3/100,000 is likely to be inaccurate, but increased disease awareness and the centralization of specialist pancreaticobiliary services seem to have been associated with an increase in overall diagnoses since 2004.
- Extrapancreatic disease, in particular IgG4-SC, appears to be frequently associated with AIP in UK patients.
- An initial course of oral prednisolone has been the usual treatment approach for AIP in the UK, but relapse is common, particularly in those patients with associated IgG4-SC. Azathioprine appears to have an effective role in maintaining remission in patients who relapse after a course of steroids.

- International multicenter randomized trials for the management of AIP/IgG4-SC are warranted.

## References


1. Kamisawa T, Funata N, Hayashi Y, Eishi Y, Koike M, Tsuruta K, Okamoto A, Egawa N, Nakajima H. A new clinicopathological entity of IgG4-related autoimmune disease. J Gastroenterol. 2003;38:982–4.
2. Hirano K, Shiratori Y, Komatsu Y, Yamamoto N, Sasahira N, Toda N, Isayama H, Tada M, Tsujino T, Nakata R, Kawase T, Katamoto T, Kawabe T, Omata M. Involvement of the biliary system in autoimmune pancreatitis: a follow-up study. Clin Gastroenterol Hepatol. 2003;1:453–64.
3. Kamisawa T, Funata N, Hayashi Y. Lymphoplasmacytic sclerosing pancreatitis is a pancreatic lesion of IgG4-related systemic disease. Am J Surg Pathol. 2004;28:1114.
4. Kamisawa T, Nakajima H, Egawa N, Funata N, Tsuruta K, Okamoto A. IgG4-related sclerosing disease incorporating sclerosing pancreatitis, cholangitis, sialadenitis and retroperitoneal fibrosis with lymphadenopathy. Pancreatology. 2006;6:132–7.
5. Kamisawa T, Okamoto A. Autoimmune pancreatitis: proposal of IgG4-related sclerosing disease. J Gastroenterol. 2006;41:613–25.
6. Bjornsson E, Chari ST, Smyrk TC, Lindor K. Immunoglobulin G4 associated cholangitis: description of an emerging clinical entity based on review of the literature. Hepatology. 2007;45:1547–54.
7. Sarles H, Sarles JC, Muratore R, Guien C. Chronic inflammatory sclerosis of the pancreas–an autonomous pancreatic disease? Am J Dig Dis. 1961;6:688–98.
8. Bartholomew LG, Cain JC, Woolner LB, Utz DC, Ferris DO. Sclerosing cholangitis: its possible association with Riedel's struma and fibrous retroperitonitis. Report of two cases. N Engl J Med. 1963;269:8–12.
9. Yoshida K, Toki F, Takeuchi T, Watanabe S, Shiratori K, Hayashi N. Chronic pancreatitis caused by an autoimmune abnormality. Proposal of the concept of autoimmune pancreatitis. Dig Dis Sci. 1995;40:1561–8.
10. Varadarajulu S, Cotton PB. Autoimmune pancreatitis: is it relevant in the west? Gastroenterology. 2003;125:1557.
11. Chari ST, Smyrk TC, Levy MJ, Topazian MD, Takahashi N, Zhang L, Clain JE, Pearson RK, Petersen BT, Vege SS, Farnell MB. Diagnosis of autoimmune pancreatitis: the Mayo Clinic experience. Clin Gastroenterol Hepatol. 2006;4:1010–6. quiz 934.
12. Church NI, Pereira SP, Deheragoda MG, Sandanayake N, Amin Z, Lees WR, Gillams A, Rodriguez-Justo M, Novelli M, Seward EW, Hatfield AR, Webster GJ. Autoimmune pancreatitis: clinical and radiological features and objective response to steroid therapy in a UK series. Am J Gastroenterol. 2007;102:2417–25.
13. Frulloni L, Scattolini C, Falconi M, Zamboni G, Capelli P, Manfredi R, Graziani R, D'Onofrio M, Katsotourchi AM, Amodio A, Benini L, Vantini I. Autoimmune pancreatitis: differences between the focal and diffuse forms in 87 patients. Am J Gastroenterol. 2009;104:2288–94.
14. Sutton R. Autoimmune pancreatitis–also a Western disease. Gut. 2005;54:581–3.
15. Otsuki M, Chung JB, Okazaki K, Kim MH, Kamisawa T, Kawa S, Park SW, Shimosegawa T, Lee K, Ito T, Nishimori I, Notohara K, Naruse S, Ko SB, Kihara Y. Asian diagnostic criteria for autoimmune pancreatitis: consensus of the Japan-Korea symposium on autoimmune pancreatitis. J Gastroenterol. 2008;43:403–8.
16. Ghazale A, Chari ST, Zhang L, Smyrk TC, Takahashi N, Levy MJ, Topazian MD, Clain JE, Pearson RK, Petersen BT, Vege SS, Lindor K, Farnell MB. Immunoglobulin G4-associated cholangitis: clinical profile and response to therapy. Gastroenterology. 2008;134:706–15.
17. Huggett MT, Tang M, Johnson GJ, Hatfield A, Pereira S, Webster G. Disease profile and long-term outcome of patients with autoimmune pancreatitis/IgG4 systemic disease. Gastroenterology. 2011;140:S-545.
18. Deheragoda MG, Church NI, Rodriguez-Justo M, Munson P, Sandanayake N, Seward EW, Miller K, Novelli M, Hatfield AR, Pereira SP, Webster GJ. The use of immunoglobulin g4 immunostaining in diagnosing pancreatic and extrapancreatic involvement in autoimmune pancreatitis. Clin Gastroenterol Hepatol. 2007;5:1229–34.
19. Waldram R, Kopelman H, Tsantoulas D, Williams R. Chronic pancreatitis, sclerosing cholangitis, and sicca complex in two siblings. Lancet. 1975;1:550–2.
20. Parkes M, Booth JC, Pillai G, Mee AS. Do steroids help jaundice caused by primary sclerosing cholangitis? J Clin Gastroenterol. 2001;33:319–22.
21. Sandanayake NS, Church NI, Chapman MH, Johnson GJ, Dhar DK, Amin Z, Deheragoda MG, Novelli M, Winstanley A, Rodriguez-Justo M, Hatfield AR, Pereira SP, Webster GJ. Presentation and management of post-treatment relapse in autoimmune pancreatitis/immunoglobulin G4-associated cholangitis. Clin Gastroenterol Hepatol. 2009;7:1089–96.
22. Erdogan D, Kloek JJ, ten Kate FJ, Rauws EA, Busch OR, Gouma DJ, van Gulik TM. Immunoglobulin G4-related sclerosing cholangitis in patients resected for presumed malignant bile duct strictures. Br J Surg. 2008;95:727–34.
23. Weber SM, Cubukcu-Dimopulo O, Palesty JA, Suriawinata A, Klimstra D, Brennan MF, Conlon K. Lymphoplasmacytic sclerosing pancreatitis: inflammatory mimic of pancreatic carcinoma. J Gastrointest Surg. 2003;7:129–37. discussion 137–9.
24. Kamisawa T, Imai M, Yui Chen P, Tu Y, Egawa N, Tsuruta K, Okamoto A, Suzuki M, Kamata N. Strategy for differentiating autoimmune pancreatitis from pancreatic cancer. Pancreas. 2008;37:e62–7.
25. Chari ST, Takahashi N, Levy MJ, Smyrk TC, Clain JE, Pearson RK, Petersen BT, Topazian MA, Vege SS.

A diagnostic strategy to distinguish autoimmune pancreatitis from pancreatic cancer. Clin Gastroenterol Hepatol. 2009;7:1097–103.
26. Sugumar A, Levy MJ, Kamisawa T, JMW G, Kim MH, Enders F, Kim MH, Amin Z Z, Baron TH, Chapman MH, Church NI, Clain JE, Egawa N, Johnson GJ, Okazaki K, Pearson RK, Pereira SP, Petersen BT, Read S, Sah RP, Sandanayake NS, Takahashi N, Topazian MD, Uchida K, Vege SS, Chari ST. Endoscopic retrograde pancreatography criteria to diagnose autoimmune pancreatitis: an international multicentre study. Gut. 2011;60:666–70.
27. Kalaitzakis E, Levy M, Kamisawa T, Johnson G, Baron TH, Topazian M, Takahashi H, Kanno A, Okazaki K, Egawa N, Uchida K, Sheikh K, Amin Z, Shimosegawa T, Sandanayake N, Church NI, Chapman MH, Pereira S, Chari S, Webster G. Endoscopic retrograde cholangiography does not reliably distinguish IgG4-associated cholangitis from PSC or cholangiocarcinoma. Clin Gastroenterol Hepatol. 2011;9:800–803.
28. Sugumar A, Chari ST. Distinguishing pancreatic cancer from autoimmune pancreatitis: a comparison of two strategies. Clin Gastroenterol Hepatol. 2009;7:S59–62.
29. Department of Health. The NHS cancer plan and the new NHS. London: COI Communications; 2004.
30. Nishimori I, Tamakoshi A, Otsuki M. Prevalence of autoimmune pancreatitis in Japan from a nationwide survey in 2002. J Gastroenterol. 2007;42 Suppl 18:6–8.
31. Sandanayake N, Chapman MH, Kalaitzakis E, Amin Z, Novelli M, Winstanley A, Rodriguez-Justo M, Hatfield AR, Pereira SP, Webster GJ. Do steroids improve the long-term outcome of autoimmune pancreatitis? Gut. 2010;59:A1.
32. Raina A, Yadav D, Krasinskas AM, McGrath KM, Khalid A, Sanders M, Whitcomb DC, Slivka A. Evaluation and management of autoimmune pancreatitis: experience at a large US center. Am J Gastroenterol. 2009;104:2295–306.
33. Kamisawa T, Shimosegawa T, Okazaki K, Nishino T, Watanabe H, Kanno A, Okumura F, Nishikawa T, Kobayashi K, Ichiya T, Takatori H, Yamakita K, Kubota K, Hamano H, Okamura K, Hirano K, Ito T, Ko S, Omata M. Standard steroid therapy for autoimmune pancreatitis. Gut. 2009;58:1504–7.
34. Sah RP, Pannala R, Chari ST, Sugumar A, Clain JE, Levy MJ, Pearson RK, Smyrk TC, Petersen BT, Topazian MD, Takahashi N, Vege SS. Prevalence, diagnosis, and profile of autoimmune pancreatitis presenting with features of acute or chronic pancreatitis. Clin Gastroenterol Hepatol. 2010;8:91–6.
35. Hamano H, Arakura N, Muraki T, Ozaki Y, Kiyosawa K, Kawa S. Prevalence and distribution of extrapancreatic lesions complicating autoimmune pancreatitis. J Gastroenterol. 2006;41:1197–205.
36. Fujinaga Y, Kadoya M, Kawa S, Hamano H, Ueda K, Momose M, Kawakami S, Yamazaki S, Hatta T, Sugiyama Y. Characteristic findings in images of extra-pancreatic lesions associated with autoimmune pancreatitis. Eur J Radiol. 2010;76:228–38.
37. Webster GJ, Deheregoda MG, Church NI. Extrapancreatic manifestations in autoimmune pancreatitis. Minerva Gastroenterol Dietol. 2009;55:41–51.
38. Nishino T, Oyama H, Hashimoto E, Toki F, Oi I, Kobayashi M, Shiratori K. Clinicopathological differentiation between sclerosing cholangitis with autoimmune pancreatitis and primary sclerosing cholangitis. J Gastroenterol. 2007;42:550–9.
39. Okazaki K, Kawa S, Kamisawa T, Ito T, Inui K, Irie H, Irisawa A, Kubo K, Notohara K, Hasebe O, Fujinaga Y, Ohara H, Tanaka S, Nishino T, Nishimori I, Nishiyama T, Suda K, Shiratori K, Shimosegawa T, Tanaka M. Japanese clinical guidelines for autoimmune pancreatitis. Pancreas. 2009;38:849–66.
40. Sadler R, Chapman RW, Simpson D, Soonawalla ZF, Waldegrave EL, Burden JM, Misbah SA, Ferry BL. The diagnostic significance of serum IgG4 levels in patients with autoimmune pancreatitis: a UK study. Eur J Gastroenterol Hepatol. 2011;23:139–45.
41. Kamisawa T, Tu Y, Nakajima H, Egawa N, Tsuruta K, Okamoto A. Usefulness of biopsying the major duodenal papilla to diagnose autoimmune pancreatitis: a prospective study using IgG4-immunostaining. World J Gastroenterol. 2006;12:2031–3.
42. Kamisawa T, Egawa N, Nakajima H, Tsuruta K, Okamoto A. Morphological changes after steroid therapy in autoimmune pancreatitis. Scand J Gastroenterol. 2004;39:1154–8.
43. Nishino T, Toki F, Oyama H, Shimizu K, Shiratori K. Long-term outcome of autoimmune pancreatitis after oral prednisolone therapy. Intern Med. 2006; 45:497–501.
44. Ito T, Nishimori I, Inoue N, Kawabe K, Gibo J, Arita Y, Okazaki K, Takayanagi R, Otsuki M. Treatment for autoimmune pancreatitis: consensus on the treatment for patients with autoimmune pancreatitis in Japan. J Gastroenterol. 2007;42 Suppl 18:50–8.
45. Kamisawa T, Okamoto A, Wakabayashi T, Watanabe H, Sawabu N. Appropriate steroid therapy for autoimmune pancreatitis based on long-term outcome. Scand J Gastroenterol. 2008;43:609–13.
46. Webster G, Pereira S. Mesh-metal stents for hilar cholangiocarcinoma. Gastrointest Endosc. 2009; 70:817–8.
47. Kamisawa T, Yoshiike M, Egawa N, Nakajima H, Tsuruta K, Okamoto A. Treating patients with autoimmune pancreatitis: results from a long-term follow-up study. Pancreatology. 2005;5:234–8. discussion 238–40.
48. Kamisawa T, Egawa N, Inokuma S, Tsuruta K, Okamoto A, Kamata N, Nakamura T, Matsukawa M. Pancreatic endocrine and exocrine function and salivary gland function in autoimmune pancreatitis before and after steroid therapy. Pancreas. 2003; 27:235–8.

49. Nishimori I, Tamakoshi A, Kawa S, Tanaka S, Takeuchi K, Kamisawa T, Saisho H, Hirano K, Okamura K, Yanagawa N, Otsuki M. Influence of steroid therapy on the course of diabetes mellitus in patients with autoimmune pancreatitis: findings from a nationwide survey in Japan. Pancreas. 2006;32:244–8.
50. Kim KP, Kim MH, Song MH, Lee SS, Seo DW, Lee SK. Autoimmune chronic pancreatitis. Am J Gastroenterol. 2004;99:1605–16.
51. Kalaitzakis E, Webster GJ. Review article: autoimmune pancreatitis – management of an emerging disease. Aliment Pharmacol Ther. 2010. doi:10.1111/j.1365-2036.2010.04526.x.
52. Johnson PJ, McFarlane IG, Williams R. Azathioprine for long-term maintenance of remission in autoimmune hepatitis. N Engl J Med. 1995; 333:958–63.
53. Hegarty JE, Nouri Aria KT, Portmann B, Eddleston AL, Williams R. Relapse following treatment withdrawal in patients with autoimmune chronic active hepatitis. Hepatology. 1983;3:685–9.

# Japanese Experience

# 22

Kazuichi Okazaki and Kazushige Uchida

## Introduction

Autoimmune pancreatitis (AIP) is accepted worldwide as a distinctive type of pancreatitis [1–4]. Recent studies suggested two subtypes of AIP, type 1 related with IgG4 (lymphoplasmacytic sclerosing pancreatitis; LPSP) [5] and type 2 related with a granulocytic epithelial lesion (idiopathic duct-centric pancreatitis; IDCP) [6, 7]. In Japan, most cases of AIP are type 1, whereas type 2 AIP has been rarely reported. Features of type 1 AIP include increased serum IgG4 levels, abundant infiltration of IgG4+plasmacytes and lymphocytes, fibrosis, and steroid responsiveness, which suggest an autoimmune process. In addition to pancreatic manifestations, patients with type 1 AIP often have accompanying extrapancreatic lesions such as biliary lesions, sialadenitis, retroperitoneal fibrosis, enlarged celiac and hilar lymph nodes, chronic thyroiditis, and interstitial nephritis, suggesting that type 1 AIP may be a component of a multiorgan disorder [8–10], and the novel concept of IgG4-related disease has been proposed. On the other hand, patients with type 2 AIP rarely have organ involvement (OOI) except for ulcerative colitis. Although the pathogenesis of AIP still remains unknown, it is suspected that an autoimmune mechanism may be involved, although some debate whether type 2 AIP should be classified as an autoimmune disease [11]. The most important issue in the management of both types of AIP is to differentiate them from pancreatic and biliary tract malignancy. At the international consensus meeting for AIP sponsored by the International Association of Pancreatology (IAP) 2010 held in Fukuoka, international consensus criteria for both AIP subtypes were proposed [12]. Here, we present the Japanese experience of AIP in Japan.

K. Okazaki, M.D., Ph.D. (✉) • K. Uchida, M.D., Ph.D.
Department of Gastroenterology and Hepatology,
Kansai Medical University, 2-3-1, Shinmachi
Hirakata, Osaka, Japan 573-1191
e-mail: okazaki@takii.kmu.ac.jp

## Clinical Findings of Autoimmune Pancreatitis in Japan

1. Subtypes of AIP and Demographic Findings in Japan

   In Japan, most patients with AIP have type 1 (LPSP), whereas type 2 AIP (IDCP) is rarely observed. The Japanese Research Committee for Intractable Disease, supported by the Japanese Ministry of Labor, Health and Welfare, surveyed 546 cases of AIP from Japan in a nationwide study in 2007 [13] (Table 22.1) and predicted the incidence of 2.87 cases in 100,000 population (about 2,800 patients in Japan) with type 1 AIP, but only 7 cases of type 2 AIP have been histologically confirmed. The mean age at diagnosis was 62.6 years and the ratio of male to female was 4–1.

M.J. Levy and S.T. Chari (eds.), *Autoimmune (IgG4-related) Pancreatitis and Cholangitis*,
DOI 10.1007/978-1-4419-6430-4_22, 

**Table 22.1** Autoimmune pancreatitis in Japan (Ref. [13])

| Pancreas imaging | % in total | Diffuse (1/3<) | Focal (<1/3) | Unknown |
|---|---|---|---|---|
| Parenchyma on CT/MRI | | | | |
| Swelling | 88 | 68 % | 29 % | 3 % |
| Not swelling | 12 | ND | ND | ND |
| Pancreatic main duct on ERCP | | | | |
| Narrowing | 86 | 66 % | 32 % | 2 % |
| Without narrowing | 14 | | | |
| Serology | | High (%) | Normal (%) | Unknown (%) |
| Serum IgG (<1,800 mg/dl) | | 54 | 40 | 6 |
| Serum IgG4 (<134 mg/dl) | | 71 | 10 | 19 |
| Eosinophilia (< %) | | 3 | 58 | 39 |
| ANA (<x40) | | 28 | 56 | 16 |
| RF | | 16 | 42 | 42 |
| AMA | | 2 | 34 | 64 |
| Anti-SSa/SSb | | 2 | 50 | 48 |
| Histology | | | % in the total cases | |
| Confirmed LPSP | | | 43 | |
| With EUS-FNA | | | 16.8 | |
| With EUS-TCB | | | 0.7 | |
| With percutaneous biopsy | | | 7.9 | |
| Resected pancreas | | | 9.3 | |
| Other organs | | | | |
| Duodenal papilla | | | 1.1 | |
| Salivary gland | | | 3.3 | |
| Bile duct | | | 6.4 | |
| OOI | | Definite (%) | Probable (%) | None (%) |
| Sclerosing cholangitis | | 52.9 | 3.8 | 43.2 |
| Sclerosing sialadenitis | | 13.9 | 2.6 | 83.5 |
| Swelling of lachrymal glands | | 6.6 | 1.3 | |
| Retroperitoneal fibrosis | | 8.1 | 1.6 | 92.1 |
| Chronic thyroiditis | | 2.6 | 0.5 | 90.2 |
| Interstitial pneumonia | | 3.7 | 1.1 | 96.8 |
| Interstitial nephritis | | 2.6 | 1.8 | 95.2 |
| Swelling of lymph node | | 12.6 | 0.5 | 86.8 |
| Pseudotumor | | 1.5 | 0.7 | 97.8 |
| Steroid and treatment | | With (%) | Without (%) | Unknown (%) |
| Steroid | | | | |
| Diagnostic trial | | 6.6 | 89.9 | 3.4 |
| For treatment | | 83 | 16.7 | 0.4 |
| Other treatment | | | | |
| Biliary drainage for jaundice | | 41.4 | 52.9 | 5.7 |
| Surgical resection | | 9.2 | 86.8 | 4 |

**Table 22.2** Clinical symptoms in autoimmune pancreatitis

| | |
|---|---|
| Obstructive jaundice | 33–59 % |
| Abdominal pain | 32 % |
| Back pain | 15 % |
| Body weight loss | 15 % |
| Anorexia | 9 % |
| General fatigue | 9 % |
| Abnormal stool | 7 % |
| Fever | 6 % |
| No symptoms | 15 % |

Ref. [14]

2. Clinical Symptoms of AIP in Japan (Table 22.2)

   Although most patients show mild or no abdominal pain, a few cases of acute or severe pancreatitis have been reported. In Japan, one third to one half of the patients show obstructive jaundice or mild abdominal pain, and 15 % have shown back pain or weight loss [14–16]. More than half of the cases are associated with sclerosing cholangitis, diabetes mellitus, sclerosing sialadenitis/dacryoadenitis, or retroperitoneal fibrosis, showing, in some cases, obstructive jaundice, polydipsia/polyuria or malaise, xerostomia/xerophthalmia, or hydronephrosis, respectively.
3. Pancreas Imaging of AIP in Japan with Special Reference to Diffuse and Segmental/Focal Mass Type

   Since most cases in Japan show a diffusely enlarged pancreas and narrowing of the main pancreatic duct (MPD), it is believed that typical AIP lesions involve more than one third of the pancreas; however, there are also cases of focal, segmental, or mass-forming types [11, 14]. In the Japanese nationwide study [13] (Table 22.1), diffuse enlargement involving more than one third of the entire pancreas on CT/MRI was observed in 67 % and focal enlargement with less than one third in 30 %. Irregular narrowing of the MPD on ERCP images was observed in 86 % of patients, in which 66 % had diffuse narrowing involving more than one third of the gland.
4. Serological Findings of AIP in Japan

   Immunological examinations show high incidences of hypergammaglobulinemia (43 %), increased levels of serum total IgG (62–80 %), increased levels of serum

IgG4(68–92 %) [14–16], antinuclear antibodies (28–64 %), and rheumatoid factor (25 %) [15, 18], although these are not disease specific. Some reports have shown the presence of autoantibodies, such as anti-carbonic anhydrase II antibodies (55 %) or anti-lactoferrin antibodies (75 %), in patients with AIP in high frequency, and these tests are not readily obtainable and their utility has not been validated [11–18]. Anti-SSa/SSb antibodies or antimitochondrial antibodies, on the other hand, are rarely seen [11–13]. Among all serological diagnostic tests, the serum IgG4 level offers the highest diagnostic utility, providing a sensitivity and specificity of 80 % and 98 %, respectively [19]. The test is limited by the lack of disease specificity. The sensitivity and specificity of serum total IgG are 70 % and 75 %, respectively, and antinuclear antibodies (ANA) and rheumatoid factor (RF) are detected in 60 % and 20–30 % of patients, respectively [19]. Even when the result of serum total IgG is combined with ANA or RF, the sensitivity is 91 %, but the specificity is 61 %. While the specificity of serum total IgG is lower than that of serum IgG4, the sensitivity of both tests is comparable (Table 22.3) [19].

In the Japanese nationwide study (Table 22.1), increased serum levels of IgG (2,066 mg/dl on average) and IgG4 (522 mg/dl on average) were observed in 54 % and 71 % of patients, respectively [13]. ANA and RF were positive in 28 % and 16 % of the cases, respectively. On the other hand, antimitochondrial antibody (AMA) or anti-SSa/SSb antibody was identified only 1.6 % and 1.3 %, respectively. Peripheral blood shows eosinophilia in 13 % of patients. Histological findings were confirmed as LPSP in 43 % of the cases.

5. Other Organ Involvement (OOI) in Japan

A variety of extrapancreatic lesions are associated with AIP including lachrymal and salivary gland lesions [20], hilar lymphadenopathy [21], sclerosing cholangitis [22, 23], retroperitoneal fibrosis [24], and tubulointerstitial nephritis [25]. These extrapancreatic lesions share the same pathological conditions and showed favorable response to corticosteroid therapy, indicating the presence of a common pathophysiological background. The prevalence of extrapancreatic lesions (Table 22.4) [26–29] suggests that AIP may represent one component of a multiorgan disorder referred to as IgG4-related diseases (IgG4-RD). Manifestations of extrapancreatic lesions may precede or occur after the clinical onset of AIP and may lead to diagnostic uncertainty. However, recognition of these extrapancreatic lesions may also aid in the diagnosis of AIP.

In the Japanese nationwide study [13], the rates for specific sites of OOI were 52.9 % in sclerosing cholangitis, 13.9 % in sclerosing sialadenitis, 6.6 % for lachrymal gland involvement, 8.1 % in retroperitoneal fibrosis, 2.6 % in chronic thyroiditis, 3.7 % in interstitial pneumonia, 2.6 % in interstitial nephritis, 12.6 % for benign lymphadenopathy, and 1.5 % for pseudotumor formation.

6. Diagnostic Procedure in Japan by Using JPS-2006 and Asian Criteria

Various diagnostic criteria for AIP have been proposed, including those from Japan [30], Korea [31, 32], Mayo [33], and Asia [34]. As corticosteroid therapy is usually effective, a steroid response is included in the diagnostic

**Table 22.3** Comparison of various markers in the differentiation between autoimmune pancreatitis and pancreatic cancer using identical sera

| | Sensitivity (AIP $n=100$) (%) | Specificity (vs. PC $n=80$) (%) | Accuracy (vs. PC) (%) |
|---|---|---|---|
| IgG4 | 86 | 96 | 91 |
| IgG | 69 | 75 | 72 |
| ANA(antinuclear antibody) | 58 | 79 | 67 |
| RF(rheumatoid factor) | 23 | 94 | 54 |
| IgG4+ANA | 95 | 76 | 87 |
| IgG+ANA | 85 | 63 | 75 |
| IgG4+IgG+ANA | 95 | 94 | 81 |
| IgG4+RF | 90 | 90 | 90 |
| IgG+RF | 78 | 73 | 76 |
| IgG4+IgG+RF | 91 | 71 | 82 |
| ANA+RF | 69 | 60 | 78 |
| IgG4+ANA+RF | 97 | 73 | 86 |
| IgG+ANA+RF | 91 | 61 | 78 |
| IgG4+IgG+ANA+RF | 97 | 61 | 81 |

Ref. [15]

*AIP* autoimmune pancreatitis, *PC* pancreatic cancer

**Table 22.4** Extrapancreatic lesions complicated with autoimmune pancreatitis

| |
|---|
| Close association |
| Lachrymal gland inflammation |
| Sialadenitis |
| Hilar lymphadenopathy |
| Interstitial pneumonitis |
| Sclerosing cholangitis |
| Retroperitoneal fibrosis |
| Tubulointerstitial nephritis |
| Possible association |
| Hypophysitis |
| Autoimmune neurosensory hearing loss |
| Uveitis |
| Chronic thyroiditis |
| Pseudotumor (breast, lung, liver) |
| Gastric ulcer |
| Swelling of papilla of vater |
| IgG4 hepatopathy |
| Aortitis |
| Prostatitis |
| Schonlein-Henoch purpura |
| Autoimmune thrombocytopenia |

Ref. [15]

**Table 22.5** Clinical diagnostic criteria of autoimmune pancreatitis 2006 (JPS-2006) (Proposed by the Research Committee of Intractable Diseases of the Pancreas supported by the Japanese Ministry of Health, Labor and Welfare and Japan Pancreas Society)

| |
|---|
| I. Clinical diagnostic criteria |
| 1. Diffuse or segmental narrowing of the main pancreatic duct with irregular wall and diffuse or localized enlargement of the pancreas by imaging studies, such as abdominal ultrasonography (US), computed tomography (CT), and magnetic resonance imaging (MRI) |
| 2. High serum γ-globulin, IgG or IgG4, or the presence of autoantibodies, such as antinuclear antibodies and rheumatoid factor |
| 3. Marked interlobular fibrosis and prominent infiltration of lymphocytes and plasma cells in the periductal area, occasionally with lymphoid follicles in the pancreas |
| For diagnosis, criterion 1 must be present, together with criterion 2 and/or 3 |
| Diagnosis of autoimmune pancreatitis is established when criterion 1 together with criterion 2 and/or 3 is fulfilled |
| However, it is necessary to exclude malignant diseases such as pancreatic or biliary cancers |

Ref. [30]

criteria proposed by Korea and Mayo but is excluded from the Japanese criteria [14–16].

(i) JPS-2006 Criteria

The Japan Pancreas Society proposed the world's first clinical diagnostic criteria for AIP in 2002, which was later revised in 2006 by the joint efforts of the Research Committee of the Intractable Pancreatic Diseases, supported by the Ministry of Health, Labor and Welfare of Japan and the Japan Pancreas Society [30] (Table 22.5, Fig. 22.1). The basic concepts were established based on the following minimal consensus criteria: (1) the criteria may be applied not only by a pancreatologist or gastroenterologist but also by the primary care physician; (2) the criteria are used to distinguish and exclude malignant disorders such as pancreatic cancer or bile duct cancer as much as possible; (3) in terms of pathology, the criteria are applied to clinical cases showing evidence of LPSP; (4) the criteria are used to diagnose pancreatic lesions, although the disease may be systemic; and (5) a diagnostic trial of steroid therapy is not recommended. The decision tree for the diagnosis is based on (1) specific image findings (a mandatory requirement), along with (2) hematological and/or (3) histopathological evidence [2–4, 14].

According to the clinical diagnostic criteria 2006, the pancreatic images used to evaluate AIP may include those previously obtained [14, 30]. Although some patients with pancreatic cancer show high levels of serum IgG4, patients with AIP tend to demonstrate higher levels of serum IgG4, although overlap may exist [14, 15, 30–34]. Diagnostic criteria for AIP have also been proposed by Korea [32] and the Mayo Clinic in the United States [33]. The Asian diagnostic criteria were proposed jointly by researchers in Japan and Korea [34] (Table 22.6,

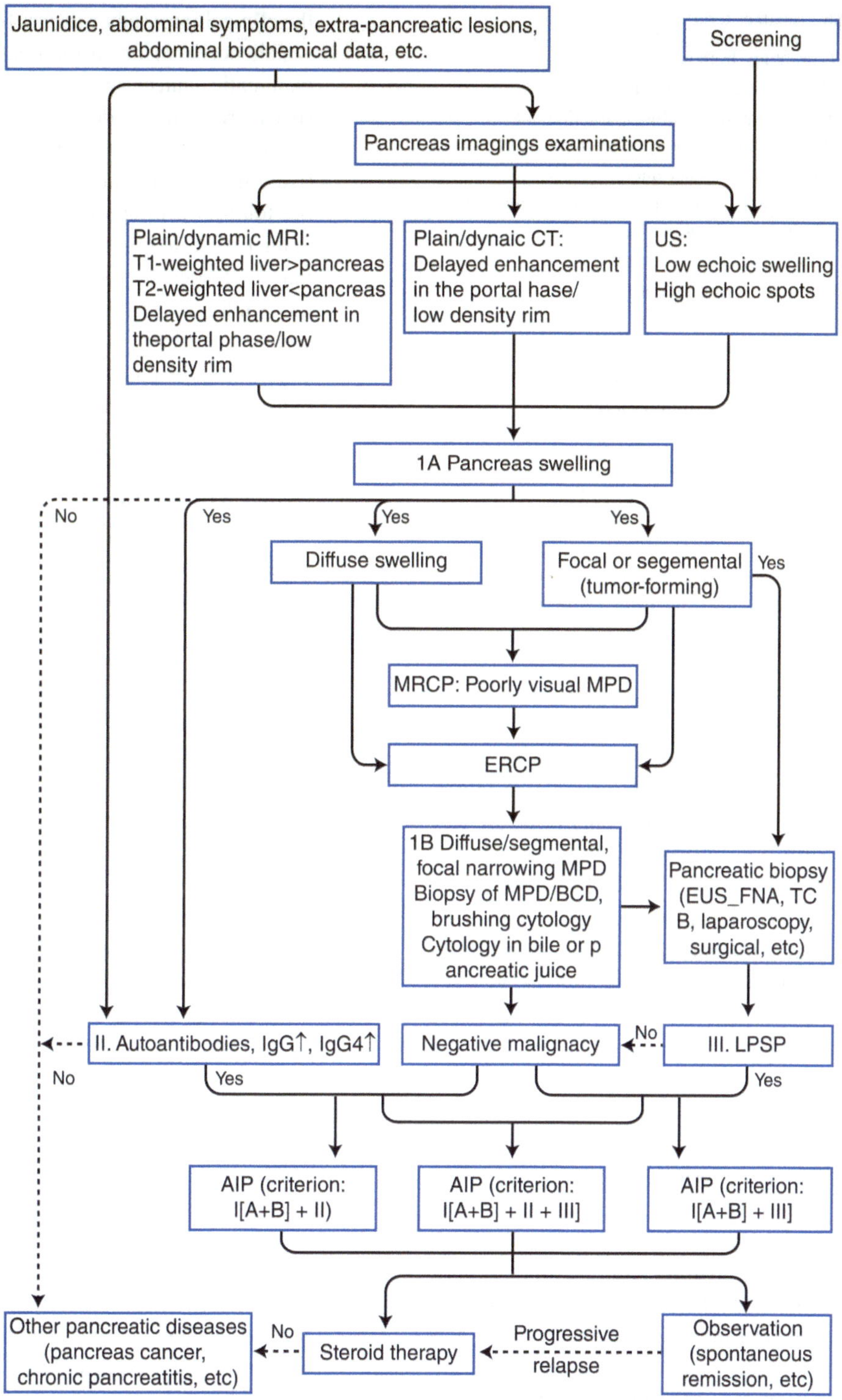


**Fig. 22.1** Algorithm of diagnosis and management of AIP by the Japanese diagnostic criteria 2006 (Ref. [14])

**Table 22.6** Asian criteria

| |
|---|
| Criterion I. Imaging (both required) |
| Imaging of pancreatic parenchyma |
| Diffusely/segmentally/focally enlarged gland, occasionally with mass and/or hypoattenuation rim |
| Imaging of pancreaticobiliary ducts |
| Diffuse/segmental/focal pancreatic ductal narrowing, often with the stenosis of bile duct |
| Criterion II. Serology (one required) |
| Elevated level of serum IgG or IgG4 |
| Detected autoantibodies |
| Criterion III. Histopathology of pancreatic biopsy lesion |
| Lymphoplasmacytic infiltration in fibrosis, common with abundant IgG4-positive cell infiltration |
| *Option: response to steroids |
| Diagnostic trial of steroid therapy could be done carefully in patients fulfilling criterion 1 alone with negative workup for pancreatobiliary cancer by experts |
| Diagnosis of AIP is made when any two criteria including criterion I are satisfied or histology of lymphoplasmacytic sclerosing pancreatitis is present in the *resected pancreas* |

Ref. [34]

Fig. 22.2). Use of the response to steroid treatment as a diagnostic option is permitted for specialists only in Japan. Key differences between Japan and Western approaches to AIP are the role of ERCP images, response to steroid treatment, and extrapancreatic lesions in establishing the diagnosis. Although the presence of extrapancreatic lesions is not formally listed as a diagnostic tool in the Japanese diagnostic criteria 2006 or the Asian diagnostic criteria, a complete examination is important because the presence of extrapancreatic lesions may be indicative of AIP.

In Japanese criteria, steroid effects on pancreatic and extrapancreatic lesions are excluded from AIP diagnosis for the following reasons: (i) the effect of steroid treatment as a diagnostic criterion for autoimmune diseases is not used except for autoimmune hepatitis; (ii) the disease that needs to be differentiated from autoimmune hepatitis is chronic hepatitis of other pathogenesis; the clinical importance differs from AIP, which needs to be differentiated from pancreatic cancer or bile duct cancer; (iii) there is no evidence to show that steroid administration does not negatively impact the outcome of surgery or the long-term prognosis; (iv) there is a danger that a diagnostic steroid trial may be too easily performed foregoing more intense efforts to exclude a pancreatic cancer; (v) the standards were established for pancreatologists, gastroenterologists, and primary care physicians; (vi) in Japan, the prime objective of the diagnostic criteria is not so much to find AIP but rather to eliminate the misdiagnosis of malignant tumors; and (vii) there have been reports of AIP associated with pancreatic cancer [2].

(ii) Asian Criteria

The Asian diagnostic criteria proposed by Japanese and Korean specialists in 2008 [34] state that if pancreatic cancer has been rigorously sought and excluded by efforts such as endoscopic ultrasonography (EUS)-guided fine-needle aspiration (EUS-guided FNA), the steroid trial may be used as optional diagnostic criteria. However, one must be mindful of the false negative rate of EUS-FNA that may be as high as 10–40 %. In addition, there are reports of pancreatic cancers occurring in the setting of AIP. It is unclear if there is any causal role of AIP in pancreatic cancer, or if patients developed both entities separately, or if these patients had a false diagnosis of AIP. Therefore, if a patient responds to steroid treatment, it may suggest that he/she has AIP; however, it does not exclude the coexistence of malignant tumors such as pancreatic cancer or biliary cancer [15, 16].

(iii) JPS-2011 Criteria [35, 36]

In response to the proposal of International Consensus of Diagnostic Criteria (ICDC) for AIP, the JPS has

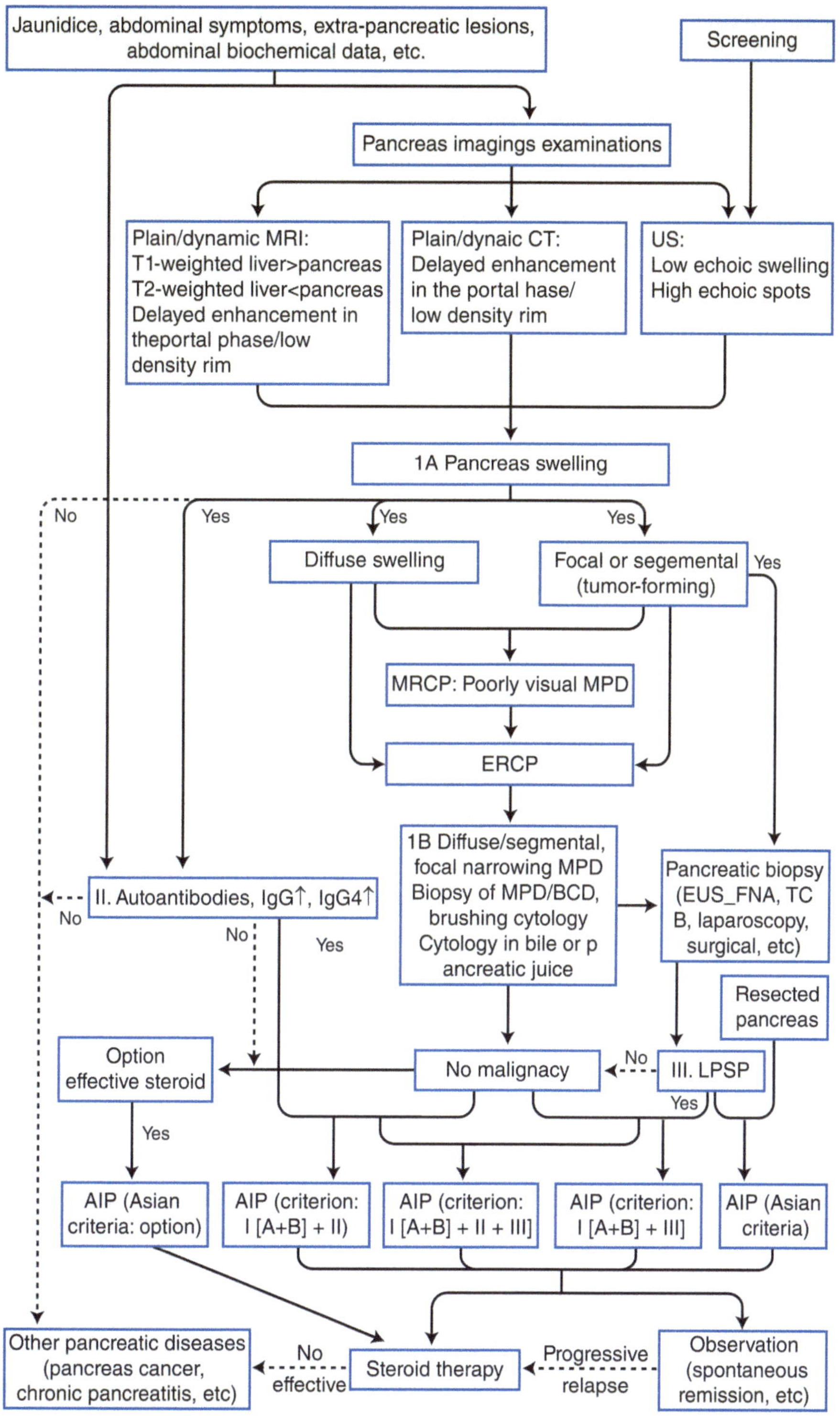


**Fig. 22.2** Algorithm of diagnosis and management of AIP by Asian diagnostic criteria (Ref. [14])

most recently proposed the JPS-2011 for type 1 AIP (Table 22.7).

(iv) Comparison of Diagnostic Criteria

In Japan, patients have been diagnosed with AIP using revised JPS criteria from 2006 or Asian criteria proposed in 2008. In a prospective study for the comparison of diagnostic criteria, the Korean or Asian criteria were most sensitive. In Kansai Medical University, 30 of 275 patients with pancreatic diseases were prospectively screened by at least 2 of the following including the elevation of pancreatic enzymes; swelling of the pancreas by US, CT, or MRI; and abnormal immunological findings. Twenty-one of 30 patients (M/F 13/8, mean 62 year) were diagnosed as having "definite AIP" at the time of initial evaluation with 9 patients diagnosed with "suspected AIP" that was confirmed based on their subsequent course. The sensitivity of Japanese-2006, Korean, and the original Mayo criteria were 71.4 %, 76.2 %, and 52.3 %, respectively, with 100 % of specificity for all sets of criteria. The Korean criteria are believed to provide the greatest diagnostic sensitivity. These findings suggest that if steroid response and autoantibody are included in the criteria, then diagnostic sensitivity should be increased.

Most recently, the ICDC for both types of AIP and JPS-2011 for type 1 AIP have been proposed. Although a prospective study is needed to validate these criteria, our previous cases showed that the sensitivity of ICDC (95.1 % for both types) and JPS-2011 (93.4 % for type1) is superior to other criteria [36].

7. Pancreatic Exocrine and Endocrine Function in AIP

While pancreatic exocrine and endocrine dysfunctions have been reported to improve with steroid therapy when clinically evident pancreatic dysfunction occurred, we believe that steroid therapy provided minimal improvement in function. Pancreatic exocrine dysfunction is seen in 83 to 88 % of the cases and diabetes mellitus in 42–78 % [37, 38]. By the national survey of the Japanese Research Committee, 66.5 % of AIP cases were associated with diabetes mellitus; of those, 33.3 % had diabetes mellitus diagnosed prior to the onset of AIP and 51.6 % thereafter. Among those patients having diabetes mellitus, 14 % developed diabetes after steroid treatment [37–40], suggesting that such diabetes may be caused by long-term steroid treatment. However, it is also possible that diabetes is a part of the natural disease course.

In AIP, the mechanisms of exocrine and endocrine dysfunction have not been clearly elucidated. However, pancreatic exocrine dysfunction is assumed to develop secondary to decreased pancreatic enzyme secretion associated with collapsed acinar cells caused by pronounced cellular infiltration mainly of plasmacytes and fibrosis and by obstructed flow of pancreatic juice due to inflammatory cell infiltration and the resulting narrowing around the pancreatic ducts [37–40]. In contrast, diabetes mellitus is assumed to develop secondary to impaired blood flow in the islets glands and damaged function of the islets of Langerhans due to fibrosis and inflammation.

8. Steroid Trial and Treatment

Facile steroid trial is not recommended in the Japanese criteria but is acceptable only by experts after a workup of malignancy in Asian, ICDC, and JPS-2011 criteria. In the nationwide study, a steroid trial was performed in 6.6 % of all cases. On the other hand, steroids were administered in 83 % of the patients after diagnosing AIP. The indications for steroid therapy in AIP patients are symptoms such as obstructive jaundice, abdominal and back pain, and the presence of symptomatic extrapancreatic lesions. In cases with obstructive jaundice due to bile duct stenosis, endoscopic or transhepatic biliary drainage should be performed. Cytological examination of the bile duct is necessary to help exclude malignancy. Steroid therapy can be started without biliary drainage in cases with mild jaundice, but such patients should be followed closely. Blood glucose levels should be controlled in patients

**Table 22.7** Clinical diagnostic criteria for autoimmune pancreatitis 2011 [35]

*A. Diagnostic criterion*

I. Enlargement of the pancreas
- (a) Diffuse enlargement
- (b) Segmental/focal enlargement

II. ERP (endoscopic retrograde pancreatography) shows irregular narrowing of the main pancreatic duct

III. Serological findings
Elevated levels of serum IgG4 (≥135 mg/dl)

IV. Pathological findings among i) ~ iv) listed below
- (a) Three or more are observed
- (b) Two are observed
- (i) Prominent infiltration and fibrosis of lymphocytes and plasmacytes
- (ii) Ten or more diffuse IgG4-positive plasmacytes per high-power microscope field
- (iii) Storiform fibrosis
- (iv) Obliterative phlebitis

V. Other organ involvement (OOI): sclerosing cholangitis, sclerosing dacryoadenitis/sialadenitis, retroperitoneal fibrosis
- (a) Clinical lesions
Extrapancreatic sclerosing cholangitis, sclerosing dacryoadenitis/sialadenitis (Mikulicz disease), or retroperitoneal fibrosis can be diagnosed with clinical and image findings
- (b) Pathological lesions
Pathological examination shows characteristic features of sclerosing cholangitis, sclerosing dacryoadenitis/sialadenitis, or retroperitoneal fibrosis

<Option> Effectiveness of steroid therapy

A specialized facility may include in its diagnosis the effectiveness of steroid therapy, once pancreatic or bile duct cancers have been ruled out. When it is difficult to differentiate from malignant conditions, it is desirable to perform cytological examination using an endoscopic ultrasound-guided fine-needle aspiration (EUS-FNA). Facile therapeutic diagnosis by steroids should be avoided unless the possibility of malignant tumor has been ruled out by pathological diagnosis

*B. Diagnosis*

I. Definite diagnosis
1. Diffuse type: I a + <III/IVb/V(a/b)>
2. Segmental/focal type:
I b + II + two or more of <III/IV b/V (a/b)>
I b + II + <III/IV b/V (a/b)> + option
3. Definite diagnosis by histopathological study: IV a

II. Probable diagnosis
Segmental/focal type: I b + II + <III/IVb/V (a/b)>

III. Possible diagnosis[a]
Diffuse type: I a + II + option
Segmental/focal type: I b + II + option

When a patient with a focal/segmental image of AIP on CT/MRI without ERCP findings fulfills more than one of III, IVb, and V(a/b) criteria, he/she can be diagnosed as possible AIP only after the negative workup for malignancy by EUS-FNA and confirmed as probable one by an optional steroid response

[a]A case may be possibly type 2, although it is extremely rare in Japan

"+" refers to "and", and "/" refers to "or"

with diabetes mellitus before steroid therapy [41]. Since there was no correlation between the degree of morphological improvement of the pancreatic and bile ducts and the initial prednisolone dose (30 or 40 mg/day), it is recommended that the initial oral prednisolone dose is 0.6 mg/kg/day, with a gradual taper after 2–4 weeks [42]. After 2–4 weeks at the initial dose, the dose is tapered by 5 mg every 1–2 weeks, based on changes in the clinical manifestations, biochemical blood tests (such as liver enzymes and IgG or IgG4 levels), and repeated imaging findings (US, CT, MRCP, ERCP, etc.). The dose is tapered to a maintenance

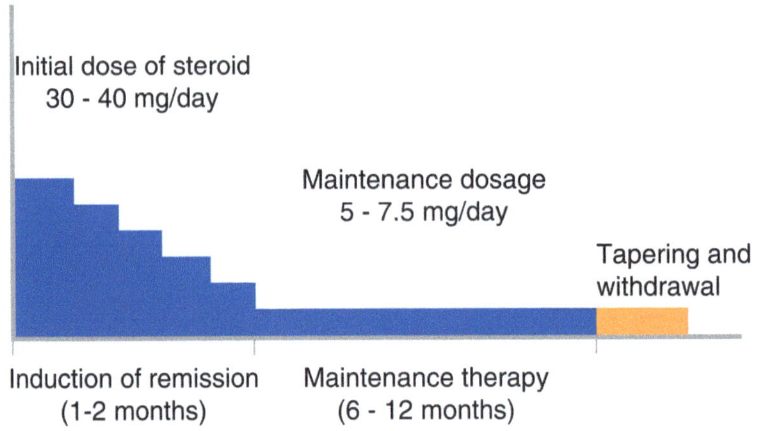


**Fig. 22.3** Treatment of AIP (Ref. [46])

dose over a period of 2–3 months. Maintenance therapy is effective to prevent relapse (Fig. 22.3). However, since AIP patients are typically elderly and are at high risk of developing steroid-related complications such as osteoporosis and diabetes mellitus, an effort to discontinue the medication should be made. Stopping of maintenance therapy should be planned within at least 3 years in cases with radiological and serological improvement. After stopping medication, patients should be followed for evidence of disease relapse. Biliary drainage for jaundice and surgical resection is preformed in 41.4 % and 9.2 %, respectively.

9. Prognosis of AIP in Japan

Swelling of the pancreas or irregular narrowing of the main pancreatic duct improves spontaneously without steroid therapy in some AIP patients. It has been reported that most AIP cases that improved spontaneously did not have bile duct stenosis [43, 44]. According to Kamisawa et al [43], spontaneous improvement was detected in 2 of 21 non-jaundiced AIP patients. Kubota et al. compared the clinicopathological parameters in 8 AIP patients with remission in the absence of steroid therapy and 12 patients with remission after steroid therapy. They found an association between remission in the absence of steroid therapy and seronegativity for IgG4, absence of obstructive jaundice, absence of diabetes mellitus, and the presence of focal pancreatic swelling [44]. The prognosis of AIP appears to be good over the short term with steroid therapy. Japanese patients with AIP frequently (<6 M,32 %; <1 year,56 %; <3 year,92 %) show relapse of the disease after or during the steroid therapy [42]. It is unclear whether the long-term outcome is good, because there are many unknown factors such as relapse, pancreatic exocrine or endocrine dysfunction, and associated malignancy [45–47].

**Acknowledgments** This study was partially supported by (1) Grant-in-Aid for Scientific Research (C) of the Ministry of Culture and Science of Japan (23591017, 24591020), (2) Research Program Intractable Diseases, from Minister of Labor and Welfare of Japan, and (3) grants-in-aid from the Ministry of Education, Culture, Sports, Science and Technology of Japan, from CREST Japan Science and Technology Agency.

## References

1. Yoshida K, Toki F, Takeuchi T, et al. Chronic pancreatitis caused by an autoimmune abnormality. Proposal of the concept of autoimmune pancreatitis. Dig Dis Sci. 1995;40:1561–8.
2. Okazaki K, Chiba T. Autoimmune-related pancreatitis. Gut. 2002;51:1–4.
3. Pickartz T, Mayerle J, Lerch MM. Autoimmune pancreatitis. Nat Clin Pract Gastroenterol Hepatol. 2007;4(6):314–23.

4. Gardner TB, Chari ST. Autoimmune pancreatitis. Gastroenterol Clin North Am. 2008;37:439–60.
5. Kawaguchi K, Koike M, Tsuruta K, et al. Lymphoplasmacytic sclerosing pancreatitis with cholangitis: a variant primary sclerosing cholangitis extensively involving pancreas. Hum Pahtol. 1991;22: 387–95.
6. Notohara K, Burgart LJ, Yadav D, et al. Idiopathic chronic pancreatitis with periductal lymphoplasmacytic infiltration: clinicopathologic features of 35 cases. Am J Surg Pathol. 2003;27:1119–27.
7. Zamboni G, Luttges J, Capelli P, et al. Histopathological features of diagnostic and clinical relevance in autoimmune pancreatitis: a study on 53 resection specimens and 9 biopsy specimens. Virchows Arch. 2004;445:552–63.
8. Kamisawa T, Funata N, Hayashi Y, et al. A new clinicopathological entity of IgG4-related autoimmune disease. J Gastroenterol. 2003;38:982–4.
9. Yamamoto M, Takahashi H, Ohara M, et al. Mod Rheumatol. 2006;16:335–40.
10. Masaki Y, Dong L, Kurose N, et al. Proposal for a new clinical entity, IgG4-positive multi-organ lymphoproliferative syndrome: analysis of 64 cases of IgG4-related disorders. Ann Rheum Dis. 2009;68:1310–5.
11. Chari ST, Kloeppel G, Zhang L, et al. Histopathologic and clinical subtypes of autoimmune pancreatitis: the Honolulu consensus document. Pancreas. 2010; 39(5):549–54.
12. Shimosegawa T, Chari ST, Frulloni L, et al. International consensus diagnostic criteria for autoimmune pancreatitis. Pancreatology. 2011;40:352–8.
13. Nishimori I, Shimosegawa T, et al. Nationwide survey for autoimmune pancreatitis in Japan. Annual reports of research committee of intractable pancreatic diseases supported by Ministry of Health, Labour and Welfare of Japan. 2010;125–36. (In Japanese).
14. Okazaki K, Kawa S, Kamisawa T, Shimosegawa T, Tanaka M, Research Committee for Intractable Pancreatic Disease and Japan Pancreas Society. Japanese consensus guidelines for management of autoimmune pancreatitis: I. Concept and diagnosis of autoimmune pancreatitis. J Gastroenterol. 2010; 45(3):249–65.
15. Kawa S, Okazaki K, Kamisawa T, Shimosegawa T, Tanaka M, Working members of Research Committee for Intractable Pancreatic Disease and Japan Pancreas Society. Japanese consensus guidelines for management of autoimmune pancreatitis: II. Extrapancreatic lesions, differential diagnosis. J Gastroenterol. 2010;45(4):355–69.
16. Kamisawa T, Okazaki K, Kawa S, Shimosegawa T, Tanaka M, Research Committee for Intractable Pancreatic Disease and Japan Pancreas Society. Japanese consensus guidelines for management of autoimmune pancreatitis: III. Treatment and prognosis of AIP. J Gastroenterol. 2010;45(5):471–7.
17. Hamano H, Kawa S, Horiuchi A, et al. High serum IgG4 concentrations in patients with sclerosing pancreatitis. N Engl J Med. 2001;344:732–8.
18. Okazaki K, Uchida K, Ohana M, et al. Autoimmune-related pancreatitis is associated with autoantibodies and a Thl/Th2-type cellular immune response. Gastroenterology. 2000;118:573–81.
19. Kawa S. Immunological aspects of autoimmune pancreatitis. Nippon Shokakibyo Gakkai Zasshi. 2008; 105(4):494–501. in Japanese.
20. Kamisawa T, Funata N, Hayashi Y, et al. Close relationship between autoimmune pancreatitis and multifocal fibrosclerosis. Gut. 2003;52:683–7.
21. Yoshimura Y, Takeda S, Ieki Y, et al. IgG4-associated prostatitis complicating autoimmune pancreatitis. Intern Med. 2006;45:897–901.
22. Erkelens GW, Vleggaar FP, Lesterhuis W, et al. Sclerosing pancreato-cholangitis responsive to steroid therapy. Lancet. 1999;354:43–4.
23. Nakazawa T, Ohara H, Yamada T, et al. Atypical primary sclerosing cholangitis cases associated with unusual pancreatitis. Hepatogastroenterology. 2001;48:625–30.
24. Hamano H, Kawa S, Ochi Y, et al. Hydronephrosis associated with retroperitoneal fibrosis and sclerosing pancreatitis. Lancet. 2002;359:1403–4.
25. Takeda S, Haratake J, Kasai T, et al. IgG4-associated idiopathic tubulointerstitial nephritis complicating autoimmune pancreatitis. Nephrol Dial Transplant. 2004;19:474–6.
26. van der Vliet HJ, Perenboom RM. Multiple pseudotumors in IgG4-associated multifocal systemic fibrosis. Ann Intern Med. 2004;141:896–7.
27. Komatsu K, Hamano H, Ochi Y, et al. High prevalence of hypothyroidism in patients with autoimmune pancreatitis. Dig Dis Sci. 2005;50:1052–7.
28. Ohara H, Nakazawa T, Sano H, et al. Systemic extra-pancreatic lesions associated with autoimmune pancreatitis. Pancreas. 2005;31:232–7.
29. Hamano H, Arakura N, Muraki T, et al. Prevalence and distribution of extrapancreatic lesions complicating autoimmune pancreatitis. J Gastroenterol. 2006; 41:1197–205.
30. Okazaki K, Kawa S, Kamisawa T, et al. Clinical diagnostic criteria of autoimmune pancreatitis: revised proposal. J Gastroenterol. 2006;41:626–31.
31. Kim K, Kim MW, Kim JC, et al. Diagnostic criteria for autoimmune pancreatitis revisited. World J Gastroenterol. 2006;12:2487–96.
32. Kim MH, Lee TY. Diagnostic criteria for autoimmune pancreatitis (AIP); A proposal of revised Kim criteria. J Gastroenterol Hepatol. 2007;22 Suppl 2:A104.
33. Chari ST, Smyrk TC, Levy MJ, et al. Diagnosis of autoimmune pancreatitis: the Mayo Clinic experience. Clin Gastroenterol Hepatol. 2006;4:1010–6.
34. Otsuki M, Chung JB, Okazaki K, et al. Asian diagnostic criteria for autoimmune pancreatitis: consensus of the Japan-Korea symposium on autoimmune pancreatitis. J Gastroenterol. 2008;43:403–8.
35. The Japan Pancreas Society, the Ministry of Health and Welfare Investigation Research Team for Intractable Pancreatic Disease. Clinical diagnostic for autoimmune pancreatitis 2011 (Proposal) (in Japanese with English abstract). J Jpn Pancreas (Suizo). 2012; 27:17–25.

36. Sumimoto K, Uchida K, Mitsuyama T, et al. A proposal of a diagnostic algorithm with validation of International Consensus Diagnostic Criteria for autoimmune pancreatitis in a Japanese cohort. Pancreatology. 2013;13:230–7.
37. Nishimori I, Tamakoshi A, Kawa S, et al. Influence of steroid therapy on the course of diabetes mellitus in patients with autoimmune pancreatitis: findings from a nationwide survey in Japan. Pancreas. 2006;32:244–8.
38. Kamisawa T, Egawa N, Inokuma S, et al. Pancreatic endocrine and exocrine function and salivary gland function in autoimmune pancreatitis before and after steroid therapy. Pancreas. 2003;27:235–8.
39. Ito T, Kawabe K, Arita Y, et al. Evaluation of pancreatic endocrine and exocrine function in patients with autoimmune pancreatitis. Pancreas. 2007;34:254–9.
40. Tanaka S, Kobayashi T, Nakanishi K, et al. Corticosteroid-responsive diabetes mellitus associated with autoimmune pancreatitis. Lancet. 2000;356:910–1.
41. Ito T, Nishimori I, Inoue N, et al. Treatment for autoimmune pancreatitis: consensus on the treatment for patients with autoimmune pancreatitis in Japan. J Gastroenterol. 2007;42 Suppl 18:50–8.
42. Kamisawa T, Shimosegawa T, Okazaki K, et al. Standard steroid therapy for autoimmune pancreatitis. Gut. 2009;58(11):1504–7.
43. Kamisawa T, Yoshiike M, Egawa N, et al. Treating patients with autoimmune pancreatitis: results from a long-term follow-up study. Pancreatology. 2005;5: 234–40.
44. Kubota K, Iida H, Fujisawa T, et al. Clinical factors predictive of spontaneous remission or relapse in cases of autoimmune pancreatitis. Gastrointest Endosc. 2007;66:1142–51.
45. Kamisawa T, Okamoto A, Wakabayashi T, et al. Appropriate steroid therapy for autoimmune pancreatitis based on long-term outcome. Scand J Gastroenterol. 2008;43:609–13.
46. Hirano K, Tada M, Isayama H, et al. Long-term prognosis of autoimmune pancreatitis with and without corticosteroid treatment. Gut. 2007;56:1719–24.
47. Uchida K, Yazumi S, Nishio A, Kusuda T, Koyabu M, Fukata M, Miyoshi H, Sakaguchi Y, Fukui T, Matsushita M, Takaoka M, Okazaki K. Long-term outcome of autoimmune pancreatitis. J Gastroenterol. 2009;44(7):726–32.

# Korean Experience

# 23

Myung-Hwan Kim and Sung-Hoon Moon

## Introduction

The first case of autoimmune pancreatitis (AIP) was diagnosed in Korea in 2002 [1]. Since then, increasing numbers of cases have been described nationwide [2–4]. The prevalence of AIP in Korea was reported to be 5.4 % among 315 patients with chronic pancreatitis [5]. Till date, more than 200 cases with AIP have been diagnosed in Korea. The sudden increase in reported cases may reflect the growing awareness of AIP, rather than a true rise in the incidence of AIP [2]. To improve the diagnosis of AIP in Korea, "Kim criteria" were proposed in 2006 [6, 7]. The following year, Korean diagnostic criteria were proposed by the Korean Pancreato Biliary Association based on Kim criteria [3]. As a first step to establish an international consensus diagnostic criteria for AIP, Korean and Japanese pancreatologists published consensus Asian criteria in 2008 [8].

M.-H. Kim, M.D., Ph.D. (✉)
Department of Internal Medicine,
University of Ulsan College of Medicine,
Asan Medical Center, 388-1, Pungnap-2done,
Songpa-gu, Seoul 138-736, South Korea
e-mail: mhkim@amc.seoul.kr

S.-H. Moon, M.D.
Department of Internal Medicine, Hallym
University Sacred Heart Hospital, Hallym University
College of Medicine, Anyang-si, South Korea

## Cardinal Features of Autoimmune Pancreatitis in Korean Patients

Among the reported cases of AIP in Korea, 125 are registered in the prospectively collected database of the Asan Medical Center, Seoul, South Korea (Table 23.1).

### Demographics and Clinical Features

AIP was diagnosed in 125 patients (101 men and 24 women) during the 8-year period (from 2003 to 2010) at the Asan Medical Center. The average age at diagnosis was 56 years (range 18–81). Most of the patients (70 %) were older than 50 years of age, and a male predominance (81 %) was noted. The frequency of symptoms included jaundice (49 %), abdominal pain (39 %), and weight loss (42 %). Some patients had severe abdominal pain (15 %) or a presentation as acute pancreatitis (7 %). Diabetes was found in 41 % of the patients.

### Imaging Features

On CT, 71 % of the patients had diffuse pancreatic enlargement, while 29 % of the patients had segmental/focal pancreatic enlargement. A pancreatic mass, defined as a lesion that had a different density compared with the surrounding pancreatic tissue by CT scan, was suspected in 17 % of the patients. A capsule-like low-density

M.J. Levy and S.T. Chari (eds.), *Autoimmune (IgG4-related) Pancreatitis and Cholangitis*,
DOI 10.1007/978-1-4419-6430-4_23, © Springer Science+Business Media New York 2013

**Table 23.1** Autoimmune pancreatitis in Korea

| | | | |
|---|---|---|---|
| *Pancreas imaging* | Diffuse (>2/3) | Segmental/focal | |
| Parenchyma (enlargement[a]) | 71 % | 29 % | Mass[a] 17 % |
| Pancreatic main duct | 65 % | 35 % | |
| *Serology* | % in the total cases | | |
| Serum IgG (≥1,800 mg/dL) | 47 % | | |
| Serum IgG4 (≥135 mg/dL) | 53 % | | |
| *Pancreas histology* | | | |
| LPSP | 30 % | | |
| IDCP | 12 % | | |
| Unavailable or indeterminate | 58 % | | |
| *OOI* | | | |
| Hilar/intrahepatic biliary stricture | 15 % | | |
| Renal involvement | 15 % | | |
| Retroperitoneal fibrosis | 10 % | | |
| Sclerosing sialadenitis | 8 % | | |
| *Treatment* | | | |
| Surgery | 10 % | | |
| Steroids | 90 % | | |
| Endoscopic biliary drainage | 61 % | | |

*LPSP* lymphoplasmacytic sclerosing pancreatitis, *IDCP* idiopathic duct-centric pancreatitis, *OOI* other organ involvement
[a]Mass was defined as a lesion that had a different density compared with the surrounding pancreatic tissue by CT scan. Pancreatic enlargement was defined as an increase in the size of the gland.

rim was found in 31 % of patients. On endoscopic retrograde cholangiopancreatography (ERCP) or magnetic resonance cholangiopancreatography (MRCP), 65 % of the patients showed diffuse irregular narrowing of the main pancreatic duct, while 35 % showed segmental/focal main pancreatic ductal narrowing.

## Serologic Features

An increase in serum IgG level (≥1,800 mg/dL) and serum IgG4 level (≥135 mg/dL) was observed in 47 % and 53 % of the patients, respectively. Either elevated serum IgG or IgG4 level was observed in 68 % of our patients. The serum CA 19–9 level was elevated (>37 U/mL) in 24 % of the patients, in whom it was measured.

## Other Organ Involvement

AIP is a pancreatic lesion reflecting a multiorgan disorder referred to as IgG4-related disease (IgG4-RD). The most commonly involved extra-pancreatic organs include the proximal bile duct, kidney, retroperitoneum, and salivary gland. Evidence of other organ involvement was seen in 39 % of patients, including hilar/intrahepatic biliary stricture (15 %), retroperitoneal fibrosis with or without ureteral obstruction (10 %), sclerosing sialadenitis (8 %), and a renal mass (15 %). Although biliary stents were temporarily placed in 61 % of the patients for a distal common bile duct (CBD) stricture, involvement of the distal CBD alone was not included as evidence of other organ involvement. This feature was excluded because narrowing of the intrapancreatic CBD may represent a secondary phenomenon due to extrinsic compression resulting from AIP-related pancreatic enlargement [9].

## Clinicopathologic Subtype: Idiopathic Duct-Centric Pancreatitis (IDCP)

Until recently, IDCP or AIP with granulocytic epithelial lesions (GEL) has been reported mostly in the USA and Europe, and it thought to be very rare in Asia. However, the prevalence of IDCP in AIP in

Korea may not be as rare as previously thought. After histologic review of pancreatic resection specimens and of materials obtained by core biopsy (percutaneous ultrasound-guided or endoscopic ultrasound (EUS)-guided), 15 of 125 AIP patients (12 %) were diagnosed with IDCP. Patients with IDCP were younger (median 34 years) and had more frequent severe abdominal pain (60 %), normal serum IgG4 levels, and an association with ulcerative colitis (33 %). No other extrapancreatic involvement was found in patients with IDCP.

Only 7 cases (1 %) of IDCP had been confirmed in 546 Japanese cases of AIP by the Japanese nationwide study in 2007. Core biopsy from the pancreas (percutaneous ultrasound-guided or EUS-guided) has likely been more often performed in Korea than in Japan, which may contribute to the relatively higher incidence of IDCP in Korea.

## Treatment and Relapse

As an initial treatment, surgical resection was performed in 12 of 125 (10 %) patients. All remaining patients were diagnosed as having AIP without laparotomy and treated with steroids. They showed complete clinical and radiological remission. Our treatment protocol is prednisolone 0.5 mg/kg per day for 1–2 months followed by a gradual taper of 5–10 mg per month to the maintenance dose of 2.5–7.5 mg/day, which is continued for an average of 6 months [10]. In our patients who had a follow-up period of more than 2 years after initial diagnosis, 30 % of the patients experienced a disease relapse. In order to decrease the relapse rate of AIP, it would seem reasonable to confirm remission before steroid tapering or determining the end point of treatment [11].

## Evaluation and Management Algorithm for Autoimmune Pancreatitis in Korea

The Korean algorithm of evaluation and management for patients with obstructive jaundice and/or pancreatic mass/enlargement is shown in Fig. 23.1. This algorithm is a revised form of our original management algorithm [12] that takes new findings into account [13–15]. The main characteristics of our algorithm are as follows. Patients are stratified on the basis of CT features (typical versus atypical imaging). ERCP is not essential for the diagnosis of AIP, but tailored to CT findings. In patients with atypical imaging, exclusion of malignancy is an essential step in the diagnosis of AIP and EUS plays a pivotal role for this purpose.

## Substantial Evidence for Suspicion of AIP Based on Imaging Findings

The diagnosis of AIP requires a high index of suspicion based on imaging findings. The cardinal imaging features of AIP (versus pancreatic adenocarcinoma) are defined as follows [12]: (1) diffuse pancreatic enlargement with or without a capsule-like rim and non-dilated pancreatic duct on CT (versus upstream parenchymal atrophy and pancreatic duct dilatation); (2) homogenous enhancement of the pancreatic mass (versus poorly enhanced low-density mass); (3) a diffusely attenuated main pancreatic duct with an irregular wall or multifocal strictures of main pancreatic duct with normal-looking intervening duct (versus a single localized stricture); (4) no to mild upstream duct dilatation despite a long stricture (versus marked upstream duct dilatation); (5) double duct sign without a discrete pancreatic mass on CT in a patient with obstructive jaundice (versus a visible mass); (6) association of hilar or intrahepatic duct strictures (versus common bile duct stricture alone); (7) other organ involvement unusual for pancreatic cancer such as salivary gland, kidney, or retroperitoneal fibrosis (versus no involvement of these organs); or (8) diffuse or multifocal FDG uptake in the pancreas on PET with or without concomitant extrapancreatic uptake by the salivary glands (versus localized uptake) [16].

## Typical Versus Atypical Imaging Features

The typical pancreatic imaging findings of AIP are diffuse enlargement of the pancreas (CT) and diffuse/segmental irregular narrowing of the

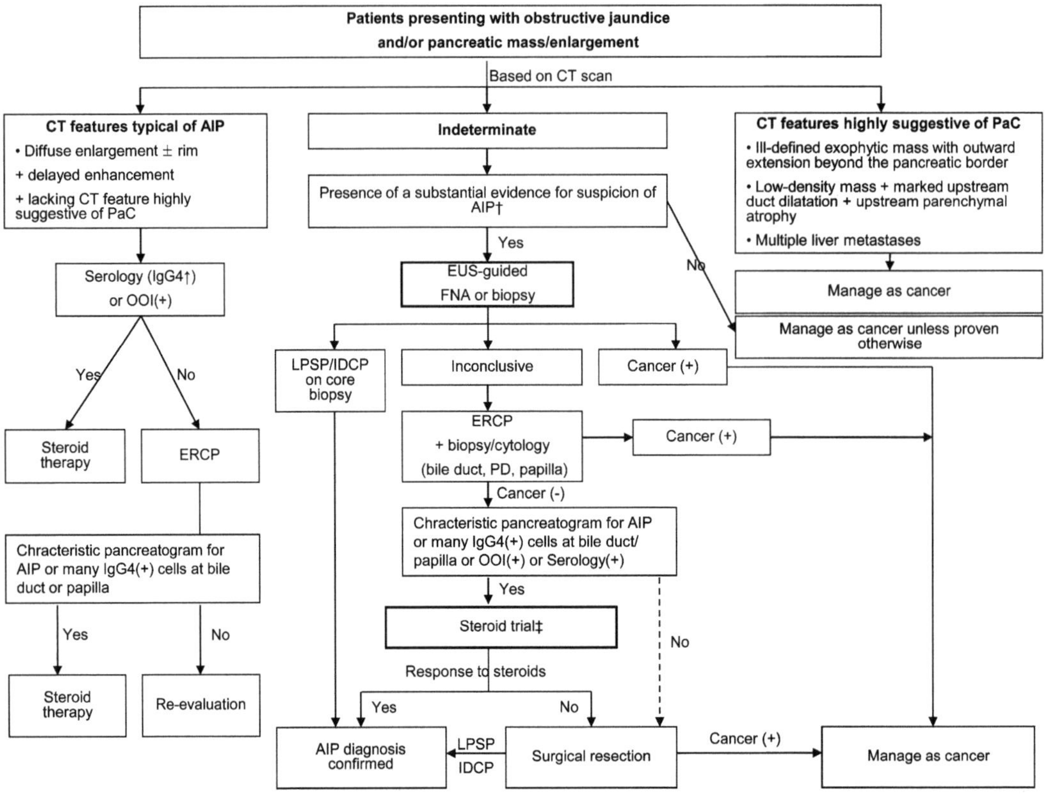


**Fig. 23.1** An evaluation and management algorithm for autoimmune pancreatitis in Korea. *AIP* autoimmune pancreatitis, *PaC* pancreatic cancer, *OOI* other organ involvement, *LPSP* lymphoplasmacytic sclerosing pancreatitis, *IDCP* idiopathic duct-centric pancreatitis, *PD* pancreatic duct. † CT findings for suspicion of AIP: (1) diffuse pancreatic enlargement (without peripancreatic stranding), (2) presence of a capsule-like rim, (3) homogenous enhancement of the low-density pancreatic mass, (4) double duct sign without a discrete pancreatic mass on CT in a patient with obstructive jaundice, (5) presence of multifocal lesion, and (6) characteristic OOI such as proximal bile duct stricture, kidney, or retroperitoneal fibrosis. ‡ Steroid trial: Steroid trial should be performed carefully only by specialists in pancreatology. Steroid responsiveness should be assessed 2 weeks after steroids administration

main pancreatic duct without upstream duct dilatation (ERCP). The concurrence of these two imaging features is exceedingly rare in other pancreatic disorders and is highly specific for AIP. With the increasing number of AIP cases reported, however, various atypical imaging findings in AIP—such as a discrete pancreatic mass, focal pancreatic enlargement, and focal narrowing of the main pancreatic duct with or without upstream duct dilatation—are being encountered. For clinical purpose, imaging should be classified into typical and atypical features: with atypical imaging features, a higher level of collateral evidence is required for diagnosis [13, 15].

Our management algorithm divides the imaging findings into (1) typical of AIP, (2) indeterminate (or atypical), and (3) highly suggestive of pancreatic cancer.

## Management of Patients with Typical AIP Imaging Findings

In patients with typical findings of AIP (diffuse enlargement, delayed enhancement, and a lack of CT features highly suggestive of pancreatic cancer), the diagnosis of AIP can be made by the presence of any collateral evidence including serology (elevated IgG4) or other organ involvement (typical radiological features described in association with AIP or compatible histology). According to Japanese guidelines, serologic criteria include elevated serum total IgG, or IgG4, or the presence of autoantibodies such as antinuclear antibodies or rheumatoid factor [17, 18]. However, there has been controversy over the use of serum total IgG or autoantibodies because of their low specificity.

In patients without serologic evidence or other organ involvement, ERCP should be performed in order to obtain a pancreatogram, and biopsy specimens should be taken from the major duodenal papilla or bile ducts for the purpose of IgG4 immunostaining. According to recent studies [19–21], IgG4 immunostaining of duodenal papillary and bile duct biopsy specimens may be useful for supporting a diagnosis of AIP.

## Management of Patients with Imaging Findings Highly Suggestive of Pancreatic Cancer

Patients with imaging findings that are highly suggestive of pancreatic cancer (low-density mass, marked upstream duct dilatation, and upstream parenchymal atrophy) or evidence of metastasis should be managed as cancer. Clinical features that are highly suggestive of pancreatic cancer are (1) weight loss and severe pain necessitating narcotics or (2) markedly elevated serum CA 19–9 or CEA levels which do not decrease even after biliary decompression.

## Management of Patients with Indeterminate Imaging Findings

Investigation of patients with indeterminate imaging findings might be difficult and requires a substantial amount of experience. Such patients should be referred to a tertiary center with clinicians and radiologists who are familiar with both AIP and pancreatic cancer. Unless substantial evidence for suspicion of AIP exists, patients with indeterminate CT findings should be considered as cancer: this is because AIP is a rare disease (much less common than pancreatic adenocarcinoma or cholangiocarcinoma) [22].

### The Role of EUS and ERCP

In patients suspected of having AIP with the continued need for differentiation from pancreatic cancer due to indeterminate CT findings, EUS should be considered as a first step. EUS is superior to other radiologic modalities including CT scans in the detection of a pancreatic mass, having the negative predictive value for pancreatic tumor detection of nearly 100 % [23]. EUS-guided fine-needle aspiration (FNA) or Tru-Cut biopsy (TCB) should generally be performed for patients with indeterminate imaging. The role of pathologic examination is twofold in the diagnosis of AIP, especially with indeterminate imaging. The first is the pathologic confirmation of AIP and the second is the exclusion of malignancy [12, 24, 25].

Histopathological characteristics of lymphoplasmacytic sclerosing pancreatitis (LPSP) are the combination of periductal lymphoplasmacytic infiltrate, storiform fibrosis, and obliterative phlebitis. While tissue samples collected via FNA do not have a preserved tissue architecture, EUS-TCB may provide sufficient tissue samples to allow adequate histologic examination and diagnosis of AIP [26, 27]. However, EUS-TCB is only available at specialized centers and technically difficult when the lesion is located on the pancreatic head [26]. The technical difficulty of EUS-TCB in accessing a pancreatic head lesion represents its largest drawback because tumor-forming AIP most often involves the pancreatic head [28]. EUS-FNA is an established and widely used technique to evaluate pancreatic mass and is both safe and provides high diagnostic specificity for malignancy [27, 29]. Therefore, the role of a preoperative histopathological examination of the pancreas in patients with suspected AIP may be to exclude malignancy rather than provide definite evidence for a diagnosis of AIP [5, 24]. However, the diagnostic sensitivity of EUS-FNA remains a problem, and a negative FNA result should not be considered definitive evidence to exclude a malignancy. If the diagnosis is inconclusive, even after EUS-FNA/TCB, ERCP should be performed to exclude malignancy in order to obtain biopsy specimen from bile duct, pancreatic duct, and papilla. Endoscopic retrograde pancreatographic findings (multifocal narrowing or a long attenuated segment of the pancreatic duct without upstream duct dilatation) may also aid in the diagnosis of AIP.

Because serum IgG4 levels are elevated in 5–10 % of patients with pancreatic cancer, elevations in serum IgG4 alone cannot be used to distinguish AIP from pancreatic cancer [30, 31]. Because AIP is much less common than pancreatic cancer, serum IgG4 elevations in patients with low pretest probability of having AIP are likely to represent false positive [31].

Even after such a thorough work-up including CT, EUS, ERCP, serology, and pathology, in patients suspected of having AIP with the continued need of differentiation from pancreatic cancer, a "steroid trial" can be used as a diagnostic tool to differentiate AIP from pancreatic cancer.

## Steroid Trial

Steroid therapy is more than a treatment modality for AIP. The dramatic response to steroids is reassuring and typically confirms the diagnosis of AIP [32]. In our algorithm, "steroid therapy" and "steroid trial" are used separately. In patients with "typical" imaging of AIP, the diagnosis of AIP is made before steroid administration; as such, they are "treated" with steroids. In such patients, follow-up imaging is usually performed 4–6 weeks after the initiation of "steroid therapy." In patients with "indeterminate" imaging of AIP, regardless of the fulfillment of diagnostic criteria and/or negative work-up for malignancy, there still exists a possibility of pancreaticobiliary malignancy. In such cases, a complete steroid response is a reliable test to confirm the diagnosis; this diagnostic use of steroids is termed "steroid trial" in our algorithm.

Predictors of steroid responsiveness must be objectively monitored and must be interpreted with caution [22]. In a broad sense, response to steroids may include improvement in clinical symptoms, normalization of elevated levels of serum IgG4, and reversion of abnormal pancreatic imaging. Due to anti-inflammatory effect of steroids, pancreatic enlargement developed by obstructive pancreatitis associated with ductal adenocarcinoma may be relieved with steroid therapy. Steroid responsiveness should be defined not simply as an improvement in pancreatic swelling but, more stringently, as a relief of the main pancreatic duct/common bile duct narrowing and resolution of a pancreatic mass.

Given the error inherent in fine-needle aspiration of the pancreas or intraductal biopsy, particularly in patients with atypical CT finding, the assessment of steroid responsiveness should be done 2 weeks after the initiation of steroids. The reasons for assessing steroid responsive after a short duration (2 weeks) are as follows [12]: (1) radiological improvement of AIP can occur as early as 1–2 weeks after steroid therapy, and (2) given the aggressiveness of pancreatic cancer biology, possible cancer progression in resectable patients is a concern during a more prolonged steroid trial. Moreover, if the tumor becomes unresectable during this delay (2 weeks), it is highly unlikely that earlier surgery would have changed the prognosis of such an aggressive tumor dramatically [25].

Due to clinical and radiological mimicry between AIP and pancreaticobiliary malignancy, there exists a risk of misdiagnosis of AIP as malignancy or vice versa. Inappropriate pancreatic resection may be performed for AIP, and steroids may be given to patients with resectable pancreatic cancer. Multidisciplinary investigations and steroid trial according to our algorithm may minimize the risk of misdiagnosis.

## References

1. Kim JY, Chang HS, Kim MH, et al. A case of autoimmune chronic pancreatitis improved with oral steroid therapy. Korean J Gastroenterol. 2002;39:304–8.
2. Kim KP, Kim MH, Lee SS, Seo DW, Lee SK. Autoimmune pancreatitis: it may be a worldwide entity. Gastroenterology. 2004;126(4):1214.
3. Ryu JK, Chung JB, Park SW, et al. Review of 67 patients with autoimmune pancreatitis in Korea: a multicenter nationwide study. Pancreas. 2008;37(4):377–85.

4. Park SJ, Kim MH, Moon SH, et al. Clinical characteristics, recurrence features, and treatment outcomes of 55 patients with autoimmune pancreatitis. Korean J Gastroenterol. 2008;52(4):230–46.
5. Kim KP, Kim MH, Song MH, Lee SS, Seo DW, Lee SK. Autoimmune chronic pancreatitis. Am J Gastroenterol. 2004;99(8):1605–16.
6. Kim KP, Kim MH, Kim JC, Lee SS, Seo DW, Lee SK. Diagnostic criteria for autoimmune chronic pancreatitis revisited. World J Gastroenterol. 2006;12(16): 2487–96.
7. Kwon S, Kim MH, Choi EK. The diagnostic criteria for autoimmune chronic pancreatitis: it is time to make a consensus. Pancreas. 2007;34(3):279–86.
8. Otsuki M, Chung JB, Okazaki K, et al. Asian diagnostic criteria for autoimmune pancreatitis: consensus of the Japan-Korea symposium on autoimmune pancreatitis. J Gastroenterol. 2008;43(6):403–8.
9. Park do H, Kim MH. Intrapancreatic common bile duct involvement of autoimmune pancreatitis: is it really IgG4-associated cholangitis? Gastroenterology. 2008;135(1):324–5. author reply 325.
10. Park do H, Kim MH, Oh HB, et al. Substitution of aspartic acid at position 57 of the DQbeta1 affects relapse of autoimmune pancreatitis. Gastroenterology. 2008;134(2):440–6.
11. Kim MH, Moon SH. The need for a consensus on the definition of remission of autoimmune pancreatitis after steroid treatment. Gut. 2010;59(12):1730.
12. Moon SH, Kim MH, Park DH, et al. Is a 2-week steroid trial after initial negative investigation for malignancy useful in differentiating autoimmune pancreatitis from pancreatic cancer? A prospective outcome study. Gut. 2008;57(12):1704–12.
13. Chari ST, Takahashi N, Levy MJ, et al. A diagnostic strategy to distinguish autoimmune pancreatitis from pancreatic cancer. Clin Gastroenterol Hepatol. 2009;7(10):1097–103.
14. Kamisawa T, Imai M, Yui Chen P, et al. Strategy for differentiating autoimmune pancreatitis from pancreatic cancer. Pancreas. 2008;37(3):e62–7.
15. Sugumar A, Chari ST. Distinguishing pancreatic cancer from autoimmune pancreatitis: a comparison of two strategies. Clin Gastroenterol Hepatol. 2009;7(11 Suppl):S59–62.
16. Lee TY, Kim MH, Park do H, et al. Utility of 18F-FDG PET/CT for differentiation of autoimmune pancreatitis with atypical pancreatic imaging findings from pancreatic cancer. AJR Am J Roentgenol. 2009;193(2):343–8.
17. Okazaki K, Kawa S, Kamisawa T, et al. Clinical diagnostic criteria of autoimmune pancreatitis: revised proposal. J Gastroenterol. 2006;41(7):626–31.
18. Okazaki K, Kawa S, Kamisawa T, Shimosegawa T, Tanaka M. Japanese consensus guidelines for management of autoimmune pancreatitis: I. Concept and diagnosis of autoimmune pancreatitis. J Gastroenterol. 2010;45(3):249–65.
19. Kamisawa T, Tu Y, Egawa N, Tsuruta K, Okamoto A. A new diagnostic endoscopic tool for autoimmune pancreatitis. Gastrointest Endosc. 2008;68(2):358–61.
20. Kawakami H, Zen Y, Kuwatani M, et al. IgG4-related sclerosing cholangitis and autoimmune pancreatitis: histological assessment of biopsies from Vater's ampulla and the bile duct. J Gastroenterol Hepatol. 2010;25(10):1648–55.
21. Moon SH, Kim MH, Park do H, et al. IgG4 immunostaining of duodenal papillary biopsy specimens may be useful for supporting a diagnosis of autoimmune pancreatitis. Gastrointest Endosc. 2010;71(6):960–6.
22. Gardner TB, Levy MJ, Takahashi N, Smyrk TC, Chari ST. Misdiagnosis of autoimmune pancreatitis: a caution to clinicians. Am J Gastroenterol. 2009;104(7):1620–3.
23. Klapman JB, Chang KJ, Lee JG, Nguyen P. Negative predictive value of endoscopic ultrasound in a large series of patients with a clinical suspicion of pancreatic cancer. Am J Gastroenterol. 2005;100(12):2658–61.
24. Finkelberg DL, Sahani D, Deshpande V, Brugge WR. Autoimmune pancreatitis. N Engl J Med. 2006;355(25):2670–6.
25. Levy P, Hammel P, Ruszniewski P. Diagnostic challenge in autoimmune pancreatitis: beware of shipwreck! Gut. 2008;57(12):1646–7.
26. Levy MJ, Reddy RP, Wiersema MJ, et al. EUS-guided trucut biopsy in establishing autoimmune pancreatitis as the cause of obstructive jaundice. Gastrointest Endosc. 2005;61(3):467–72.
27. Mizuno N, Bhatia V, Hosoda W, et al. Histological diagnosis of autoimmune pancreatitis using EUS-guided trucut biopsy: a comparison study with EUS-FNA. J Gastroenterol. 2009;44(7):742–50.
28. Bang SJ, Kim MH, Kim do H, et al. Is pancreatic core biopsy sufficient to diagnose autoimmune chronic pancreatitis? Pancreas. 2008;36(1):84–9.
29. Sreenarasimhaiah J. Efficacy of endoscopic ultrasound in characterizing mass lesions in chronic pancreatitis. J Clin Gastroenterol. 2008;42(1):81–5.
30. Song TJ, Kim MH, Moon SH, et al. The combined measurement of total serum IgG and IgG4 may increase diagnostic sensitivity for autoimmune pancreatitis without sacrificing specificity, compared with IgG4 alone. Am J Gastroenterol. 2010;105(7):1655–60.
31. Ghazale A, Chari ST, Smyrk TC, et al. Value of serum IgG4 in the diagnosis of autoimmune pancreatitis and in distinguishing it from pancreatic cancer. Am J Gastroenterol. 2007;102(8):1646–53.
32. Ghazale A, Chari ST. Optimising corticosteroid treatment for autoimmune pancreatitis. Gut. 2007;56(12):1650–2.

# 24 Summary and Look to the Future

William R. Brugge and Markus M. Lerch

This book, dedicated to autoimmune pancreatitis (AIP) and IgG4-related sclerosing cholangitis, (IgG4-SC) has covered all presently known aspects regarding the pathogenesis, diagnosis, imaging procedures, and therapy of these largely overlapping disorders. AIP with IgG4-SC is a puzzling disease. Although the cardinal features were first reported in Europe [1], it seemed for a long time an Asian phenomenon, which many Western clinicians felt they could safely ignore [2, 3]. With time, more case series were reported from Europe and the USA, and it became increasingly clear that AIP affects patients throughout the world from various ethnic backgrounds. AIP shares features with two other disorders of the pancreas from which a distinction is critical and determines appropriate treatment and clinical outcome. The first is chronic pancreatitis of either the environmentally induced (alcohol or tobacco) or the hereditary variety [4–7]. The most important difference in terms of treatment, prognosis, and, to a lesser degree, diagnosis is that AIP rapidly responds to the administration of steroids [8] and other types of pancreatitis do not. The same is true for IgG4-SC, which often mimics primary sclerosing cholangitis (PSC) on imaging studies such as ERCP and MRCP but is highly responsive to steroids whereas PSC is not. Our current knowledge regarding the optimal dose and duration of steroid treatment as well as the probability of recurrence following therapy are outlined in Chap. 20. What will have to be solved in future studies is the effectiveness of alternatives to steroids. While a case report suggests that rituximab may provide an alternative treatment option [9], little experience is presently available on more common types of immunosuppressive agents such as azathioprine, tacrolimus, sirolimus, mycophenolate mofetil, and cyclosporine, for how long they would have to be administered, and to what extent they can replace steroids.

When it comes to making the diagnosis, reports from Japan suggested that AIP can be distinguished from chronic pancreatitis by serological markers alone, most prominently serum IgG4 levels [10]. Unfortunately, this serologic marker was quickly found to be much less reliable in Caucasian patients [11]. The reason behind this difference lies in two subtypes of AIP with different prevalence in Europe and Asia (see also Chap. 3). The first subtype, and by far the most common in Asia, has recently been termed lymphoplasmacytic sclerosing pancreatitis (LPSP or type 1 AIP) according to its histological features [12]. It is commonly associated with immunological changes such as elevated IgG4 serum levels or various autoantibodies of lesser diagnostic value. A second disease variety, termed idiopathic duct-centric pancreatitis (IDCP or type 2 AIP), accounts for a significant percentage of Western

W.R. Brugge, M.D.
Harvard Medical School, Massachusetts General Hospital, Boston, MA, USA

M.M. Lerch, M.D., FRCP (✉)
Department of Medicine, University Hospital Greifswald, Friedrich-Coeffer Str. 23 A, Greifswald 17475, Germany
e-mail: lerch@uni-greifswald.de

M.J. Levy and S.T. Chari (eds.), *Autoimmune (IgG4-related) Pancreatitis and Cholangitis*, DOI 10.1007/978-1-4419-6430-4_24, © Springer Science+Business Media New York 2013

patients with AIP but is rarely found in Japan. Type 2 AIP displays often none of the immunological changes of AIP type 1 and is characterized histologically by granulocytic epithelial lesions [13]. These clinical characteristics limit the diagnostic options for type 2 AIP to either histology from resection specimens, core biopsies obtained by endoscopic ultrasound, or cross-sectional diagnostic imaging. The features of diagnostic imaging, however, are not nearly as well defined or universally established as one would wish. Nevertheless, it appears that both types of AIP are remarkably sensitive to relative short courses of systemic corticosteroids.

This brings us to the second disease that AIP needs to be distinguished from, namely, pancreatic cancer. The characteristic imaging appearance of AIP has been reported to include diffuse swelling of the entire organ (the "sausage-shaped" pancreas) and a diffuse narrowing of the pancreatic duct, often combined with similar changes in the bile ducts when occurring as part of the multiorgan disorder termed IgG4-related disease (IgG4-RD) [14]. The latter appearance can easily mimic the "double duct" sign of pancreatic cancer [15]. When inflammatory infiltrates manifest themselves as focal pancreatic enlargement, a distinction between cancer and AIP becomes even more difficult. A focal enlargement or mass lesion was found in up to 40 % of AIP patients in a recent trial [16]. This difficulty in distinguishing between pancreatic cancer and AIP, particularly of the IDCP, type 2 variety, remains the principal reason why many patients with AIP still undergo pancreatic resection, only to learn after histological examination that surgery was neither required nor will it cure their disease (see also Chap. 9). Until specific immunological tests become available for the diagnosis of type 2 AIP, antigens such as UBR2 [17] or trypsin [18, 19], or until better imaging modalities permit more accurate diagnosis, the need for surgical resection or intervention in AIP patients will not be completely eliminated. The question about the best diagnostic imaging modality to distinguish AIP from either more common pancreatitis varieties or from pancreatic cancer remains unresolved. One issue that remains particularly controversial is the use of diagnostic ERCP. In a recent study [16], it was suggested that four distinct ductal features can be used to differentiate cancer from AIP. Long strictures involving more than one third of the duct length, strictures that do not result in an upstream dilatation of the duct, or strictures from which side branches arise are more likely to be caused by AIP than by cancer. The fourth characteristic is the presence of multiple strictures in the duct. Two questions remained unanswered in this study. The first is to what extent simultaneously occurring changes in the bile duct, particularly when AIP and IgG4-SC coexist, require ERCP as a diagnostic test or help to distinguish between AIP and cancer. The other question regards the relative diagnostic utility of ERCP for the two types of AIP. The current paradox is the following: the Japanese consensus guidelines have made ERCP a mandatory diagnostic criterion although an alternative test (serum IgG4) would aid diagnosis in the majority of Japanese patients [20]. Conversely, the HISORt criteria from the Mayo Clinic [21], derived from experience with mostly Caucasian patients, do not include ERCP as a mandatory diagnostic test although Caucasian patients with AIP often present without diagnostic lab tests. The diagnosis may be facilitated in these patients by performing ERCP because core biopsy is the only alternative test for confirming the diagnosis (short of obtaining resection specimens) in the prevalent type 2 AIP. Not surprisingly, a study including mostly Japanese patients attempted to differentiate cancer and AIP based on a protocol that included ERCP [22], whereas a Western study addressing the same issue made do without [23]. What remains to be addressed in future studies is how well the ERP criteria of Sugumar et al. work specifically in type 2 AIP (IDCP). Type 2 is the subgroup which potentially benefits the most from diagnostic ERCP and in which ERCP may prevent most of the unnecessary pancreatic resections. Future studies also need to clarify whether concerns about post-ERCP pancreatitis in patients with suspected AIP are unfounded. The most recent study [16] supports the Japanese consensus which strongly recommends ERCP for the diagnosis of AIP [20] and argues against the Mayo view [21] which does not make it a requirement. If the ductal changes reported recently [16] can be confirmed in their specificity for type 2 AIP, as well as the superiority of ERCP over MRCP in detecting them, then as for PSC, AIP may be a condition in which diagnostic ERCP cannot yet be replaced by less invasive diagnostic test. Whether ERCP can serve in a similar role for monitoring treatment response in AIP will also have to be addressed in future trials. While the use of EUS TCB may obviate the need for ERP, the relative safety and specificity of TCB findings needs to be further clarified. Regardless of the diagnostic accuracy of EUS TCB, the difficulty in obtaining tissue will continue to limit use in most centers.

The last issue that needs mentioning in the context of future perspectives is the option of alternative imaging techniques. The most sensitive imaging modality for any pancreatic disorder at this point in time is probably endoscopic ultrasound. Much progress has recently been made in differentiating AIP from other, more common varieties of chronic pancreatitis by endoscopic ultrasound [24, 25]. Whether the sensitivity and specificity of EUS in distinguishing AIP is equally good for type 1 and type 2 AIP needs to be confirmed in additional studies. The promising finding that a simple endoscopic biopsy of the papilla of Vater (more simple than obtaining an EUS-guided core biopsy of the pancreas itself) can be diagnostic for AIP when IgG- or IgG4-positive plasma cells are identified [26] in the papilla will also need confirmation from additional studies that carefully distinguish between type 1 and type 2 AIP (IDCP). There are few emerging diseases in gastroenterology that have captured the imagination of clinicians and stimulated a large number of high-quality studies on pathogenesis and treatment. We remain optimistic that the remaining open issues outlined above shall be addressed in the near future, and many of the questions will be solved for the benefit of affected patients.

**Acknowledgment** Some of the points discussed here have recently been reviewed in a commentary in the journal Gut (2011 May;60(5):565–6). The authors thank Julia Mayerle for helpful discussions.

## References

1. Sarles H, Sarles JC, Muratore R, Guien C. Chronic inflammatory sclerosis of the pancreas – an autonomous pancreatic disease? Am J Dig Dis. 1961;1:688–98.
2. Yoshida K, Toki F, Takeuchi T, Watanabe S, Shiratori K, Hayashi N. Chronic pancreatitis caused by an autoimmune abnormality. Proposal of the concept of autoimmune pancreatitis. Dig Dis Sci. 1995;40:1561–8.
3. Varadarajulu S, Cotton PB. Autoimmune pancreatitis: is it relevant in the west? Gastroenterology. 2003;125:1557.
4. Pickartz T, Mayerle J, Lerch MM. Autoimmune pancreatitis. Nat Clin Pract Gastroenterol Hepatol. 2007;4:314–23.
5. Keim V, Bauer N, Teich N, Simon P, Lerch MM, Mössner J. Clinical characterization of patients with hereditary pancreatitis and mutations in the cationic trypsinogen gene. Am J Med. 2001;111:622–6.
6. Gress TM, Müller-Pillasch F, Lerch MM, Friess H, Büchler M, Beger HG, Adler G. Balance of expression of genes coding for extracellular matrix proteins and extracellular matrix degrading proteases in chronic pancreatitis. Z Gastroenterol. 1994;32:221–5.
7. Ellis I, Lerch MM, Whitcomb DC. Genetic testing for hereditary pancreatitis: guidelines for indications, counselling, consent and privacy issues. Pancreatology. 2001;1:405–15.
8. Moon SH, Kim MH, Park DH, Hwang CY, Park SJ, Lee SS, Seo DW, Lee SK. Is a 2-week steroid trial after initial negative investigation for malignancy useful in differentiating autoimmune pancreatitis from pancreatic cancer? A prospective outcome study. Gut. 2008;57:1704–12.
9. Topazian M, Witzig TE, Smyrk TC, Pulido JS, Levy MJ, Kamath PS, Chari ST. Rituximab therapy for refractory biliary strictures in immunoglobulin G4-associated cholangitis. Clin Gastroenterol Hepatol. 2008;6:364–6.
10. Hamano H, Kawa S, Horiuchi A, Unno H, Furuya N, Akamatsu T, Fukushima M, Nikaido T, Nakayama K, Usuda N, Kiyosawa K. High serum IgG4 concentrations in patients with sclerosing pancreatitis. N Engl J Med. 2001;344:732–8.
11. Aparisi L, Farre A, Gomez-Cambronero L, Martinez J, De Las HG, Corts J, Navarro S, Mora J, Lopez-Hoyos M, Sabater L, Ferrandez A, Bautista D, Perez-Mateo M, Mery S, Sastre J. Antibodies to carbonic anhydrase and IgG4 levels in idiopathic chronic pancreatitis: relevance for diagnosis of autoimmune pancreatitis. Gut. 2005;54:703–9.
12. Chari ST, Kloeppel G, Zhang L, Notohara K, Lerch MM, Shimosegawa T; Autoimmune Pancreatitis International Cooperative Study Group (APICS). Histopathologic and clinical subtypes of autoimmune pancreatitis: the Honolulu consensus document. Pancreas. 2010;39:549–54.

13. Klöppel G, Detlefsen S, Chari ST, Longnecker DS, Zamboni G. Autoimmune pancreatitis: the clinicopathological characteristics of the subtype with granulocytic epithelial lesions. J Gastroenterol. 2010;45:787–93.
14. Ghazale A, Chari ST, Zhang L, Smyrk TC, Takahashi N, Levy MJ, Topazian MD, Clain JE, Pearson RK, Petersen BT, Vege SS, Lindor K, Farnell MB. Immunoglobulin G4-associated cholangitis: clinical profile and response to therapy. Gastroenterology. 2008;134:706–15.
15. Menges M, Lerch MM, Zeitz M. The double duct sign in patients with malignant and benign pancreatic lesions. Gastrointest Endosc. 2000;52:74–7.
16. Sugumar A, Levy MJ, Kamisawa T, Webster GJM, Kim MH, Enders F, Amin Z, Baron TH, Chapman MH, Church NI, Clain JE, Egawa N, Johnson GJ, Okazaki K, Pearson RK, Pereira SP, Petersen BT, Read S, Sah RP, Sandanayake NS, Takahashi N, Topazian MD, Uchida K, Vege SS, Chari ST. Endoscopic retrograde pancreatography criteria to diagnose autoimmune pancreatitis: an international multicenter study. Gut. 2011;60:666–70.
17. Frulloni L, Lunardi C, Simone R, Dolcino M, Scattolini C, Falconi M, Benini L, Vantini I, Corrocher R, Puccetti A. Identification of a novel antibody associated with autoimmune pancreatitis. N Engl J Med. 2009;361:2135–42.
18. Halangk W, Krüger B, Ruthenbürger M, Stürzebecher J, Albrecht E, Lippert H, Lerch MM. Trypsin activity is not involved in premature, intrapancreatic trypsinogen activation. Am J Physiol Gastrointest Liver Physiol. 2002;282:G367–74.
19. Löhr JM, Faissner R, Koczan D, Bewerunge P, Bassi C, Brors B, Eils R, Frulloni L, Funk A, Halangk W, Jesnowski R, Kaderali L, Kleeff J, Krüger B, Lerch MM, Lösel R, Magnani M, Neumaier M, Nittka S, Sahin-Tóth M, Sänger J, Serafini S, Schnölzer M, Thierse HJ, Wandschneider S, Zamboni G, Klöppel G. Autoantibodies against the exocrine pancreas in autoimmune pancreatitis: gene and protein expression profiling and immunoassays identify pancreatic enzymes as a major target of the inflammatory process. Am J Gastroenterol. 2010;105:2060–71.
20. Kamisawa T, Okazaki K, Kawa S, Shimosegawa T, Tanaka M. Research Committee for Intractable Pancreatic Disease and Japan Pancreas Society. Japanese consensus guidelines for management of autoimmune pancreatitis: III. Treatment and prognosis of AIP. J Gastroenterol. 2010;45:471–7.
21. Chari ST. Diagnosis of autoimmune pancreatitis using its five cardinal features: introducing the Mayo Clinic's HISORt criteria. J Gastroenterol. 2007;42 Suppl 18:39–41.
22. Kamisawa T, Imai M, Yui Chen P, Tu Y, Egawa N, Tsuruta K, Okamoto A, Suzuki M, Kamata N. Strategy for differentiating autoimmune pancreatitis from pancreatic cancer. Pancreas. 2008;37:e62–7.
23. Chari ST, Takahashi N, Levy MJ, Smyrk TC, Clain JE, Pearson RK, Petersen BT, Topazian MA, Vege SS. A diagnostic strategy to distinguish autoimmune pancreatitis from pancreatic cancer. Clin Gastroenterol Hepatol. 2009;7:1097–103.
24. Farrell JJ, Garber J, Sahani D, Brugge WR. EUS findings in patients with autoimmune pancreatitis. Gastrointest Endosc. 2004;60:927–36.
25. Finkelberg DL, Sahani D, Deshpande V, Brugge WR. Autoimmune pancreatitis. N Engl J Med. 2006;355:2670–6.
26. Sepehr A, Mino-Kenudson M, Ogawa F, Brugge WR, Deshpande V, Lauwers GY. IgG4+ to IgG+ plasma cells ratio of ampulla can help differentiate autoimmune pancreatitis from other "mass forming" pancreatic lesions. Am J Surg Pathol. 2008;32:1770–9.

# Index



M.J. Levy and S.T. Chari (eds.), *Autoimmune (IgG4-related) Pancreatitis and Cholangitis*, DOI 10.1007/978-1-4419-6430-4, © Springer Science+Business Media New York 2013

**I**

MIX
Papier aus verantwortungsvollen Quellen
Paper from responsible sources
FSC® C105338

If you have any concerns about our products,
you can contact us on
**ProductSafety@springernature.com**

In case Publisher is established outside the EU,
the EU authorized representative is:
**Springer Nature Customer Service Center GmbH**
**Europaplatz 3, 69115 Heidelberg, Germany**

Printed by Libri Plureos GmbH
in Hamburg, Germany